CURRENT REVIEW OF
RHINITIS

CURRENT REVIEW OF
RHINITIS

Edited by

MICHAEL A. KALINER, MD

Professor
Department of Medicine
George Washington University Medical School
Chief, Allergy Division
Washington Hospital Center
Washington, DC

With 28 contributors

Current Medicine, Inc., Philadelphia

Current Medicine, Inc.

400 Market Street
Suite 700
Philadelphia, PA 19106

Developmental Editor .... *Teresa M. Giuliana*
Commissioning Supervisor .... *Annmarie D'Ortona*
Illustrator .... *Wieslawa Langenfeld, Maureen Looney*
Cover Design.. *William Whitman, Jr.*
Design and Layout .... *Christine Keller-Quirk*
Indexing .... *Prottsman Indexing Services, Inc.*

ISBN 1-57340-179-X
ISSN 1535-6582

Although every effort has been made to ensure that drug doses and other information are presented accurately in this publication, the ultimate responsibility rests with the prescribing physician. Neither the publishers nor the author can be held responsible for errors or for any consequences arising from the use of the information contained therein. Any product mentioned in this publication should be used in accordance with the prescribing information prepared by the manufacturers. No claims or endorsements are made for any drug or compound at present under clinical investigation.

Current Medicine Inc. grants authorization to photocopy items for educational, classroom, or internal use, and to republish in print, Internet, CD-ROM, slide, or other media, provided that the appropriate fee is paid directly to Copyright Clearance Center Inc. (CCC), 222 Rosewood Drive, Danvers, MA 01923, USA (Tel: (978) 750-8400; Fax: (978) 750-4470; E-mail: info@copyright.com; Website: http://www.copyright.com). For permission for other uses, please contact the Permissions Department, Current Medicine Inc., 400 Market Street, Suite 700, Philadelphia, PA 19106-2514, USA.

Printed in the United States by IPC.
5 4 3 2 1

Preface

Rhinitis is a universally experienced medical problem. However, because problems involving the nose are more an annoyance rather than a life-threatening situation, rhinitis is often trivialized. After reading this extraordinary book focusing on rhinitis, the reader will appreciate the scope, cost, significance, and complexity of this set of diseases. Few books are devoted to rhinitis, and none have been written this concisely, with this degree of focus, and with the timeliness of this text. The book was developed and written by acknowledged experts for a clinical audience, and should prove invaluable to practitioners caring for patients.

The book covers all of the major causes of rhinitis, explores pathophysiology and treatment options, and discusses the major advances in rhinitis, all in a concise clinically-relevant format. The practitioner who wants to treat his rhinitis patients more effectively could not read any text which would compare in usefulness to this one. It has been a labor of love to create this text so quickly and efficiently. I hope that it is appreciated for what it offers, and that the readers enjoy its lessons as much as the authors enjoyed providing these clinical pearls.

Michael A. Kaliner, MD
Chevy Chase, Maryland

Contributors

Patrick Ambrosio, DO

Fellow
Department of Allergy and Immunology
University of Medicine and Dentistry of New Jersey
Newark, New Jersey

James N. Baraniuk, MD

Associate Professor
Department of Medicine
Georgetown University
Washington, DC

William E. Berger, MD, MBA

Clinical Professor
Department of Pediatrics
Division of Allergy and Immunology
University of California, Irvine
Irvine, California
Medical Director
Allergy and Asthma Associates of Southern California
Mission Viejo, California

Leonard Bielory, MD

Associate Professor
Departments of Medicine, Pediatrics, and Ophthalmology
University of Medicine and Dentistry of New Jersey
Newark, New Jersey

Michael S. Blaiss, MD

Clinical Professor
Departments of Pediatrics and Medicine
University of Tennessee, Memphis
Memphis, Tennessee

Jaime Castillo, MD

Fellow
Department of Medicine
Division of Allergy and Immunology
University of Texas Medical Branch
Galveston, Texas

Terence M. Davidson, MD

Professor
Department of Surgery/Head and Neck Surgery
Associate Dean for Continuing Medical Education
University of California, San Diego School of Medicine
Section Chief
San Diego VA Healthcare System
San Diego, California

G. Paul Digoy, MD

Resident
Department of Surgery/Head and Neck Surgery
University of California, San Diego School of Medicine
San Diego VA Healthcare System
San Diego, California

Kerry L. Drain, MD

Allergy-Immunology Fellow
Departments of Allergic Diseases and Internal Medicine
Mayo Medical School
Rochester, Minnesota

Athena Economides, MD

Medical Associate
Institute for Asthma and Allergy
Chevy Chase, Maryland

Deborah A. Gentile, MD

Assistant Professor
Department of Pediatrics
Section of Allergy and Immunology
University of Pittsburgh
Assistant Professor
Children's Hospital of Pittsburgh
Pittsburgh, Pennsylvania

John W. Georgitis, MD

Clinical Professor
Department of Pediatrics
Wake Forest University
Physician
Piedmont Allergy and Asthma Associates
Winston-Salem, North Carolina

J. Andrew Grant, MD

Professor
Department of Medicine
Division of Allergy and Immunology
University of Texas Medical Branch at Galveston
Physician
University of Texas Medical Branch
Galveston, Texas

Elizabeth Juniper, MCSP, MSc

Professor Emeritus
Department of Clinical Epidemiology and Biostatistics
McMaster University Faculty of Health Sciences
Hamilton, Ontario
Canada

Michael A. Kaliner, MD

Professor
Department of Medicine
George Washington University Medical School
Chief, Allergy Division
Washington Hospital Center
Washington, DC

James T.C. Li, MD

Professor
Department of Medicine
Mayo Medical School
Rochester, Minnesota

Phillip Lieberman, MD

Clinical Professor
Departments of Medicine and Pediatrics
University of Tennessee
Memphis, Tennessee

Eli O. Meltzer, MD

Clinical Professor
Department of Pediatrics
University of California, San Diego
Co-Director
Allergy and Asthma Medical Group and Research Center
San Diego, California

Robert A. Nathan, MD

Clinical Professor
Department of Medicine
University of Colorado Health Sciences Center
Denver, Colorado
President
Asthma and Allergy Associates Research Center
Colorado Springs, Colorado

David B. Peden, MD, MS

Associate Professor
Department of Pediatrics
University of North Carolina
Chapel Hill, North Carolina

Muhammad Rais, MD

Clinical Postdoctoral Fellow
Department of Pediatric Pulmonology
Baylor College of Medicine
Houston, Texas

Mark Scarupa, MD

Physician
Department of Medicine
Washington Hospital Center
Washington, DC

William F. Schoenwetter, MD

Clinical Professor
Department of Medicine
University of Minnesota
Park Nicollet Clinic
Minneapolis, Minnesota

Guy A. Settipane, MD

Clinical Professor
Department of Medicine
Brown Medical School
Providence, Rhode Island

Russell A. Settipane, MD

Clinical Professor
Department of Medicine
Brown Medical School
Providence, Rhode Island

David P. Skoner, MD

Associate Professor
Departments of Pediatrics and Otolaryngology
Chief, Section of Allergy and Immunology
Children's Hospital of Pittsburgh
Pittsburgh, Pennsylvania

Richard J. Sveum, MD

Clinical Professor
Departments of Medicine and Pediatrics
University of Minnesota
Consultant
Park Nicollet Clinic
Minneapolis, Minnesota

Ann K. Thompson, MBA, BSN

Kansas City, Kansas

Contents

CHAPTER 1

Costs of Allergic Rhinitis

Michael S. Blaiss

Allergic disorders affect a large percentage of the population, and allergic rhinitis is one of the most common chronic medical conditions. Not only does allergic rhinitis lead to high expenditures for medical care; it also generates high indirect costs from work and school absences and decreases in productivity. With the changes occurring in the health care arena and continued decreases in resources, cost considerations must be assessed in addition to clinical efficacy and safety in the management of allergic rhinitis.

This chapter reviews the cost aspects of allergic rhinitis and discusses cost-effective approaches to its treatment.

ALLERGIC RHINITIS

About 20% of the population suffers from allergic rhinitis [1,2]. A majority of allergic rhinitis patients are children and young adults; the prevalence rate in this group is estimated to be as much as 30% [3]. Allergic rhinitis sufferers are rarely, if ever, hospitalized and rarely require surgery or other sophisticated interventions. Because allergic rhinitis does not threaten the patients' day-to-day survival, it may be seen only as a minor nuisance. This is, however, not true. Of allergic rhinitis patients, 50% experience symptoms more than 4 months out of every year and 20% are symptomatic at least 9 months out of the year. This disease accounts for over 10 million office visits to physicians yearly in the United States. It has a major impact on the productivity of the population, leading to an estimated 28 million days of restricted activity yearly in the United States alone. Allergic rhinitis accounts for over 2 million days of school missed yearly in the United States. This means that on a typical school day, 10,000 children are absent because of allergic rhinitis.

Economic impact

Allergic rhinitis is now recognized as a costly condition in the managed-care setting. Costs of allergic rhinitis can be divided into two major categories: direct and indirect. Direct costs are due to monies consumed in the care of the patient, whereas indirect costs are monies lost due to the disease. An important aspect of allergic rhinitis costs is that this condition can lead to or complicate other high-cost disorders, such as asthma, sinusitis, otitis media with effusion, and nasal polyposis. These conditions can be classified as "hidden" direct costs and account for a significantly increased economic burden associated with allergic rhinitis (Table 1-1) [4].

Recently, several studies evaluated the cost of allergic rhinitis in the United States. Each of these studies assessed cost in different ways, leading to different cost estimates. McMenamin [4] assessed the costs and prevalence of this condition in 1990 using the National Health Interview Survey to estimate the number of patients with allergic rhinitis and the National Ambulatory Medical Care Survey to estimate the type of physician treatments provided. His results suggested that the prevalence rate of allergic rhinitis was 9.3%, with total costs in 1990 to be $1.8 billion. Direct costs totaled $1.16 billion—$881 million from physician costs and $276 million from medication costs. Indirect costs from allergic rhinitis came to $639 million, estimated from a loss of 3.4 million work days.

Ross [5] assessed the indirect cost of allergic rhinitis in the workplace. Using data from the United States Public Health Survey, he calculated that allergic rhinitis affected 12.6 million people in the United States work-

force in 1989. Next, Ross extrapolated the increase in the workforce through 1993 and determined that the loss of productivity in the labor force due to allergic rhinitis in 1993 was $2.39 billion in men and $1.4 billion in women. Because of the prevalence of allergic rhinitis, it is estimated that lost productivity due to hay fever may cost $1000 for each worker in the United States each year.

Malone et al. [6] produced another study addressing the burden of allergic rhinitis on the national economy. Using the data from the 1987 National Medical Expenditure Survey, they calculated estimates of resource use, medical expenditures, and lost productivity from allergic rhinitis and extrapolated the data in 1994 dollars. They estimated that 39 million Americans had allergic rhinitis in 1987, but only 12.3% obtained medical care from physicians. Allergic rhinitis accounted for 811,000 missed work days, 824,000 missed school days, and 4,230,000 reduced-activity days in 1987. The total cost of allergic rhinitis in 1994 dollars was $1.23 billion.

Storms et al. [7] conducted a nationwide survey in 1993 to evaluate the costs related to the management of allergic rhinitis in the United States. Patients with ocular or nasal symptoms for 7 days or longer during the previous 12 months were assessed for the amount of health care services, including spending on medication, over that 12-month period. Of the respondents, 63% had consulted a physician in the past 12 months with an estimated cost of $1.1 billion dollars. The average per-person expenditure for prescription medications was $56 per year. The same amount was spent on nonprescription medications yearly, giving an estimated total cost in medications for allergic rhinitis to be in the range of $2.4 billion.

Mackowiak [8] developed an employer cost/benefit economic model for allergic rhinitis. Looking at pharmaceutical costs, he obtained data on drug sales from various pharmaceutical companies for his model. The

TABLE 1-1. DIRECT AND INDIRECT COSTS OF ALLERGIC RHINITIS

Direct costs

Physician/provider consultation
Laboratory testing: allergy skin tests, RAST, etc.
Costs of specific allergy therapy: environmental control, prescription and OTC medications, immunotherapy

"Hidden" direct costs

Costs for antibiotics, radiographs for treatment, and emergency department visits for complicating sinusitis
Surgical costs for nasal polyposis and sinusitis
Antibiotic costs for treatment of sinusitis
Medical and surgical costs for otitis media with effusion
Costs of worsening asthma and frequent URIs
Orthodontics costs
Evaluation and treatment of ocular symptoms

Indirect costs

Sleep disorders and neuropsychiatric abnormalities
Activity limitation due to symptoms and effects of first-generation antihistamines
Decreased decision-making capacity
Impaired psychomotor function
Poor concentration
Irritability
Fatigue
Decreased functioning at work and school
Increased motor vehicle accidents and school and workplace injuries

OTC—over the counter; RAST—radioallergosorbent test; URI—upper respiratory infection.
Adapted from Blaiss et al. [39].

TABLE 1-2. ECONOMIC EVALUATIONS IN HEALTHCARE

Cost-effectiveness
Costs are compared to clinical effects produced between different programs or treatments

Cost benefit
Costs are compared with benefits from a program or treatment as defined by society

Cost identification
Costs are compared between different programs or treatments

Cost utility
Costs are compared to quality-adjusted life years attained between different programs or treatment

preliminary data shows direct costs of allergic rhinitis at $4.48 billion and indirect costs at $3.37 billion.

Ray *et al.* [9•] assessed direct expenditures for treatment of allergic rhinoconjunctivitis in 1996, along with calculating the "hidden" direct costs of rhinitis, such as sinusitis, asthma, acute upper respiratory infection, pharyngitis and tonsillitis, nonatopic conjunctivitis, and chronic otitis media and eustachian tube disorders. The authors found that rhinitis as the primary diagnosis led to direct costs of $1.86 billion (in 1996 dollars). Costs for rhinitis as a secondary diagnosis were estimated at $4.0 billion.

Yawn *et al.* [10••] evaluated the cost implications for patients with allergic rhinitis and asthma versus rhinitis alone in Minnesota. Medication costs were not assessed in this study. The authors concluded that yearly medical costs were on average 46% higher for patients with concomitant allergic rhinitis and asthma compared to asthma alone, even when controlled for sex and age.

These economic studies do not take into consideration complications and secondary costs of rhinitis, such as asthma, sinusitis, otitis media with effusion, and nasal polyposis. Although all of these studies took distinct approaches and used different methodologies to determine costs related to allergic rhinitis, it is clear that this disease has a significant economic impact on the health care system. Because many patients with allergic rhinitis do not seek medical care, most of the data probably underreported the true costs of this disease [11•].

Cost-effective management

In allergic rhinitis, treatment consists of a threefold approach. First, avoidance procedures are instituted to decrease exposure to harmful allergens. Next, appropriate pharmaceutical agents are prescribed to help alleviate and prevent chronic symptoms. Last, allergen immunotherapy may be necessary to desensitize or possibly eliminate symptoms due to specific allergens. There are many different economic methods used to assess costs between different treatments or programs in the health care field (Table 1-2). With the large population of allergic rhinitis patients and its high total cost, it is important to be able to determine what treatment measures are truly cost effective in the management of this disease.

Avoidance procedures are probably the most cost-effective means in treating many patients with allergic rhinitis. If one can avoid the allergens that are triggering symptoms, then no other treatments are warranted. Animal allergy can be significantly improved by removing the pet from the house. Measures shown to decrease animal dander in homes where pets cannot be removed include use of a filtering device, keeping the pet out of the patient's bedroom, and removing carpet from that room. A major cause of perennial allergic

rhinitis is house dust mites [12]. Dust mites grow in hot, humid environments, with the highest concentrations found in carpeting and bedding. Avoidance procedures that have been demonstrated to decrease house dust mite levels include removing all feather objects and wall-to-wall carpeting from the patient's bedroom; encasing the pillow, mattress, and box springs with zipped, impermeable covers; and washing all bedding regularly with hot water.

Medical management

The mainstays of pharmacologic therapy for allergic rhinitis are oral and topical antihistamines and intranasal corticosteroids. Table 1-3 lists some first- and second-generation antihistamines and their daily cost, calculated from their average wholesale cost and recommended daily usage. First-generation antihistamines have been in use for many years. These drugs are all very effective in decreasing the symptoms of allergic rhinitis, such as rhinorrhea, sneezing, nasal itching, and ocular symptoms, and are the least expensive daily pharmacologic therapy in the management of allergic rhinitis. These agents may not be the most cost effective, however, because many patients experience significant side effects that may impair productivity. These antihistamines cross the blood–brain barrier and may cause significant central nervous system sedation, including depression [13]. This sedation may be so pronounced that, in many states, it is illegal to operate heavy machinery or a motor vehicle while using these medications. Weiler *et al.* [14•] determined that a person driving a car under the influence of diphenhydramine, a first-generation antihistamine, was more impaired than a person using alcohol or fexofenadine, a nonsedating second-generation antihistamine. The first-generation sedating antihistamines have been shown to have a detrimental effect on learning in children [15–17]. Fireman [18], using pharmacy data from a health management organization (HMO), determined that first-generation antihistamine use was associated with statistically significantly elevated work-related injuries compared to control groups. The author estimated the annual cost of lost productivity to employers and society due to allergic rhinitis and use of over-the-counter sedating antihistamines to be greater than $4 billion.

The second-generation antihistamines, which are also shown in Table 1-3, are often thought of as the nonsedating antihistamines. These agents are as effective in relief of symptoms as the first-generation antihistamines [19,20]. The advantages these antihistamines have over the first-generation agents include rare sedation (no higher than placebo at the indicated dosage except cetirizine), no anticholinergic effects, lack of tolerance with prolonged use, and decreased dosing frequency [21,22].

An antihistamine nasal spray (Table 1-3) is available for treatment of seasonal allergic rhinitis and nonallergic vasomotor rhinitis. The cost is equivalent to the cost of second-generation antihistamines and has been shown to be equal in efficacy [23,24]. The side effects observed with this agent include somnolence and bitter taste.

Intranasal corticosteroids

Another important modality in the treatment of allergic rhinitis has been the intranasal corticosteroids. Table 1-4 summarizes the preparations available, along with their daily cost based on the average wholesale price. These drugs have been shown to be extremely effective in patients with moderate to severe allergic rhinitis because of the direct delivery of corticosteroid to the nasal mucosa. Intranasal corticosteroids have been shown to reduce sneezing, nasal itching, nasal congestion, and rhinorrhea. With chronic use at the recommended dose, there is no evidence of systemic corticosteroid side effects, such as adrenal suppression, weight gain, or cataracts. Disadvantages of these medications include local irritation and epistaxis in selected patients; rare complications, such as nasal septal perforation; and patient dislike for corticosteroids in any form.

Comparative studies in pharmacologic management

In general, the daily cost of intranasal corticosteroids is less than that of second-generation antihistamines (Tables 1-2 and 1-3). Several studies have evaluated the cost effectiveness and quality of life of these two major treatments for allergic rhinitis. Bronsky *et al.* [25] compared an intranasal corticosteroid (fluticasone), a second-generation antihistamine (terfenadine), and placebo for treatment of seasonal allergic rhinitis in 348 patients. Patient-rated total nasal symptom scores throughout treatment and total nasal airflow measured by rhinomanometry were significantly improved ($P < 0.05$) in the fluticasone group compared with the terfenadine group. Other clinical studies have shown that adults and adolescents with seasonal allergic rhinitis had significantly better improvement with fluticasone nasal spray than loratadine tablets [26•]. Kozma *et al.* [27] compared cost-efficacy ratios for intranasal fluticasone propionate and terfenadine tablets within a sample of patients with seasonal allergic rhinitis symptoms due to mountain cedar allergy. Costs measured were the direct costs of the drugs used for therapy; efficacy was assessed using patient ratings of symptoms and their overall assessment of response to treatment. The cost-efficacy ratios for intranasal fluticasone once daily were more favorable than the ratios for terfenadine 60 mg twice daily.

Other intranasal corticosteroids and second-generation antihistamines have been compared in assessing clinical efficacy. Bernstein *et al.* [28] conducted a multicenter, double-blind, parallel-group study in 239 patients who were randomized to receive either triamcinolone acetonide nasal spray or astemizole tablets. Overall, triamcinolone acetonide spray was more effective than astemizole in reducing total nasal symptoms, nasal stuffiness, nasal itching, and sneezing. Schoenwetter

---

TABLE 1-3. COST PER DAY FOR ANTIHISTAMINES AT RECOMMENDED DOSAGES

First generation

Drug	Cost, $
Diphenhydramine 50 mg	$0.56 per day
Clemastine fumerate 2.68 mg (Tavist)	$1.35 per day

Second generation (available in U.S.)

Drug	Cost, $
Fexofenadine 180 mg (Allegra; Aventis Pharmaceuticals, Parsippany, NJ)	$2.07 per day
Loratadine 10 mg (Claritin; Schering, Kenilworth, NJ)	$2.44 per day
Cetirizine 10 mg (Zyrtec; Pfizer, New York, NY)	$1.96 per day

Nasal spray

Drug	Cost, $
Azelastine (Astelin; Wallace Laboratories, Cranbury, NJ)	$1.98 per day

Data from reference [40], based on average wholesale price on H1 antagonists at the recommended daily dosage.

et al. [29] compared the safety and efficacy of intranasal triamcinolone acetonide with oral loratadine in relieving symptoms of ragweed-induced seasonal allergic rhinitis. Improvement in all rhinitis symptoms was significantly greater with triamcinolone acetonide than with loratadine. Physicians' global evaluations indicated that triamcinolone acetonide provided moderate-to-complete relief in 78% of patients, compared with 58% of loratadine-treated patients ($P \leq 0.0001$). Schulz *et al.* [30] assessed quality of life in patients with allergic rhinitis using triamcinolone nasal spray versus loratadine; at day 14, the patients using triamcinolone spray were significantly better ($P < 0.05$) in several different components and overall quality of life.

Weiner *et al.* [31••] performed a meta-analysis of articles comparing intranasal corticosteroids and nonsedating H_1 antagonists in the management of allergic rhinitis. The conclusions gained from this study point out the greatest improvement in allergic rhinitis symptoms with intranasal corticosteroids, except in eye symptoms, for which both agents were equal. The authors were not able to truly analyze cost-effectiveness from the studies but did compare the mean daily cost of oral corticosteroids in Australia (by asking pharmacists in four Australian states) with the mean daily cost of intranasal corticosteroids. Their surveillance data found that H_1 antagonists were 4.5 times more expensive daily than intranasal corticosteroids.

In general, these studies tend to indicate that the intranasal corticosteroids are more cost effective than the second-generation antihistamines. It is important to remember that convenience and compliance are factors in chronic use of medication. Oral medications have a higher compliance rate than inhaler agents [32]. Also, these studies evaluated chronic use of these different medications, and many patients only use these agents on an as-needed basis. Informing patients on the pros and cons of each type of medication and allowing them to participate in deciding pharmacologic management may be the best approach for highest compliance.

Role of allergen immunotherapy

Allergen immunotherapy is the administration of low, then sequentially increasing, doses of allergens by subcutaneous injection in patients with IgE-mediated diseases, such as allergic rhinitis, allergic asthma, and insect-sting anaphylaxis [33]. It has been shown to be efficacious in treatment of patients with allergic rhinitis by decreasing or eliminating the condition [34,35••]. Sullivan [36] reported that the average direct cost for immunotherapy at Emory University was $800 for the first year and $170 for the next 2 to 4 years.

In determining the cost effectiveness of allergen immunotherapy, Kumar *et al.* [37] looked at costs of treatment and quality of life in allergic rhinitis prior to allergen immunotherapy and then assessed these variables yearly over 3 years of immunotherapy. The cost of care in the year prior to immunotherapy was $1129±321 and for the third year of allergen immunotherapy it was $950±352. This study suggests that allergen immunotherapy by the third year is no more costly than allergy treatment without immunotherapy, with significant improvement in quality of life. Another pharmacoeconomic analysis estimated that pharmacotherapy for allergic rhinitis (using a second-generation antihistamine and an intranasal corticosteroid) would cost about $6000 over a 5-year period, while immunotherapy would cost approximately $2000 over the same period. If patients can decrease medication by half while on immunotherapy, total costs would decrease by $1000 dollars over the 5-year period and more saving would occur as immunotherapy continued and medication use declined [38].

TABLE 1-4. COST PER DAY FOR INTRANASAL CORTICOSTEROIDS AT RECOMMENDED DOSAGE

Drug	Cost, $
Fluticasone propionate (Flonase; Glaxo Wellcome, Research Triangle Park, NC)	$1.87 per day
Triamcinolone acetonide (Nasacort; Aventis Pharmaceuticals, Parsippany, NJ)	$1.41 per day
Flunisolide (Nasarel; Dura Pharmaceuticals, San Diego, CA)	$1.74 per day
Budesonide (Rhinocort Aqua; Astra Pharmaceuticals, Wayne, PA)	$1.66 per day
Momentasone (Nasonex; Schering, Kenilworth, NJ)	$1.83 per day

Data from reference [40], based on average wholesale price on intranasal corticosteroids at the recommended daily dosage.

REFERENCES AND RECOMMENDED READING

Recently published papers of particular interest have been highlighted as:
- • Of interest
- •• Of outstanding interest

1. Sibbald B, Rink E: Epidemiology of seasonal and perennial rhinitis: clinical presentation and medical history. *Thorax* 1991, 46:895–901.

2. Naclerio R: Allergic rhinitis. *N Engl J Med* 1991, 325:860–869.

3. Arrighi HM, Maler WC, Redding GJ: The impact of allergic rhinitis in Seattle school children [abstract]. *J Allergy Clin Immunol* 1995, 95:192.

4. McMenamin P: Costs of hay fever in the United States in 1990. *Ann Allergy* 1994, 73:35–39.

5. Ross RN: The costs of allergic rhinitis. *Am J Manag Care* 1996, 2:285–290.

6. Malone DC, Lawson KA, Smith DH, *et al.*: A cost of illness study of allergic rhinitis in the United States. *J Allergy Clin Immunol* 1997, 99:22–27.

7. Storms W, Meltzer EO, Nathan RA, Selner JC: The economic impact of allergic rhinitis. *J Allergy Clin Immunol* 1997, 97:S820–S824.

8. Mackowiak J: The health and economic impact of rhinitis: a roundtable discussion. *Am J Managed Care* 1997, 3:S8–S18.

9.• Ray N, Baraniuk J, Thamer M: Direct expenditures for the treatment of allergic rhinoconjunctivitis in 1996, including the contributions of related airway illnesses. *J Allergy Clin Immunol* 1999, 103:401–407.
This paper documents for the first time the high cost of allergic rhinitis as a secondary condition to other diseases, such as asthma, otitis media, and sinusitis.

10.•• Yawn BP, Yunginger JW, Wollan PC, *et al.*: Allergic rhinitis in Rochester, Minnesota residents with asthma: frequency and impact on health care charges. *J Allergy Clin Immunol* 1999, 103:54–59.
This is the first study to prove that patients with allergic rhinitis and asthma have significantly higher medical costs than patients with allergic rhinitis alone, even when medication costs are not included.

11.• Weiss KB, Sullivan SD: The health economics of asthma and rhinitis. I. Assessing the economic impact. *J Allergy Clin Immunol* 2001, 107:3–8.
This publication gives an important general overview of the costs associated with allergic conditions.

12. Platts-Mills TA: How environment affects patients with allergic disease: indoor allergens and asthma. *Ann Allergy* 1994, 72:381–384.

13. Storms WW: Treatment of allergic rhinitis: effects of allergic rhinitis and antihistamines on performance. *Allergy Asthma Proc* 1997, 18:59–61.

14.• Weiler JM, Bloomfield JR, Woodworth GG, *et al.*: Effects of fexofenadine, diphenhydramine, and alcohol on driving performance. A randomized, placebo-controlled trial in the Iowa driving simulator. *Ann Intern Med* 2000, 132(5):354–363.
This article illustrates the tremendous impairment on driving abilities caused by first-generation antihistamines, even when the patients did not perceive sedation.

15. Kemp JP: Special considerations in the treatment of seasonal allergic rhinitis in adolescents: the role of antihistamine therapy. *Clin Pediatr* 1996, 35:383–389.

16. Simons FE: Learning impairment and allergic rhinitis. *Allergy Asthma Proc* 1996, 17:185–189.

17. Vuurman EF, van Veggel LM, Uiterwijk MM, *et al.*: Seasonal allergic rhinitis and antihistamine effects on children's learning. *Ann Allergy* 1993, 71:121–126.

18. Fireman P: Treatment of allergic rhinitis: effect on occupation productivity and work force costs. *Allergy Asthma Proc* 1997, 18:63–67.

19. Busse WW: Role of antihistamines in allergic disease. *Ann Allergy* 1994, 72:371–375.

20. Du Buske LM: Clinical comparison of histamine H₁-receptor antagonist drugs. *J Allergy Clin Immunol* 1996, 98:S307–S318.

21. Adelsberg BR: Sedation and performance issues in the treatment of allergic conditions. *Arch Intern Med* 1997, 157:494–500.

22. Pedinoff AJ: Approaches to the treatment of seasonal allergic rhinitis. *South Med J* 1996, 89:1130–1139.

23. Conde Hernandez DJ, Palma Aqilar JL, Delgado Romero J: Comparison of azelastine nasal spray and oral ebastine in treating seasonal allergic rhinitis. *Curr Med Res Opin* 1995, 13:299–304.

24. Gastpar H, Nolte D, Aurich R, *et al.*: Comparative efficacy of azelastine nasal spray and terfenadine in seasonal and perennial rhinitis. *Allergy* 1994, 49:152–158.

25. Bronsky EA, Dockhorn RJ, Meltzer EO, *et al.*: Fluticasone propionate aqueous nasal spray compared with terfenadine tablets in the treatment of seasonal allergic rhinitis. *J Allergy Clin Immunol* 1996, 97:915–921.

26.• Gehanno P, Desfougeres JL: Fluticasone propionate aqueous nasal spray compared with oral loratadine in patients with seasonal allergic rhinitis. *Allergy* 1997, 52:445–450.
The effectiveness and safety of fluticasone propionate aqueous nasal spray (200 µg once daily for 4 weeks) were compared with those of loratadine (10 mg once daily for 4 weeks) in 114 adults and adolescents with seasonal allergic rhinitis in this multicenter, double-blind, double-dummy, randomized, parallel-group study. In both physician-based and patient-based scoring of clinical symptoms, fluticasone was significantly better than loratadine.

27. Kozma CM, Schulz RM, Sclar DA, *et al.*: A comparison of costs and efficacy of intranasal fluticasone propionate and terfenadine tablets for seasonal allergic rhinitis. *Clin Ther* 1996, 18:334–346.

28. Bernstein DI, Creticos PS, Busse WW, *et al.*: Comparison of triamcinolone acetonide nasal inhaler with astemizole in the treatment of ragweed-induced allergic rhinitis. *J Allergy Clin Immunol* 1996, 97:749–755.

29. Schoenwetter W, Lim J: Comparison of intranasal triamcinolone acetonide with oral loratadine for the treatment of patients with seasonal allergic rhinitis. *Clin Ther* 1995, 17(3):479–492.

30. Schulz RM, Smith DH, Lim J: Quality of life in patients with seasonal allergic rhinitis (SAR): triamcinolone acetonide aqueous nasal spray versus loratadine [abstract]. *Ann Allergy Asthma Immunol* 1997, 78:155.

31.•• Weiner JM, Abramson MJ, Puy RM: Intranasal corticosteroids versus oral H₁ receptor antagonists in allergic rhinitis: systematic review of randomised controlled trials. *Br Med J* 1998, 317:1624–1629.
This meta-analysis documents that the best overall improvement in allergic symptoms occurs with the use of intranasal corticosteroids. The authors conclude that intranasal corticosteroids should be considered first-line therapy for allergic rhinitis.

32. Kelloway JS, Wyatt RA, Adlis SA: Comparison of patients' compliance with prescribed oral and inhaled asthma medications. *Arch Intern Med* 1994, 154:1349–1352.

33. Hedlin G: The role of immunotherapy in pediatric allergic disease. *Curr Opin Pediatr* 1995, 7:676–682.

34. Creticos PS: The role of immunotherapy in allergic rhinitis/allergic asthma. *Allergy Proc* 1995, 16:297–302.

35.•• Ross RN, Nelson HS, Finegold I: Effectiveness of specific immunotherapy in the treatment of allergic rhinitis: an analysis of randomized, prospective, single- or double-blind, placebo-controlled studies. *Clin Ther* 2000, 22(3):342–350.
This meta-analysis uses rigorous criteria in its evaluation of the literature and validates the efficacy of allergen immunotherapy in the management of allergic rhinitis.

36. Sullivan TJ: *Expert Care and Immunotherapy for Asthma.* Chicago: American College of Allergy, Asthma, and Immunology; 1996.

37. Kumar P, Kamboj S, Rao P: The cost of care and quality of life in patients with allergic rhinitis on allergen immunotherapy. *Allergy Clin Immunol Int* 1997, 9:133–135.

38. Bernstein JA: Pharmacoeconomic considerations for allergen immunotherapy. In *Allergens and Allergen Immunotherapy.* Edited by Lockey RF, Bukantz SC. New York: Marcel Decker, 1988:445–453.

39. Blaiss M, Bukstein D, Davis M, Luskin A: Improving allergy and asthma care through outcomes management. *Managed Care Focus Series.* Edited by Davis M. Milwaukee: American Academy of Allergy, Asthma, and Immunology; 1997:11.

40. *2001 Drug Topics Red Book.* Montvale, NJ: Medical Economics Company; 2001.

CHAPTER 2

Examination of the Nasal Cavity

Michael A. Kaliner
Phillip Lieberman

The nasal cavity is a far more complex space than imagined by a naive observer (Figs. 2-1, 2-2). The anatomy allows air to travel to the lungs, while being warmed, humidified, and purified, all within the time frame of 0.1 second. The entrances from the four sets of paranasal sinuses drain into the nose and must be protected from airborne pathogens. The olfactory epithelium must have free access to airflow but be out of the mainstream. The turbinates must act as baffles to the airflow, creating turbulence without obstructing flow. Thus, the nasal anatomy is designed to cause controlled chaos of airflow, but with many purposes.

Examination of the nose is a difficult technique to master. The proper examination takes into account the color of the nasal mucosa, the texture of the mucous layer, the anatomy of the turbinates, and the nasal septum and the posterior valve area. For the purposes of this discussion, only the anterior portions of the nose from the nasal vestibule to the posterior valve will be discussed, as these are the areas visible to anterior examination with the usual equipment available to physicians. Anyone who treats sinusitis will also be familiar with the posterior portions of the nose, which are visible only with rhinoscopic equipment or with the use of mirrors.

NASAL MUCOUS MEMBRANE

The nasal mucosa is a healthy pink color, exactly as is found in the buccal mucosa, which should be examined if there is any question that the nasal mucosa is abnormal in color. Allergic disease makes the mucosa swell and pale to almost a blue-white color (Fig. 2-3). This blue-white color is best seen in black patients with allergies but is also seen in Asian and white patients. Nonallergic or vasomotor rhinitis is associated with a normal to slightly erythematous color. Upper respiratory tract infections and sinusitis may be associated with reddened mucous membranes. The most reddened and irritated-looking mucosa are seen in rhinitis medicamentosa, caused by addiction to topical nasal decongestants.

The mucous layer is usually thin and watery. Allergic mucous membranes are coated with watery mucus, often copious (note secretions on Fig. 2-3A). Vasomotor rhinitis is also associated with a watery secretion. The common cold produces a serous (yellow) secretion during the first 3 days; this secretion thickens during the next few days before resolution. Sinusitis is recognized by green secretions that reflect the presence of neutrophils and eosinophils. The thickened secretions of chronic sinusitis may also take on a deep gray color. Fungal sinusitis can be recognized by silver, orange, gray, or black secretions.

The secretions in rhinitis are seen diffusely. Sinusitis is most commonly associated with secretions found around the middle meatus, where the sinuses drain. Sometimes the patient will complain of postnasal drip and no secretions can be seen anteriorly. In these patients, examination of the posterior portion of the nose may reveal secre-

tions not visible anteriorly. Another hint of drainage is the presence of lymphoid hyperplasia of the pharynx giving a "cobblestone-like" effect.

NASAL SEPTUM

The septum is usually in the midline of the nose, separating the two sides about equally. In many adults the septum may lie to one side or the other (Fig. 2-4). This

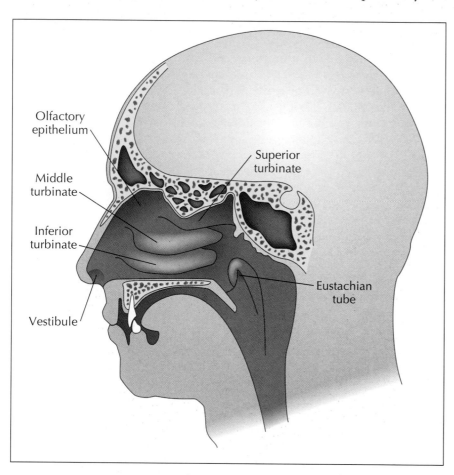

FIGURE 2-1.
Sagittal view of the inside of the nasal cavity.

Olfactory epithelium
Middle turbinate
Inferior turbinate
Vestibule
Superior turbinate
Eustachian tube

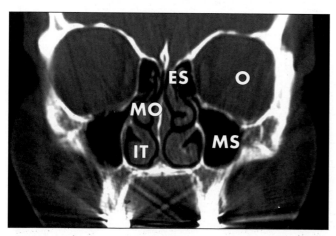

FIGURE 2-2.
Coronal plane computed tomography scan of the skull showing the nose and sinuses. ES—Ethmoid sinus; IT—inferior turbinate; MO—maxillary ostia; MS—maxillary sinus; O—orbit.

deviation of the septum is due to facial pressure exerted on the nose during talking, chewing, and respiration. Surgical repair of a deviated septum is often successful only for a limited period because these pressures are still present and can cause the septum to deviate to one side or the other again. One test to see if a deviated septum can be controlled medically is to spray the nose with a topical decongestant and see if sufficient airway appears to allow normal respirations. If it does, then the nasal obstruction from a deviated septum may be managed medically. Air passage at 20% to 50% of normal is sufficient for comfortable breathing.

Sometimes a broadened septum can obstruct both sides of the nose. In this case, a decongestant or topical corticosteroid may be tried to see if comfortable breathing returns. If this approach is insufficient and the patient is bothered by persistent nasal obstruction, then surgery may be the only solution.

NASAL TURBINATES

The inferior turbinate occupies about 50% of the internal space in the nasal passage and is designed to partly obstruct airflow in order to help humidify, warm, and filter the air. The inferior turbinate generally has a "C" shape and originates from the lateral wall of the sinus, beginning just after the vestibule (Fig. 2-5). This turbinate then continues back toward the choana.

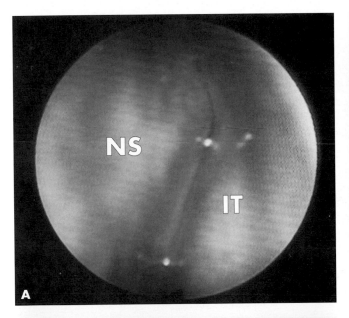

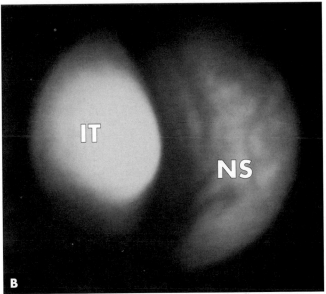

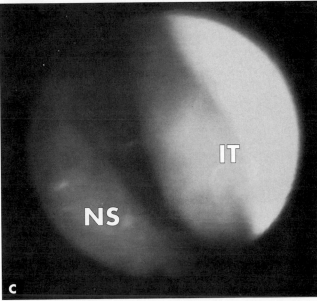

FIGURE 2-3.
Endoscopic view of the nasal mucous membrane. **A**, Swollen turbinate tightly bound to nasal septum, totally occluding all air space. **B**, Right side of another patient showing a white turbinate compared to the normal color of the septum. **C**, Left side of a third patient showing a white inferior turbinate contrasting to normal color of the septum. IT—inferior turbinate; NS—nasal septum.

The middle turbinate is found behind and superior to the inferior turbinate, often tipped at a 45° angle to the inferior turbinate in order to create turbulent airflow. Whereas the inferior turbinate is usually a healthy pink color, the middle turbinate is often lighter, nearly white (Fig. 2-6). Both the inferior and middle turbinates partly obstruct the nasal passage, but they should allow enough space for air to move freely to the back of the nose. The maxillary and ethmoid sinuses drain into the middle meatus, the space lateral to the middle turbinate. There should be adequate space between the inside wall of the middle turbinate and the outside wall of the sinuses for drainage to flow. If the turbinate is too tightly positioned to the inside wall of the meatal space, then drainage from the sinuses may be compromised, and the patient is predisposed to sinusitis.

There are a number of anatomical abnormalities of the turbinates which can obstruct the air passage or the sinus outflow track. The most common abnormality, occurring in 20% of control patients, is a concha bullosum, an extra air space within the turbinate that enlarges the size of the turbinate (Fig. 2-7). The enlarged turbinate then can obstruct airflow or block the middle meatus. These extra spaces, or sinuses, can be seen in any of the turbinates and even in the septum.

POSTERIOR VALVE AREA

The posterior valve is the area where the posterior aspects of the inferior turbinate, middle turbinate, and septum converge (Fig. 2-8). In some patients these structures come together so closely that only a small amount of free space is left. In most normal patients, a careful observer can see the posterior choana (the entrance from the nose into the pharynx). With a tight posterior valve, the posterior portions of the nose are totally blocked to the viewer and for air passage as well.

NASAL REFLEXES THAT OBSTRUCT AIRFLOW

The physiologic nasal cycle causes the nose to decongest or congest rhythmically over a 24-hour period. Ordinarily, the passage on one side is partly congested for a period of 45 to 90 minutes, while the opposite cavity is less congested. This congestion cycle reverses periodically during the day. If one side of the nose is partly blocked by an anatomical abnormality, then the physiologic cycle may worsen that congestion intermittently each day. Patients often complain of congestion alternating from one side to the other. An explanation of the nasal cycle often alleviates patients' concerns.

Other nasal reflexes result in nasal congestion. Besides the nasal cycle noted above, there is the reflex caused by recumbency. In this reaction, with the patient in the recumbent position, the side of the head on the pillow congests, while the side of the nose away from the pillow decongests. If there is an anatomical abnormality that causes partial or complete obstruction of one side, the patient usually sleeps with the partly obstructed side down in order to allow breathing through the less obstructed side.

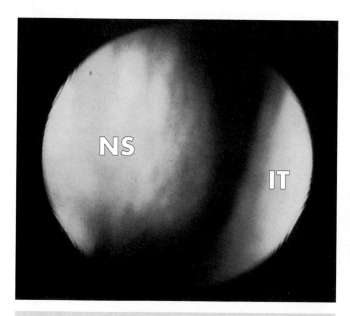

FIGURE 2-4.
Endoscopic view of deviated nasal septum bulging into the left side of patient's nose. IT—Inferior turbinate; NS—nasal septum.

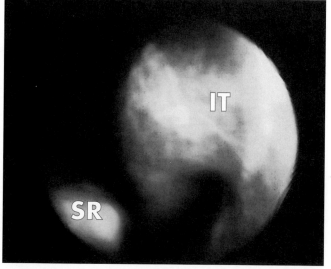

FIGURE 2-5.
Endoscopic view of inferior turbinate seen from just within the vestibule on the left side of the nose. Note curved "C" shape of the turbinate. IT—Inferior turbinate; SR—septal ridge.

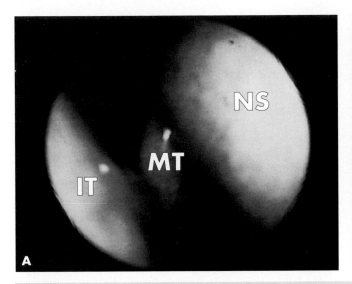

A

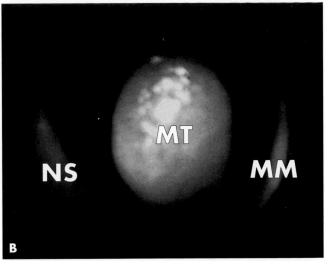

B

FIGURE 2-6.

A, Endoscopic view of the middle turbinate on the right side looking over the inferior turbinate. IT—Inferior turbinate; MT—middle turbinate; NS—nasal septum. The middle turbinate is at a 45° angle to the inferior turbinate and is a lighter color.

B, A closer view of an enlarged turbinate on the left side. NS—Nasal septum; MT—middle turbinate showing the lighter color; MM—middle meatus space lateral to the turbinate. The maxillary and ethmoid sinuses drain into this space.

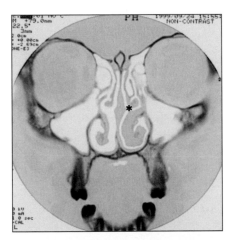

FIGURE 2-7.

Computed tomography scan of the skull showing a small concha bullosum (*), or air space, within the left middle turbinate.

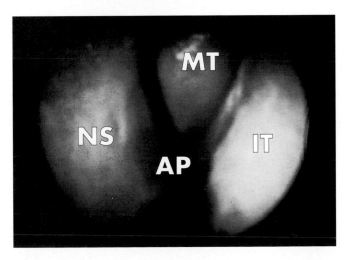

FIGURE 2-8.

Endoscopic view of the posterior valve. This patient had a very tight area on the left side where the two turbinates and septum converge, narrowing the nasal passage. AP—Air passage; IT—inferior turbinate; MT—middle turbinate; NS—nasal septum.

OLFACTORY EPITHELIUM

The sense of smell is located in the most superior aspects of the nose, where the olfactory epithelium is located (see Fig. 2-1). The olfactory epithelium is usually slightly yellow in color and easily visible to an experienced observer. In many patients with congestion, and especially when nasal polyps are present, the superior aspects of the nose are blocked by swollen mucosa and polyps, and the sense of smell is reduced.

NASAL POLYPS

Polyps usually arise from within the sinuses, and less frequently from the turbinates. They are pedunculated struc-

tures with a characteristic gray color, which contrasts uniquely with the pink colors ordinarily seen in the mucosa (Fig. 2-9). Polyps may be minute or large enough to totally obstruct the nasal passage. Polyps can be distinguished from turbinates not only by their gray color but also from their lack of pain fibers and their movability. Manipulation of polyps with a probe does not cause pain, and the polyp may be moved. Turbinates are richly endowed with pain fibers and are stationary bony structures.

A careful examination involves looking at the nose in its natural state, adding a topical decongestant, and examining again to see how the passage looks in its decongested state. Anterior otoscopy with standard equipment is adequate for most examinations.

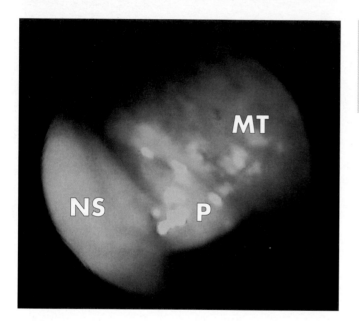

FIGURE 2-9.
Endoscopic view of a small nasal polyp seen between the turbinate and septum on the patient's left side. Polyps are usually gray in color and are movable, without pain perception. MT—middle turbinate; NS—nasal septum; P—polyp.

CHAPTER 3

Quality of Life in Patients with Allergic Rhinitis

Ann K. Thompson
Elizabeth Juniper
Eli O. Meltzer

The prevalence of allergic rhinitis in the United States is reported to be between 15% and 20% [1]. Although rhinitis symptoms are not life-threatening, they can have detrimental effects on the physical, psychologic, and social aspects of patient's lives, and can significantly decrease quality of life [2,3••]. "Quality of life" has been defined as the subjective value a person places upon satisfaction with his or her life. Within the last 10 to 15 years, there has been a move toward greater appreciation of quality of life as it relates to health status. Health-related quality of life (HRQOL) has been described by Schipper *et al.* [2] as "the functional effects of an illness and its consequent therapy upon a patient, as perceived by the patient." It is becoming increasingly accepted that to obtain a complete measure of the health status of patients with allergic rhinitis, HRQOL assessments should be made in addition to clinical measurements [4]. Indeed, the correlation between clinical measures of allergic rhinitis (*eg*, symptom severity) and patient quality of life appears to be only weak to moderate [3••,5].

Health-related quality of life is a relatively new area of investigation; nevertheless, the use of HRQOL measures in the assessment of therapeutic interventions appears to be increasing. Rigorous practical questionnaires (instruments) applicable to allergic rhinitis have been developed and validated for use in clinical research trials. Methods of correlating changes in HRQOL scores in clinical trials with clinical meaningful outcomes for individual patients have been proposed and continue to be a subject of investigation. The ease of use of many HRQOL instruments suggests they may have unity in clinical practice to document the changes in a patient's current and future health due to therapeutic decisions [6••,7–10].

This review describes the types of tools used in allergy-specific HRQOL research, the effects of allergic rhinitis on HRQOL, examples of assessment of allergy-related therapeutic interventions on HRQOL, and efforts to translate research data into useful information to guide therapeutic interventions for individual patients.

HRQOL INSTRUMENTS
Types of instruments

The quality of HRQOL data is highly dependent on the instrument with which they are gathered. Two types of instruments, generic and disease-specific, are used to assess HRQOL. Generic instruments are general measures of health status that can be used to evaluate different disease states, treatment interventions, and populations. Examples include the Sickness Impact Profile (SIP), and the generic instrument used most often in allergic rhinitis studies, the Medical Outcomes Study 36-Item Short Form Health Survey (SF-36) [11,12]. The SF-36 is a psychometric questionnaire with 36 questions in 9 domains (Table 3-1).

Generic instruments play an important role in the overall assessment of HRQOL. The breadth of coverage of these instruments may reveal important but unexpected effects on HRQOL [13,14]. Another advantage is they allow comparison of the burden of illness among different diseases. The SF-36 is not disease- or treatment-restricted [11]. Generic instruments also have disadvantages. Because they are so all-encompassing and comprehensive, they may not focus adequately on problems specific to a particular condition. Further, they may not be responsive enough to detect small but clinically meaningful changes in HRQOL in a given disease state [14].

To surmount the shortcomings of generic instruments, disease-specific HRQOL questionnaires have been developed (Table 3-2). The disease-specific instrument used most frequently in allergic rhinitis is the Rhinoconjunctivitis Quality of Life Questionnaire (RQLQ) [15]. The RQLQ measures the effect of rhinoconjunctivitis symptoms on seven disease-related domains (Table 3-3). Disease-specific instruments are more responsive than generic instruments and they can be targeted to a specific population, disease, or function. Disease-specific instruments do not allow comparisons between different medical conditions.

Generic instruments may be modified to measure disease-specific HRQOL. An instrument gaining popularity in allergic rhinitis treatment trials is the Work Productivity and Activity Impairment (WPAI) instrument. The WPAI is a generic instrument that has been validated for use in allergic rhinitis; it measures impairment of physical and occupational functioning due to allergy symptoms at work, in the classroom, and during normal daily activities [16,17•].

Developing and validating instruments

To evaluate changes in HRQOL over time in clinical trials or in clinical practice, HRQOL instruments must be responsive and valid. The RQLQ is one of the first disease-specific instruments validated to measure HRQOL in rhinitis. When developing the RQLQ, Juniper and Guyatt were guided by criteria they considered essential to a reliable instrument. Specifically, the questionnaire should (1) measure both physical and emotional func-

TABLE 3-1. HEALTH-RELATED QUALITY OF LIFE DOMAINS IN THE SF-36

Domains	Questions
Physical functioning	10
Role limitations due to physical problems	4
Bodily pain	2
General health	5
Vitality	4
Social functioning	2
Role limitations due to emotional problems	3
Mental health	5
Health transition	1

TABLE 3-2. HRQOL INSTRUMENTS USED IN ALLERGIC RHINITIS

Instrument	Questions (N)	Patient	Reference
Rhinoconjunctivitis Quality of Life Questionnaire (RQLQ)	28	Adults	15
Standardized Rhinoconjunctivitis Quality of Life Questionnaire*	28	Adults	39
Mini Rhinoconjunctivitis Quality of Life Questionnaire	14	Adults	20
Pediatric Rhinoconjunctivitis Quality of Life Questionnaire	23	6–12 y	19
Adolescent Rhinoconjunctivitis Quality of Life Questionnaire	25	12–17 y	18
Rhinitis Quality of Life Questionnaire	24	Adults	10
Nasal Comfort Index	In development	Adults	22
Nocturnal Rhinitis Quality of Life Questionnaire	In development	≥12 y	†
Work Productivity and Activity Impairment Instrument†	9	Adults	16, 17
MOS SF-36‡	36	Adults	11, 12

*Same as the original RQLQ except activities are standardized rather than specified by the patient.
†Beginning validation process [personal communication (AT, EM, EJ)].
‡Generic instrument validated for use in allergic rhinitis.

tion; (2) reflect areas of function important to patients with rhinoconjunctivitis; (3) provide summary scores amenable to statistical analysis; (4) provide reproducible scores when the clinical state is stable; (5) be responsive to clinically important changes, even small ones; (6) be valid (*ie*, actually measure subjective aspects of health status); and (7) be relatively short to optimize cost and efficiency [15].

All instruments used to evaluate HRQOL in allergic rhinitis comprise one or more of four broad domains: physical and occupational function, psychologic state, social interaction, and somatic sensation (*ie*, problems patients experience as a result of disease symptoms) [2].

TABLE 3-3. LIST OF FUNCTIONAL IMPAIRMENTS MOST IMPORTANT TO ADULTS WITH RHINOCONJUNCTIVITIS

Practical problems
  Need to blow nose repeatedly
  Need to rub nose/eyes
  Inconvenience of having to carry tissues
Nasal symptoms
  Stuffy/blocked
  Sneezing
  Runny
  Itchy
Eye symptoms
  Itchy
  Watery
  Swollen
  Sore
Sleep
  Lack of sleep
  Wake during night
  Difficulty getting to sleep
Non–hay fever symptoms
  Tiredness
  Fatigue
  Worn out
  Poor concentration
  Thirst
  Reduced productivity
Activity limitations
  Physical
  Social
  Occupational
Emotional function
  Irritable
  Frustrated
  Embarrassed by nose or eye symptoms
  Impatient
  Restless

Selecting relevant health-related questions to be included in an instrument is a methodical process. To create the RQLQ, the investigators drew on their personal experiences, reviewed other HRQOL instruments, and interviewed allergic patients to construct a broad list of 91 health-related items in areas of importance to patients. Rhinitis patients ranked items on the list in order of importance and the RQLQ was reduced to 28 items in 7 health-related domains. The instrument was then tested for reproducibility, responsiveness, and validity in a large clinical trial that evaluated different therapeutic regimens in patients with rhinoconjunctivitis. Reproducibility was established by administering the test on two occasions, 2 weeks apart, during a period of clinical stability. Responsiveness was proved by correlating the magnitude of changes in RQLQ scores with patient-reported symptom severity over the course of the trial. Validity was supported by correlations in deteriorating patient functionality reflected in RQLQ scores as pollen counts rose (and vice versa), as well as by correlations between changes in RQLQ dimension scores and recordings in nasal and eye symptoms diaries [15].

Disease-specific instruments can (and should) be adapted to a particular population. Juniper and colleagues developed and validated versions of the RQLQ for adolescents aged 12 to 17 years (Adol-RQLQ) and for children aged 6 to 12 years (PRQLQ) [18,19]. Adolescents with rhinoconjunctivitis experience problems similar to those identified by adults, except they have fewer sleep problems and more difficulty with concentration, particularly with schoolwork. Younger children (aged 6 to 12 years) are troubled by practical problems (*eg*, carrying tissues or taking medication) but do not report the interference with daily activities or the emotional distress experienced by adults or adolescents. This may be due to the younger child's difficulty in differentiating a healthy versus a diseased state and/or his or her inability to articulate the problem.

The RQLQ has also been shortened (the Mini-RQLQ) for use in large clinical trials, surveys, and practice monitoring, where high efficiency is important [20]. Additionally, the RQLQ has been adapted to measure only rhinitis (Rhinitis Quality of Life Questionnaire) by removing questions pertaining to eye symptoms [10].

An instrument must retain the exact wording and the validated administration technique must be used to avoid biases. Modes of administering HRQOL instruments vary; they include personal interview, telephone interview, patient self-reporting, and use of surrogate responders [14]. Each mode has advantages and disadvantages. Interviewing the patient face-to-face improves accuracy and minimizes missing information, but is resource intensive. Telephone interview removes the necessity of an office visit; however, the patient must be given a list of the appropriate responses before the interview and there is no guarantee that the interviewee is, in fact, the patient. Patient self-reporting requires fewer resources but there is a higher risk that the questionnaire may be incomplete. Use of surrogate responders is appealing with certain populations (*eg*, children), however, accuracy may be compromised [14]. In addition to the mode of administration, the increasing use of computers has introduced a new variable to HRQOL assessment: the mode of data collection. Until recently, data were collected only in paper form. Preliminary findings of a recent study suggest data collected electronically do not differ significantly from information collected on paper [21].

New rhinitis-specific instruments continue to be developed. For example, an instrument to assess patient comfort and satisfaction with nasal sprays has been developed, the Nasal Comfort Index (NCI), although this instrument has yet to be validated in a clinical trial [22].

EFFECTS OF ALLERGIC RHINITIS ON HRQOL

Allergic rhinitis symptoms may seem innocuous enough to the nonsufferer. People with allergic rhinitis, however, report that not only are symptoms of rhinorrhea, nasal congestion, sneezing, itching, and associated eye problems disturbing, but also their emotional well-being, social functioning, and quality of life are diminished. Bousquet *et al.* [8] used the SF-36 to assess HRQOL in subjects with perennial allergic rhinitis. These subjects reported significantly poorer HRQOL than nonallergic control subjects in 8 of 9 SF-36 domains. Similarly, using both the SF-36 and the RQLQ, Meltzer *et al.* [6••] found that subjects with allergic rhinitis experienced decreases in a majority of domains of the SF-36 and in all domains of the RQLQ (higher scores indicate more severe symptoms) compared with nonallergic controls (Figs. 3-1 and 3-2).

Rhinitis quality of life questionnaire responses in another large study of subjects with moderate-to-severe allergic rhinitis symptoms indicated more than 90% of untreated patients believed their ability to perform daily activities and work productivity were impaired by rhinitis symptoms (Fig. 3-3) [23]. Finally, in a recent study by Meltzer *et al.* [24•], untreated patients with moderate-to-severe allergic rhinitis reported high levels of activity, work, and classroom impairment (Fig. 3-4).

In addition to psychosocial effects, allergic rhinitis has detrimental effects on mood and cognitive function. Using the non–allergy-specific Positive Affect Negative Affect Scales (PANAS), Marshall and Colon showed atopic individuals experienced significant declines in positive affect scores during allergy seasons compared with nonallergy seasons [25]. Allergic subjects also consistently exhibit significant impairment in cognitive processing, psychomotor speed, verbal learning, and memory during allergy season compared with nonallergic control subjects [26]. Further, Vuurman and colleagues used a computer-simulated didactic simulation model to compare learning capacity of allergic children treated with an antihistamine or placebo with that of healthy controls [27]. Allergic children exhibited learning deficits compared with healthy children, regardless of prior treatment.

Nevertheless, although treatment may not completely eliminate the adverse effects of allergic inflammation, clinical trial data suggests a variety of pharmacologic therapies can significantly improve HRQOL.

EFFECTS OF ALLERGIC RHINITIS TREATMENTS ON HRQOL

It has been proposed that there are three reasons to treat patients: to prevent mortality, reduce probability of future morbidity, and improve well-being [3••]. Until

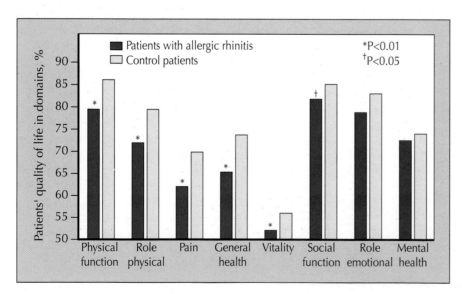

FIGURE 3-1.
Effects of allergic rhinitis on quality of life as measured with the Medical Outcomes Study 36-Item Short Form Health Survey (SF-36).

recently, the goal of treatment has been to meet the first two objectives, with improved well-being assumed to be a natural consequence of reduced symptom severity. Increasing data indicate, however, there is only a modest correlation between clinical measures and how patients feel and function [3••,5]. It is now apparent that treatments for allergic rhinitis must not only relieve symptoms but must also demonstrate the ability to improve daily functioning and maximize well-being. In fact, some national regulatory agencies are beginning to require outcomes evidence of patient benefit before approving new product submissions [3••].

Health-related quality of life data can be used to identify optimal therapeutic regimens and suggest practice guidelines for allergic disorders. Theoretically, HRQOL evaluations will provide rational comparisons of treatment alternatives and indicate the cost/benefit ratios of competing treatment options. Comparing HRQOL data from separate trials can be problematic; the case-mix of patients under study must be controlled since severity of

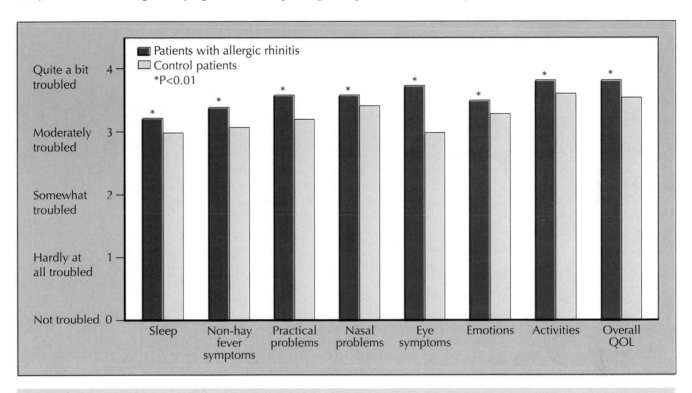

FIGURE 3-2.
Effects of allergic rhinitis on quality of life as measured with the Rhinoconjunctivitis Quality of Life Questionnaire. QOL—quality of life.

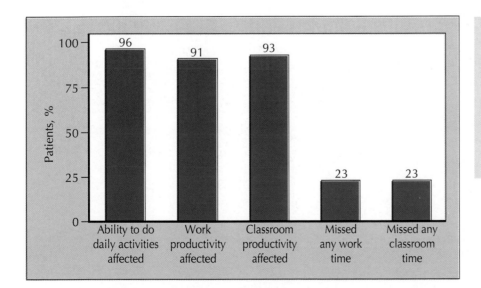

FIGURE 3-3.
Percent of patients who report impairment due to allergies as measured by the Work Productivity and Activity Impairment (WPAI) questionnaire. *Percent of patients reporting any work or classroom time missed, or any impairment in daily activities at work, or in the classroom, secondary to allergies (WPAI-AS).

disease will affect results, and patients may have comorbidities, which also must be considered. Social and financial conditions of the patient can influence outcomes as well [28].

The most common treatments for allergic rhinitis are antihistamines, decongestants, nasal steroids, and immunotherapy. Low-sedating and nonsedating antihistamines have been shown to improve HRQOL in subjects with moderate-to-severe allergic rhinitis compared with placebo [8,23,24•]. In a large health outcome study, 60 mg BID fexofenadine HCl significantly improved HRQOL as indicated by the RQLQ and performance at work and in daily activities as indicated by the WPAI in patients with moderate to severe SAR symptoms [23]. Use of these instruments in another study showed once-daily fexofenadine (120 mg and 180 mg QD) also improved patient-reported HRQOL and decreased work and activity impairment compared with placebo [24•]. Nasal steroids, including fluticasone propionate, budesonide, and beclomethasone dipropionate have also been shown to improve HRQOL in subjects with allergic rhinitis compared with placebo [9,10,29]. Finally Kumar and colleagues used the RQLQ to evaluate changes in HRQOL related to allergen immunotherapy in patients with allergic rhinitis 1 year prior to beginning immunotherapy and during the course of 3 years of treatment [30]. Health-related quality of life

was significantly improved after 1 year compared with pretreatment and at year 2 compared with year 1 (year 3 data not yet available).

Comparative HRQOL data for members of the same drug class (*eg*, antihistamines) and between drug classes (*eg*, nasal steroid versus antihistamine) are now becoming available. Results of a large multinational trial comparing the effects of fexofenadine and loratadine in SAR patients showed fexofenadine 120 mg QD significantly improved overall RQLQ scores compared with placebo (*P* < 0.01) and loratadine 10 mg QD (*P* ≤ 0.05) [31]. Similarly, a comparison of fluticasone propionate and loratadine using the RQLQ in patients with SAR indicated significantly more favorable outcomes were obtained with the nasal steroid (Fig. 3-5) [32••].

Many studies suggest various allergic rhinitis interventions are associated with statistically significant improvements in HRQOL compared with placebo. Clinical efficacy trials typically use statistical significance to indicate meaningful change; however statistical significance is not necessarily a reliable indicator in HRQOL studies. Even when HRQOL changes are statistically significant compared with placebo, perhaps the difference is so small that it has no clinical relevance. Another concern is that when a change is not statistically significant, perhaps the study has not been adequately powered to detect a meaningful change [33]. A

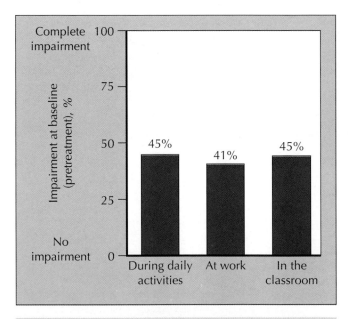

FIGURE 3-4.
Reported levels of impairment at work, in the classroom, and in daily activities due to allergic rhinitis symptoms as measured by the Work Productivity and Activity Impairment (WPAI) questionnaire. *Mean impairment levels reported by patients with seasonal allergic rhinitis (n = 845) before treatment as measured by the WPAI.

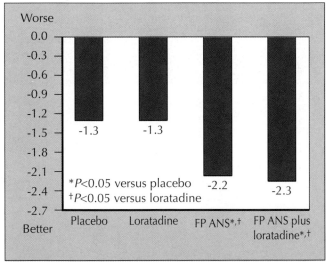

FIGURE 3-5.
Treatment comparisons made with the Rhinoconjunctivitis Quality of Life Questionnaire. FP ANS—fluticasone propionate aqueous nasal spray. (*Adapted from* Ratner *et al.* [32••].)

variety of efforts have been (and continue to be) made to interpret changes in HRQOL status in terms of their clinical relevance.

INTERPRETING HRQOL DATA

It has been proposed that any change in an HRQOL measure is clinically significant because it represents a patient's perception of their state of health [34]. Because the HRQOL assessments are perceptual and physiologic, they have been viewed as less meaningful than physiologic measures (despite the fact that subjective assessments of symptom severity are routinely used to evaluate treatment options in allergic rhinitis). Clinicians may require more experience with the HRQOL measures to trust their clinical relevance to the degree they have come to rely on changes in rhinitis symptom scores [33]. For this reason, an estimate of the difference in score on disease-specific HRQOL questionnaires that can be considered clinically meaningful has been a matter of investigation. Jaeschke et al. [35,36] developed the concept of a minimally important difference (MID), which they defined as "the smallest change in score that patients themselves perceive as important and that would justify a change in the patient's treatment in the absence of undue side effects or excessive cost." Several approaches have been suggested for determining the MID needed to signal clinical improvement (or decrement) due to therapy. A "distribution based" approach is based on statistical distribution of the results, the most commonly used statistic being "effect size," which is derived from the magnitude of change and the variability in stable subjects [3••]. The problem with this approach is it does not indicate whether the magnitude of change is of importance to the patient. Another approach is referred to as "anchor based" and involves comparing or "anchoring" changes in HRQOL measures to other patient-perceived clinically meaningful outcomes. Juniper and colleagues determined that a change in score of 0.5 on the RQLQ is the MID by anchoring RQLQ responses against patient responses on global rating of change questionnaires [3••]. Recent evidence suggests using only MID to interpret research data is not necessarily reliable. Comparing mean differences between treatment groups using only MID values may lead to erroneous conclusions. If only the mean value for the group is considered, valuable information is lost. Patients are heterogeneous in their responses to an intervention. Looking only at the mean ignores the distribution about the mean. For example, though a mean change in RQLQ score of 0.4 is less than the MID, analysis of individual scores may show more patients experienced a clinically meaningful improvement from an intervention than those whose condition worsened [37].

Using a calculation (reported elsewhere) [36] comparing the proportion of subjects benefiting from a treatment versus those not benefiting allows determination of the number needed to treat (NNT). The NNT is the number of patients who would have to be treated for one patient to experience a clinically meaningful improvement in quality of life over and above that which he or she would have experienced without the treatment (eg, with placebo) or with a different intervention. The NNT can be used either for summarizing the results of a therapeutic trial or for medical decision making about an individual patient [38]. Preliminary data suggest the NNT for some allergy and asthma treatments may be relatively low, in the single digits [37]. Single-digit NNT values strongly support the clinical relevance of an intervention. Consider, for example, that the NNTs used to justify the use of statin drugs in stroke patients are in the triple digits.

MAKING HRQOL ASSESSMENTS IN CLINICAL PRACTICE

Generic and disease-specific instruments commonly used in research have been validated in clinical trials; however, more study is needed to confirm their usefulness in individual patients. Nevertheless, a growing number of clinicians are measuring HRQOL during routine patient assessments [2]. Health-related quality of life instruments are easy to use and may provide an acceptable means of obtaining a formalized and quantitative patient history. Theoretically, the patient can complete the questionnaire in the waiting room and a quick scan of responses by the clinician might reduce consultation time and allow the clinician to quickly focus on areas of interest to the patient. Further, questionnaires may reveal problems not spontaneously volunteered by patients, particularly children [2]. Answers to questionnaires at multiple visits may indicate the effectiveness of interventions not only to the clinician, but also to the patient. Visible documentation of benefit (improvements in scores) could help to reinforce persistence with a therapeutic regimen. Evaluating the effectiveness of treatments in the "real world," and not just in highly controlled clinical studies, may also help to establish realistic practice guidelines.

CONCLUSIONS

Allergic rhinitis symptoms cause significant impairment of HRQOL. Conventional clinical indices of symptom severity do not necessarily correlate with patients' feelings and functioning. Health-related quality of life can be measured directly using generic or disease-specific instruments that have been shown to be reproducible, responsive, and valid in controlled trials, and which may be easily incorporated into clinical practice. Experience with an instrument will make determining the clinical significance of HRQOL scores easier; however, in the meantime, methods of evaluating clinical relevance of quality of life assessments are now available.

Health-related quality of life measurements can be used to indicate the risk/benefit and the cost/benefit ratios of competing treatment options. Clinicians and policy makers are already using HRQOL data to evaluate results of medical interventions to guide patient management and reimbursement decisions [2,11].

ACKNOWLEDGMENT

The authors thank Sheila Owens for assistance in the preparation of this manuscript.

REFERENCES AND RECOMMENDED READING

Papers of particular interest, published recently, have been highlighted as:
• Of importance
•• Of major importance

1. Nathan RA, Meltzer EO, Seiner JC, et al.: Prevalence of allergic rhinitis in the United States. *J Allergy Clin Immunol* 1997, 99:S808–S814.

2. Juniper EF: Rhinitis management: the patient's perspective. *Clin Exp Allergy* 1998, 28:34–38.

3.•• Juniper EF: Impact of upper respiratory allergic diseases on quality of life. *J Allergy Clin Immunol* 1998, 101:S386–S391.
This article reviews the concept of health-related quality of life and the available validated questionnaires for measuring it as related to rhinitis. The author is one of the world's experts on the development of instruments to assess quality of life in patients with airway diseases.

4. Meltzer EO, Tyrell RJ, Rich D, et al.: A pharmacologic continuum in the treatment of rhinorrhea: the clinician as economist. *J Allergy Clin Immunol* 1995, 95:1147–1152.

5. De Graff-in 't Veld T, Koenders S, Gerrelds IM, et al.: The relationships between nasal hyperactivity, quality of life, and nasal symptoms in patients with perennial allergic rhinitis. *J Allergy Clin Immunol* 1996, 98:508–513.

6.•• Meltzer EO, Nathan RA, Selner JC, et al.: Quality of life and rhinitic symptoms: results of a nationwide survey with the SF-36 and RQLQ questionnaires. *J Allergy Clin Immunol* 1997, S815–S819.
This article presents the results of a large survey of rhinitis patients. The data are derived from both a generic instrument, the SF-36, and a disease specific questionnaire, the RQLQ.

7. Blaiss MS: Quality of life in allergic rhinitis. *Ann Allergy Asthma Immunol* 1999, 83:449–454.

8. Bousquet J, Duchateau J, Pignot JC, et al: Improvement of quality of life by treatment with certirizine in patients with perennial allergic rhinitis as determined by a French version of the SF-36 questionnaire. *J Allergy Clin Immunol* 1996, 98:309–316.

9. Goodwin B, Bowers B, Hampel F: Superior improvement in disease-specific quality of life for SAR patients receiving intranasal fluticasone vs loratadine tablets. *J Allergy Clin Immunol* 1997, 99:S27D.

10. Juniper EF, Guyatt GH, Andersson B, et al.: Comparison of powder and aerosolized budesonide in perennial rhinitis: validation of rhinitis quality of life questionnaire. *Ann Allergy* 1993, 70:225–230.

11. Ware JE, Sherbourne CD: The MOS 36-item short-form health survey (SF-36). *Med Care* 1992, 30:473–483.

12. How to score the MOS 36-item short-form health survey (SF-36). SF-36 scoring rules (version 1.1) International Resource Center (IRC) for Health Care Assessment, New England Medical Center Hospitals, Copyright 1992 MOS Trust, Inc.

13. Ellis AK, Day JH, Lundie MJ: Impact of quality of life during an allergen challenge research trial. *Ann Allergy Asthma Immunol* 1999, 83:33–39.

14. Guyatt GH, Feeny DH, Patrick DL: Measuring health-related quality of life. *Ann Intern Med* 1993, 118:622–629.

15. Juniper EF, Guyatt GH: Development and testing of a new measure of health status for clinical trials in rhinoconjunctivitis. *Clin Exp Allergy* 1991, 21:77–83.

16. Reilly MC, Zbrozek AS, Dukes EM: The validity and reproducibility of a work productivity and activity impairment instrument. *PharmacoEconomics* 1993, 4:353–365.

17.• Reilly MC, Tanner A, Meltzer EO: Work, classroom, and activity impairment instruments. *Clin Drug Invest* 1996, 11:278–288.
The paper documents the discriminative and evaluative validity, reproducibility and responsiveness of the WPAI-AS measure. A simple seven question generic instrument is presented to allergic rhinitis patients to determine if it can be useful in quantifying quality of life impairment.

18. Juniper EF, Guyatt GH, Dolovich J: Assessment of quality of life in adolescents with allergic rhinoconjunctivitis: development and testing of a questionnaire for clinical trials. *J Allergy Clin Immunol* 1994, 93:413–423.

19. Juniper EF, Howland WC, Roberts NB, et al.: Measuring quality of life in children with rhinoconjunctivitis. *J Allergy Clin Immunol* 1998, 101:163–170.

20. Juniper EF, Thompson AK, Ferrie PJ, et al.: Development and validation of the mini rhinoconjunctivitis quality of life questionnaire. *Clin Exp Allergy* 2000, 30:132–140.

21. Caro JJ, Caro I, Caro J, et al.: Electronic implementation of quality of life measures in asthma [Abstract]. *Am J Respir Crit Care Med* 1999, 159:693.

22. Keresteci MA, Ungar W, Ryan N, et al.: Development of a nasal comfort index for nasal sprays in adults with seasonal allergic rhinitis [Abstract]. *Value Health* 1999, 2:181.

23. Tanner LA, Reilly M, Meltzer EO, et al.: Effect of fexofenadine on quality of life and work, classroom, and daily activity impairment in patients with seasonal allergic rhinitis. *Am J Manag Care* 1999, 5:S235–S247.

24.• Meltzer EO, Casale TB, Nathan RA, et al.: Once-daily fexofenadine HCl improves quality of life and reduces work and activity impairment in patients with seasonal allergic rhinitis. *Ann Allergy Asthma Immunol* 1999, 83:311–317.
This article demonstrates that therapeutic intervention with an antihistamine improves not only symptoms but quality of life for patients with allergic rhinitis.

25. Marshall PS, Colon EA: Effects of allergy season on mood and cognitive function. *Ann Allergy* 1993, 71:251–258.

26. Simons FER: Learning impairment and allergic rhinitis. *Allergy Asthma Proc* 1996, 17:185–189.

27. Vuurman EF, van Veggel LM, Uiterwijk MM, et al: Seasonal allergic rhinitis and antihistamine effects on children's learning. *Ann Allergy* 1993, 71:121–126.

28. Blaiss MS: Why outcomes? [editorial]. *Ann Allergy Asthma Immunol* 1995, 74:359–361.

29. Milgrom H, Biondi R, Georgitis JW, *et al.*: Comparison of ipratropium bromide 0.03% with beclomethasone dipropionate in the treatment of perennial rhinitis in children. *Ann Allergy Asthma Immunol* 1999, 83:105–111.

30. Kumar P, Kamboj S, Rao P, *et al.*: The cost of care and quality of life in patients with allergic rhinitis on allergen immunotherapy. *Allergy Clin Immunol Int* 1997, 9:133–135.

31. Van Cauwenberge P, Juniper EF, Meltzer E, Star Investigating Group: Comparison of the efficacy, safety, and quality of life provided by fexofenadine hydrochloride 120 mg, loratadine 10 mg, and placebo administered once daily for the treatment of seasonal allergic rhinitis. *Clin Exp Allergy* 2000, 30:891–899.

32.•• Ratner PH, van Bavel JH , Martin BG, *et al.*: A comparison of the efficacy of fluticasone propionate aqueous nasal spray and loratadine alone and in combination, for the treatment of seasonal allergic rhinitis. *J Fam Pract* 1998, 47:118–125.
This study demonstrates that a disease-specific measure like the Rhinoconjunctivitis Quality of Life Questionnaire can compare the degree of efficacy of various therapies. Both antihistamines and intranasal corticosteroid treatment improve the quality of life of patients suffering from allergic rhinitis.

33. Juniper EF: Quality of life questionnaires: does statistically significant equal clinically important? [editorial]. *J Allergy Clin Immunol* 1998, 102:16–17.

34. Lydick E, Epstein RS: Interpretation of quality of life changes. *Quality Life Res* 1993, 2:221–226.

35. Jaeschke R, Singer J, Guyatt GH: Measurement of health status. *Controlled Clin Trials* 1989, 10:407–415.

36. Juniper EF, Guyatt GH, Willan A, *et al.*: Determining a minimal important change in disease-specific quality of life questionnaire. *J Clin Epidemiol* 1994, 47:81–87.

37. Juniper EF: Interpreting of Quality of Life Data. Quality of Life Newsletter, September–December 1999, 2:3.

38. Chatellier G, Zapletal E, Lemaitre D, *et al.*: The number needed to treat a clinically useful nomogram in its proper context. *Br Med J* 1996, 312:426–429.

39. Juniper EF, Thompson AK, Ferrie PJ, *et al.*: Validation of the standardized version of the Rhinoconjunctivitis Quality of Life Questionnaire. *J Allergy Clin Immunol* 1999, 104:364–369.

CHAPTER 4

Pathogenesis of Allergic Rhinitis

James N. Baraniuk

The pathogenesis of allergic rhinitis can be better appreciated by understanding the numerous protective mechanisms available for mucosal defense. The system of T_H2 lymphocytes, IgE production, mast cell degranulation, eosinophil infiltration, and resident cell responses is central to our understanding and treatment of allergic rhinitis. Histamine remains pre-eminent in causing the cardinal symptoms of the immediate allergic reaction: itching, watery discharge, and nasal swelling. This chapter also reviews recruitment and activation mechanisms responsible for the late phase allergic response.

CLASSIFICATION OF RHINITIS

The differential diagnosis of rhinitis is long and complex [1–6]. The patient with rhinitis can be approached with a series of questions: Are the symptoms exaggerated normal responses or pathologic responses? Are the symptoms intermittent (seasonal) or persistent (perennial)? Are there specific signs of rhinitis? Is there a purulent or nonpurulent discharge? Is the inflammation eosinophilic or neutrophilic, or are there no changes in inflammatory leukocytes? Are anatomic factors such as septal spurs or deviated nasal septum the source of complaints [3]?

Negotiating this diagnostic algorithm requires clinical judgment to identify specific symptom complexes, the accessibility of the nostrils for inspection, and the potential need for computed tomography (CT) or rhinoscopy to identify other pathologic findings.

The diverse differential diagnosis is the product of decades of investigations of allergen and other nasal provocation studies, biopsy, nasal scraping, and lavage studies, and the explosion of information about the molecular biology of nasal, sinus, and other forms of inflammation. Many authors have examined this differential diagnosis of infectious, allergic, metabolic, vasculitic, drug-induced, atrophic, physical, chemical, and other triggers of rhinitis, and promoted algorithms for diagnosis and treatment [1–6]. More simply, rhinitis can be categorized according to inflammatory changes, neural disorders with minimal physical findings, and conditions related to hormonal, drug, and other causes (Table 4-1).

REDUCTIONIST APPROACH TO THE HISTOLOGY AND PHYSIOLOGY OF THE HUMAN NASAL MUCOSA

The functions, capabilities, and pathophysiologic changes of the human nasal mucosa can be appreciated from turbinate histology (Fig. 4-1).

A reductionist approach has been developed that identifies four major compartments within the nasal mucosa that account for the most of the signs and symptoms of rhinitis (Fig. 4-2):

1. The superficial postcapillary venules are responsible for the endothelium-directed leakage of plasma that leads to local edema and watery rhinorrhea. These endothelial cells direct leukocyte traffic by the expression of chemoattractants and adhesion markers that recruit the unique sets of neutrophils, eosinophils, basophils, lymphocytes, macrophages,

and precursor cells that characterize cellular inflammation in each form of rhinitis.

2. The deep venous sinusoids control nasal patency on the minute to minute, and longer "nasal cycle" schedules. These vasomotor processes are orchestrated by brain stem rhythms and are enacted via autonomic nerves.

3. The epithelial and glandular serous and mucous cells contribute to the sol phase antimicrobial defense factors (eg, sIgA), sticky gel phase mucopolysaccharide mucins, and ionic composition of the nasal epithelial lining fluid [1,7].

TABLE 4.1 THE SPECTRUM OF RHINOSINUSITIS

Inflammatory rhinitis			Noninflammatory rhinitis			
Predominant cellular infiltrate			**Neural dysfunction**			
Eosinophilic	Neutrophilic	Other	Irritant/ nociceptive	Cholinergic/ parasympathetic	Sympathetic	Hormones, drugs, other causes
Allergic rhinitis	Bacterial sinusitis	Viral rhinitis (mixed cellular responses)	Dry vasomotor rhinitis	Wet vasomotor rhinitis	Horner's syndrome	Pregnancy
Intermittent (seasonal)	Adenoiditis	Wegener's granulomatosis	Irritant rhinitis	Cholinergic hypersecretory rhinitis	Nonallergic rhinitis with paradoxical vasodilation instead of vasoconstriction	Hypothyroidism
Persistent (perennial)	Cystic fibrosis	Midline granuloma	MCS	Gustatory rhinitis	α-Adrenergic agonist overuse: rhinitis medicamentosa	Drugs
Allergen-specific (eg, shrimp fumes)	Foreign body	Sarcoidosis	CFS	"Skier's nose"		β-blockers and other vasodilating antihypertensives
Allergic fungal sinusitis	Immunodeficiency	Occupational and toxin reactions (eg, plicatic acid from western red cedar)	Cacosmia	"Salsa sniffles"		Cocaine
NARES	Ciliary dysfunction (eg, Kartagener's syndrome with low NO levels)	Other unusual inflammatory conditions				Trauma
CESS						Anatomical variants:
Nonallergic chronic eosinophilic mucin sinusitis						Deviated nasal septum
Nasal polyps						Concha bullosa
Aspirin sensitivity						Tumor
Triad asthma						Atrophic rhinitis

CESS—chronic eosinophilic sinusitis syndrome; CFS—chronic fatigue syndrome; MCS—multiple chemical sensitivity; NARES—nonallergic rhinitis with eosinophilia syndrome; NO—nitric oxide.

4. Nociceptive nerves are the early warning system for mucosal injury and rapidly initiate defense mechanisms via the axon response and central reflexes. Parasympathetic reflexes cause cholinergic glandular exocytosis. Sympathetic reflexes constrict venous sinusoids to regulate nasal airspace volume and nasal air flow.

Several new principles are restructuring our understanding of the various phases of allergic rhinitis: the subtypes of lymphocytes driving antigen specific inflammation; differentiation and restructuring of epithelial and other mucosal structures (eg, adhesion markers on endothelial and epithelial cells, chemoattractants, glandular changes); neurogenic mechanisms responsible for irritant syndromes that may occur in the apparent absence of mucosal inflammation

[8,9,10••]; and the human genome. Genes expressed on the distal portion of the long arm of the fifth chromosome (5q31.1-q33) play major roles in atopy, vernal keratoconjunctivitis [11], and myelodysplastic [12] and other neoplastic syndromes [13,14]. These include: interleukin (IL)-3, granulocyte-macrophage colony-stimulating factor (GM-CSF), IL-5, IL-13, IL-4, IL-9, macrophage colony-stimulating factor (M-CSF)-receptor, IL-12B p40 (40 kDa) monomer, an anonymous gene that may control the maintenance of responsiveness to IL-12, fibroblast growth factor (FGF-1) ("acidic"), early growth response gene-1 (EGRF-1), endothelial cell growth factor, platelet-derived growth factor (PDGF), feline myosarcoma viral oncogene homologue (tyrosine kinase), CD14 monocyte differentiation factors, dopamine receptor

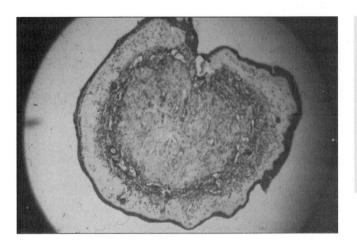

FIGURE 4-1.

Normal nasal mucosa. This cross-section of the inferior turbinate shows the outer layer of typical respiratory epithelium and its basement membrane and the superficial region of fenestrated capillaries and postcapillary venules. The latter is the region of vascular permeability and inflammatory cell diapedesis. Deep to these superficial vessels are the submucosal glands. At the center of the turbinate are the deep venous sinusoids. Dilation of the sinusoids increases the diameter of the turbinate and reduces the available airspace. Constriction of these vessels leads to nasal patency.

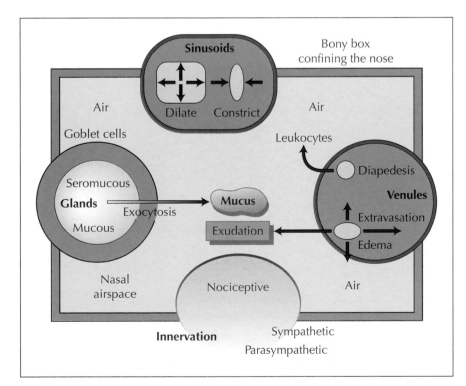

FIGURE 4-2.

Reductionist view of the nasal mucosa. This schematic separates the four functional components of the nasal mucosa as invaginations into the nasal airspace: 1) venous sinusoids; 2) postcapillary venules; 3) the "exocytosis" domain composed of surface epithelial goblet, microvilli, and ciliated cells and glandular seromucous and mucous cells; and 4) innervation by nonmyelinated type C nociceptive nerves and parasympathetic and sympathetic fibers.

type 1A, α1B-adrenergic receptor, β2-adrenergic receptor, and the glucocorticoid receptor [11–15]. Genetic modulation of the expression of these genes may become possible in this century.

GELL AND COOMBS REASSESSED

The original Gell and Coombs classification of three divisions of humoral responses and the "garbage can" division of cell-mediated immunity (segregation limited by methodology) [16] can now be expanded by including the type-1 and type-2 components of CD4 (T_H1 and T_H2) and CD8 ("T-cytotoxic" and "T-suppressor") lymphocytes and "pseudoallergic" anaphylactoid reactions that involve non–IgE-mediated mast cell degranulation and other mechanisms (Table 4-2). At present, the best rationalization for the T_H2 immune response appears to be as a prototypic antiparasite mucosal pro-

tection mechanism. This hypothesis is useful to explain sensitization by allergenic particulate material at the mucosal surface; IgE-plasma cell, mast cell, eosinophil infiltration and mediator release causing mucous secretion, smooth muscle spasm, extreme vascular permeability, and vasodilation; and neural stimulation that characterizes type I hypersensitivity reactions. This simplification explains the secretory and peristaltic intestinal responses to parasites, the pathologic "peristalsis" of the foregut-derived bronchi in asthma (bronchoconstriction with mucous plugging), and responses in other mucosal sites and the skin.

OVERVIEW OF THE NASAL ALLERGEN RESPONSE

The phases leading to chronic allergic rhinitis are defined by the standard allergen challenge model [17]. Circulating IgE binds to high-affinity Fcε-receptor I on

---

TABLE **4.2** HYPOTHETICAL MODIFICATION OF THE GELL AND COOMBS CLASSIFICATION OF IMMUNE DISEASES

Antigen presentation	Subsets of Gell and Coombs "type-IV" cellular reactions		
Gell & Coombs "cellular immunity"	Type-1–like: interferon-γ	Type-2–like: IL-3, IL4, IL-5, IL-9, IL-10, IL-13	Other
Exogenous antigen presented by class II MHC on antigen-presenting cell to T-cell receptor on CD4+ cell	DTH, T_H1 macrophage IL-12, granulomas, *eg,* TB, tuberculous leprosy	LPR, T_H2, eosinophilia, *eg,* asthma, lepromatous leprosy	Tolerance, T_H3?, TGF-β
Endogenous antigen presented by class I MHC on nucleated cells to T-cell receptor on CD8+ cell	TC-1 CD8+ cell, kill antigen presenting cell, *eg,* viral infection, neoplasia, bullous skin lesions (?)	TC-2 CD8+ cell, kill antigen-presenting cell, eosinophilia, *eg,* drug reactions, poison ivy?	
Foreign lipids and polysaccharides presented by CD1 on cutaneous (other?) Langerhans' cells	NK-1 cells (interferon-γ)	NK-2 cells (IL-5, IL-13)	CD4-, CD8-, *eg,* initiate TB immune response, ALPS (no apoptosis)
Disordered target cell receptor expression			NK cell dysfunction
Gell & Coombs "humoral immunity"	Gell and Coombs "type I" immediate hypersensitivity	Gell and Coombs "type II" hypersensitivity	Gell and Coombs "type III" hypersensitivity
Antigen in immune complexes or on cell surfaces; recognized by B-cell surface IgM; T-cell help followed by heavy chain switching to IgA1, IgA2, IgG1, IgG2, IgG3, IgG4, IgD, IgE	IgE plasma cells, IgE-mast cell, IgE-basophil, immediate degranulation with release of mediators, "anaphylaxis," T_H2 driven	Multiple antibody classes, recognition of "self" antigen with cytotoxicity (Goodpasture's syndrome) or cellular activation (long-acting thyroid-stimulating antibody), T-helper cell driven?	Immune complex formation by IgM, IgG1, IgG3; complement activation; Fc-γ and C3b-induced neutrophilia, *eg,* serum sickness, T-helper cell driven?
	Secretory IgA for muscosal defense		
Gell & Coombs "Pseudoallergic reactions": not antigen driven	Direct mast cell anaphylactoid degranulation by vancomycin, opiates, IV contrast dye, etc.	Enzyme systems: asprin sensitivity, cyclooxygenase 2 deficiency (?), ACE inhibitor cough	C3a, C5a: anaphylactotoxins, mast cell degranulation, urticaria*

A proportion of chronic idiopathic urticaria may be due to antithyroid IgG1 and IgG3 antibodies that cross-react with IgE-RIα, leading to complement binding, activation, and release of C3a and C5a.

ACE—anigiotensin-converting enzyme; ALPS—acquired lymphoproliferative syndrome; DTH—delayed-type hypersensitivity; IL—interleukin; IV—intravenous; LPR—late-phase response; MHC—major histocompatibility complex; NK—natural killer; TB—tuberculosis; TC—T-cytotoxic lymphocyte.

mast cells and basophils. It is unclear if mast cells circulate through regions of IgE production to pick up their IgE or if they passively adsorb the IgE from plasma or tissue interstitial fluids. IgE plasma cells may differentiate and synthesize IgE in the nasal mucosa [18••]. Mast cells or their precursors exit via postcapillary venules and reside in the submucosal regions. Reexposure to allergen leads to cross-linking of their Fc receptors and degranulation. The preformed and newly formed products will be described in the next section. Stimulation of type C "itch" fibers leads to neurogenic responses. After the immediate response abates, a "recruitment phase" [1] follows with the infiltration of the tissue by eosinophils, basophils, and T_H2 cells. Their activation and mediator release during the late-phase response (LPR) recapitulates much of the pathology of the immediate response. Continued allergen exposure heightens both the immediate and late-phase responses so that an exuberant chronic phase of inflammation develops.

THE CONSEQUENCES OF IMMEDIATE-PHASE MAST CELL MEDIATOR RELEASE

Deep tissue or connective tissue mast cells express chymase, tryptase, and tumor necrosis factor (TNF)–α (MC_{TC}) [19,20]. This cell population represents 85% of the IL-4–positive mast cells in the nasal lamina propria. Mast cells in the lamina propria also express IL-13,

although it is unclear if one subset or another is involved [21]. During allergen assault, the proportion of epithelial mast cells increases [22]. These mucosal mast cells produce tryptase without chymase (MC_T). MC_T cells are thought to express IL-5 and IL-6, and represent 15% of IL-4–positive mast cells [19,20]. T_H2 cytokines may inspire mucosal mast cell proliferation in allergic rhinitis [23]. Proliferation of MC_T cells occurs in the epithelium and most superficial layers of the lamina propria. Epithelial mast cell density is decreased by topical nasal glucocorticoids [22].

Allergenic proteins cross-link IgE molecules that pull their high-affinity Fcε receptors together. This induces explosive degranulation of mast cells that rapidly leads to itching, sneezing, nasal discharge, and mucosal swelling with increased nasal airways resistance [1,24,25]. Histamine plays the preeminent role in these immediate reactions (Fig. 4-3). This is clear from antihistamine studies, since these drugs reduce immediate symptoms by 50% to 60% [24]. Hence, the consequences of histamine release during the immediate phase are greater than the combined immediate effects of tryptase, prostaglandin D_2, prostaglandin F_2, leukotriene (LT) C4/D4/E4, mast cell kininogenase-mediated production of bradykinin, TNF-α, IL-4, IL-5, IL-6, transforming growth factor (TGF)–β, and IL-13 production [26]. Histamine has synergistic effects with this melange of mediators. Leukotrienes and chymase

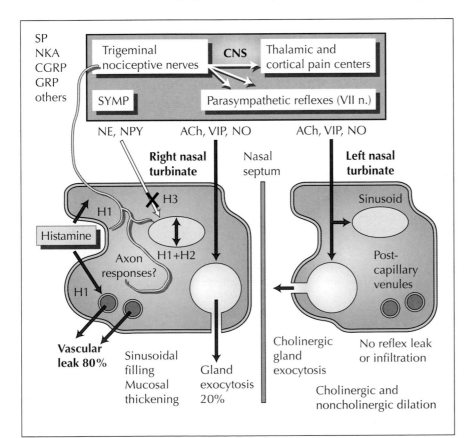

FIGURE 4-3.

How the nose runs. Histamine acts on H_1 receptors to induce vascular permeability and activate nociceptive nerves that recruit parasympathetic reflexes. Activation of nociceptive nerves may lead to axon response–mediated release of neuropeptides such as substance P and calcitonin gene–related peptide, but the most potent effects are activation of pain centers in the brain and recruitment of systemic reflexes such as sneezing and parasympathetic cholinergic reflexes that mediate glandular secretion in allergic rhinitis. ACh—acetylcholine; CGRP—calcitonin gene–related peptide; GRP—gastrin-releasing peptide; NE—norepinephrine; NKA—neurokinin A; NO—nitric oxide; NPY—neuropeptide tyrosine; SP—substance P; SYMP—sympathetic; VIP—vasoactive intestinal peptide.

stimulate glandular exocytosis and mucous secretion [27,28]. Histamine, bradykinin, LTs, and platelet-activating factor activate the endothelial cells of postcapillary venules to induce vasodilation, vascular permeability, and cellular adhesion. Contraction of postcapillary venule endothelial cells opens gaps, which permit the hydrostatic intravascular pressure to force plasma into the interstitial space. A pressure of 5 cm H_2O is capable of driving fluid from the vessels through the interstitium, across the epithelial basement membrane, and between epithelial cells and their tight junctions into the nasal lumen [29]. This is a nondamaging reversible event that may occur without significant tissue edema. Also, the nasal capillaries are fenestrated, which may allow the free exchange of plasma and interstitial fluids leading to the rapid exchange of medications and mediators to and from the lamina propria.

Histamine activates H_1 receptors on nociceptive nerve fibers to induce the sensation of itching. Histamine receptors belong to the rhodopsin receptor family with seven transmembrane segments, extracellular N-terminal, two extracellular loops, two intracellular loops, and a C-terminal tail [14]. These receptors generate intracellular messages by activating glutamyl transpeptidase (GTP)-binding protein (G-proteins). Three histamine receptors have been cloned. The H_1 receptor is the workhorse for histamine's allergic effects. The H_2 receptor participates in stomach acid production but also plays a role in vasodilation and possibly cardiac effects of histamine in anaphylaxis. H_3 receptors are present on neurons, where they appear to act as "inhibitory autoreceptors" that reduce neural activity ("shut-off" nerves). These receptors are also present in adipose tissue.

In allergic rhinitis, H_1 receptor mRNA is upregulated [30]. H_1 receptors are present on endothelial cells, where they act to induce vascular permeability and the copious watery rhinorrhea of acute allergic rhinitis [31]. H_1 receptors activate afferent nociceptive "itch" nerves leading to the appreciation of that sensation in the central nervous system. This is followed by recruitment of brain stem parasympathetic reflexes that cause glandular secretion. This reflex arc supplies the rationale for using anticholinergic drugs in allergic rhinitis.

Histamine is degraded by epithelial and endothelial histamine N-methyltransferase (HMT) [32]. This action of HMT limits the duration of action of histamine in the mucosa and explains why allergen provocation testing leads to self-limited vascular leak. Submucosal glands do not express HMT mRNA. The lack of H_1 receptors and HMT on nasal submucosal glands is consistent with the absence of histamine-induced exocytosis observed in vitro and the need for cholinergic reflex-mediated exocytosis [7].

Mast cell mediator release also participates in nonatopic disorders. Anaphylactoid reactions are similar in their immediate consequences to those of IgE-mediated mast cell degranulation. Agents acting directly on mast cells include IgE-dependent histamine releasing factor, IL-1, monocyte chemoattractant protein (MCP)-1, MCP-3, macrophage inflammatory protein (MIP)-1α, neutrophil-activating peptide (NAP)-2, connective tissue–activating peptide (CTAP)-III, opioids, mast cell–degranulating peptide, highly charged or amphipathic molecules such as intravenous contrast dye, high doses of substance P (SP), and vancomycin (red man syndrome). Factors that augment ongoing IgE-mediated degranulation include IL-1α, IL-1β, IL-3, IL-5, IL-6, IL-7, and c-kit ligand (stem cell factor). Mast cells may also be activated in immune complex diseases because complement factors such as C3a and C5a are potent anaphylatoxins. Under certain circumstances, it is possible that different IgE-independent mast cell degranulating agents may cause selective release of preformed mediators, arachidonic acid metabolites, or specific sets of cytokines. The difference between anaphylactic and anaphylactoid responses is the ability to demonstrate reproducible IgE-mediated immediate responses to picogram to nanogram amounts of allergen in immune-sensitized subjects with anaphylactic reactions, whereas anaphylactoid reactions may potentially occur in all subjects in a dose-dependent fashion provided enough of the agent is given.

NOCICEPTIVE NERVE RESPONSES

Histamine binds to H1 receptors on nociceptive type-C nerves of the first and second divisions of the trigeminal nerve [1,7]. Prostaglandins and LTs increase the sensitivity of these nerves to histamine and other agents that depolarize nociceptive nerves [33]. These neurons are extensively branched in the epithelium and submucosal regions. In the mucosa, depolarization of the neuron may lead to the release of neurotransmitters such as SP, calcitonin gene–related peptide (CGRP), neurokinin A, gastrin-releasing peptide, and possibly others by the axon response mechanism. These neuropeptides lead to local inflammatory responses termed "neurogenic inflammation." The axon response in rodents induces vascular permeability and leukocyte infiltration [34]. However, in normal humans and pigs, the axon response appears to have little if any effect on vascular leak [35–37]. In untreated, severely allergic subjects who have an increase in basal plasma extravasation as a part of their allergic pathophysiology, repeated nasal SP applications can increase leak and lavage fluid eosinophilia from 18% to 43% [38]. The cause of this increase in basal vascular leak is not known, but it does not appear to be related to neurogenic mechanisms [36,37]. This basal leak can be reduced by long-acting β2-adrenergic agonists in humans in season in vivo [39•]. Neurogenic responses are suspected in humans, because SP and CGRP are released within 3 minutes after allergen [40] and hypertonic saline nasal provocations [10••] but are not detectable after histamine challenges [40]. An alternative hypothesis is that human airway hypertonic saline–receptive nociceptive neuron axon responses and systemic reflexes may induce rapid defensive measures, such as glandular secretion to adsorb irritants and sneeze to expel them, and more delayed endothelial adhesion marker upregulation aimed at limiting an initial mucosal insult for preparation against further potential invasion. Hypertonic saline provocation leads to pain, SP release, and glandular secretion, but does not cause any changes in vascular permeability or dilation of venous sinusoids [10••]. Incubations of normal human nasal mucosal explants in vitro with SP leads to significant increases in IL-6 and IL-8 [41]. However, IL-1β, IL-2, IL-3, IL-4, IL-5, IL-6, TNF-α, and interferon-γ mRNA are induced from allergic rhinitis nasal mucosa. SP-induced cytokine production may include epithelial, endothelial, and inflammatory cells in these explants. These data indicate that in normal humans, the airway mucosal axon response induces the secretion of serous cell antibacterial enzymes such as lysozyme, lactoferrin, and secretory IgA plus mucin mucoglycoproteins from mucous and perhaps goblet cells, and induces longer-term (4 to 24 hr) changes in cytokine, chemokine, and adhesion marker expression.

Calcitonin gene–related peptide may contribute to the venous sinusoid swelling that blocks nasal airflow [42]. It is also likely the mediator of the flare responses after allergen skin testing and the Triple Response of Lewis.

In the central nervous system, trigeminal nociceptive neurons enter the pons through the sensory root and turn caudally in the trigeminal spinal tract to terminate in the pars caudalis of the nucleus of the spinal tract in the lower medulla and upper three cervical segments of the spinal cord [33]. Pars caudalis interneurons cross the midline to enter the trigeminothalamic tract and terminate in the medial part of the ventral posterior thalamic nucleus. Painful and strong thermal stimuli are appreciated at the thalamic level. Tertiary neural relays to the lower third of the parietal cortical somesthetic areas provide for localization of nasal stimuli. Glossopharyngeal afferents innervate the posterior third of the tongue, upper pharynx, tonsils, eustachian tube, and middle ear and also are of relevance to allergic rhinitis. These thermosensitive and nociceptive neurons terminate in the dorsal portion of the trigeminal spinal tract. Activation of these central registries is responsible for the sensations of itch and congestion that are the hallmarks of allergic rhinitis.

PARASYMPATHETIC REFLEXES

Connections between afferent trigeminal interneurons, the tractus solitarius, nucleus ambiguus, and salivatory nucleus of the seventh nerve serve to recruit parasympathetic reflexes. Seventh nerve motor fibers synapse in the sphenopalatine ganglia and pass with sympathetic fibers through the vidian canal to enter the nasal mucosa. These postganglionic neurons contain acetylcholine, vasoactive intestinal peptide (VIP), VIP-like peptides (eg, peptide histidine-methionine), and nitric oxide synthase (NOS, generates NO) [33]. It is possible that acetylcholine and VIP/NOS are packaged in different sets of neurons. Parasympathetic reflexes are rapidly activated after allergen challenge since VIP is released within 3 minutes after nasal allergen provocation [40].

Nociceptive nerve–parasympathetic cholinergic reflex-mediated stimulation of glandular exocytosis is probably the most important single, tonically active influence regulating glandular secretion in the respiratory tract. This reflex provides the rationale for the use of ipratropium bromide and other anticholinergic antagonists in allergic rhinitis [43]. The M_3 muscarinic receptor is the most important of the five cloned muscarinic receptors in human nasal mucosa based upon functional and in situ hybridization studies [44,45]. The M_2 receptor on nociceptive nerves may serve as an inhibitory autoreceptor. Eosinophil major basic protein and influenza virus neuraminidase may bind the M_2 receptor, inhibit its function, and promote cholinergically mediated secretion or bronchial smooth muscle constriction [46••,47]. This could be one example of eosinophil-mediated neural dysfunction.

RECRUITMENT PHASE WITH CHEMOATTRACTION OF INFLAMMATORY CELLS

Circulating leukocytes bind to postcapillary venule endothelial cell glycoprotein lectins called "selectins" (E-selectin for eosinophils, P-selectin for polymorphonuclear cells) and leukocyte glycoproteins bearing the Lewis^X blood group marker [1]. The shear forces of blood flow force these leukocytes to roll along the endothelial surface. Endothelial cells also constitutively express low levels of intercellular adhesion molecule (ICAM)-1, ICAM-2, and platelet endothelial cell adhesion molecule. When stimulated by the immediate-phase mediators, cytokines such as IL-1, TNF-α, interferon-γ, and IL-4, and eosinophil cationic proteins [48], preformed endothelial cell vesicles (Weibel-Palade bodies) fuse with the lumenal surface and greatly increase ICAM-1, vascular cell adhesion molecule–1, and other adhesion molecule expression [1]. These interact with eosinophil and basophil integrins including leukocyte function-associated antigen–1 (αLβ2), Mac-1 (αMβ2), and VLA-4 (α4β1) and Act-1 (α4β7), which causes the leukocytes to flatten and bind tightly to the endothelial surface. Glucocorticoids reduce this upregulation. In the future, drugs may be able to specifically block individual or families of these critical integrins and stop diapedesis of inflammatory cell populations from the blood.

If the adherent leukocytes receive a second, chemoattractant signal, then the characteristic allergic influx of eosinophils, basophils, and T_H2 cells will begin. These chemokines may belong to the C-X-C (α-chemokine) group from chromosome 4 that includes IL-8, platelet factor–4, NAP-2, CTAP III, lungkine, GRO-1, and GRO-2 or the C-C (β-chemokine) group from chromosome 17, which includes MCP-1, MCP-3, RANTES (regulated upon activation, normal T-cell expressed and secreted), MIP-1α, and IL-15. Additional chemokines include eotaxin and IL-13 [49–51]. The infiltrating cells become activated and release their own panoply of cytokines and mediators. After approximately 4 to 12 hours, sufficient cells may have moved into the tissue to cause symptoms of nasal blockage and obstruction. It is unclear if this is due to venous sinusoid filling, nasal secretion production, or an increase in mucosal bulk due to leukocyte invasion of the tissue. This activity constitutes the late-phase response [1]. Histamine is released without a change in tryptase, suggesting release from basophils rather than a secondary degranulation of mast cells [17]. The role of histamine in the late-phase response is less prominent than during the immediate phase since the level of itch and sneezing is low.

CHRONIC ALLERGIC RHINITIS

During prolonged, recurrent, and chronic nasal allergen exposure and repeated cycles of immediate and late-phase responses, a flood of cytokines and other mediators are released from infiltrating eosinophils (major basic protein, eosinophil cationic protein, eosinophil peroxidase, eosinophil-derived neurotoxin, halide free radicals, LTC4, IL-1, IL-4, IL-5, IL-9, TNF-α, eotaxin, GM-CSF, others), epithelial mast cells (LTC4, IL-4, IL-6, IL-13, TNF-α, TGF-β, tryptase, and other enzymes), T_H2 lymphocytes (IL-3, IL-4, IL-5, IL-9, IL-10, IL-13, and others) and resident cells such as epithelium [1,11,48–51]. Effects of these mediators in perennial rhinitis can be substantially greater than the effects of histamine, leading to symptoms that are not amenable to antihistamine therapy. Thus, glucocorticoids become the treatment of choice for persistent and severe intermittent (seasonal) rhinitis. They are most beneficial when begun before the season starts.

Fibrosis may also be a long-term consequence of chronic allergic rhinitis. Cytokines such as TGF-β from eosinophils, mast cells, and possibly other cells, insulin-like growth factor, acidic fibroblast growth factor, and platelet-derived growth factor may stimulate fibroblast proliferation, differentiation into myofibroblasts, and increased collagen deposition.

EPITHELIAL CELL CHANGES IN ALLERGIC RHINITIS

Epithelial cells become activated in chronic allergic rhinitis and express increased amounts of GM-CSF, IL-1α, IL-6, IL-8, eotaxins, RANTES, IL-1 receptors, TNF-α receptors, and class II HLA (HLA-DR) [49,52]. Cytokines and eosinophilic cationic protein also upregulate epithelial ICAM-1 expression, suggesting that rhinovirus infections may be more frequent in allergic subjects since ICAM-1 is the binding site for rhinoviruses [48]. Endothelin-1, (ET1), which is known to be expressed by epithelial and submucosal gland cells in human mucosa [53], and the enzyme that generates endothelin converting enzyme–1 are upregulated in chronic rhinitis [54].

Nitric oxide is present in exhaled nasal air (24.7 ± 2.2 ppb), and its levels are increased during allergic rhinitis (35.4 ± 2.0 ppb, $p < 0.001$) [55]. The sinuses are the greatest source of nasal NO, but the specific cellular sources in allergic rhinitis may also include endothelial cells (constitutive type III NOS), parasympathetic neurons (type I NOS and co-localized VIP), macrophages, neutrophils, mast cells, arterial smooth muscle cells, and fibroblasts (inducible type II NOS) [56]. NO may promote vasodilation, glandular secretion, and immunomodulation, and, since it is a free radical, it may have an antibacterial function or mucosal-damaging effect when present in excess.

GLANDULAR CHANGES

Submucosal gland area is increased in perennial allergic rhinitis compared with normal and hypertrophic rhinitis. The latter condition likely represents nonallergic rhinitis with increased turbinate size requiring turbinectomy. Submucosal glands represent approximately 15% of the inferior turbinate lamina propria in normal and nonallergic subjects. However, in perennial allergic rhinitis and chronic sinusitis, gland area increases to approximately 25% [57]. Mucous hypersecretion in allergic airway disease may be the result of increased submucosal gland mucous cell mucin exocytosis, goblet cell hyperplasia, plasma extravasation with formation of intralumenal albumin-fibrin-mucin globules, and, potentially, reductions in free water or the less viscous submucosal gland serous cell products. In guinea pig and rat airways, platelet-activating factor increases acidic mucin and *MUC5* gene expression [58]. This effect is potentiated by TNF-α. Epidermal growth factor may be responsible for goblet cell hyperplasia and increased *MUC5AC* mRNA and protein expression [59••]. In lower airway submucosal glands, *MUC5B* is expressed in mucous cells, whereas *MUC7* is expressed only in lysozyme-producing serous cells [60•]. Irritants such as acrolein increase *MUC5AC* mRNA [61]. IL-4 increased *MUC2*, *MUC5*, and mucous glycoconjugate expression in both NCI-H292 and mouse bronchi in vivo [62], whereas overexpression of IL-13 leads to rapid goblet cell proliferation and mucous hypersecretion in vivo [63••].

These findings are likely applicable to human nasal mucosa given the expression of mucin genes in human nasal airways. *MUC5A/C* mRNA levels were 5- to 10-fold higher than *MUC1* and *MUC2* in allergic rhinitis, cystic fibrosis and normal subjects. *MUC2* mRNA was similar in all subjects, whereas *MUC5A/C* was significantly reduced in cystic fibrosis [64]. This is in contrast to the A549 cell line where *MUC5A/C* was increased by neutrophil elastase, an inflammatory mediator of cystic fibrosis pathophysiology [65]. As in the axon response controversy mentioned above, conclusions drawn from human disease states, not in vitro or animal studies, should take precedence in developing paradigms for understanding pathogenic molecular mechanisms of mucin hypersecretion.

Treatment of mucous hypersecretion has focused on guaifenesin and related compounds. They may induce gastric nociceptive nerve irritation with recruitment of parasympathetic reflexes that increase exocytosis of low viscosity serous cell products [66,67]. Glucocorticoids may reduce mucous hypersecretion by limiting airway inflammation, the production of mediators responsible for mucin synthesis and mucous cell hyperplasia, and normalization of epithelial histology (increase in ciliated cell expression). However, prednisone has no effect on sputum volume in chronic bronchitis [68].

HYPERRESPONSIVENESS

Hyperresponsiveness is a characteristic of mucosal surfaces during inflammation. Hyperresponsiveness indicates an increased mucosal response to "nonspecific" irritants such as histamine, methacholine, bradykinin, hypertonic saline, cold, dry air, and other provocational agents [69,70]. Allergic rhinitis subjects have increased vascular innervation by SP- and VIP-containing neurons [71•,72,73] and increased nociceptive nerves sensitivity to endothelin-1, bradykinin, and lower doses of histamine that induce parasympathetic reflexes and glandular secretion [1]. Glandular responses to methacholine are also increased [74]. VIP-immunoreactive nerve fibers may be increased in density as seen in chronic bronchitis and cholinergic nonallergic rhinitis [72,73,75,76]. VIP has been proposed as an additional glandular secretagogue that participates in parasympathetic reflexes. In contrast to glandular hypersecretion, histamine-induced vascular permeability and "exudative hyperresponsiveness" do not appear to involve nociceptive axon responses or other neural effects [36].

Nociceptive nerve responses may be upregulated by neurotrophic cytokines such as IL-11, nerve growth factor, IL-6, or other members of the neurotrophin group of cytokines (leukemia inhibitory factor, CNF, oncostatin M). IL-11 may participate in the pathogenesis of viral rhinitis and asthma [77]. Nasal instillation of IL-11 in mice leads 24 hours later to cholinergic bronchial reactivity with minimal peribronchial infiltrates. Children with common colds who have elevated IL-11 concentrations in their nasal secretions are more likely to develop asthma. In addition, the asthmatic subset had significantly increased IL-11 nasal lavage levels compared with those who did not develop wheezing.

Hyporesponsiveness can also occur. For example, in chronic sinusitis, patients have high baseline secretion of glandular products, but have no reserve to exocytose additional materials when challenged with the glandular secretagogue methacholine [78]. This suggests that the glands were acting at their maximal rate of exocytosis because of high mucosal secretagogue levels or that they had developed tachyphylaxis or unresponsiveness to further muscarinic challenge.

CONCLUSIONS

Application of the new concepts of nociceptive nerve axon responses, T_H1, T_H2, and CD8 lymphocyte–related pathologic processes, molecular mechanisms of atopic disease, and general principles of leukocyte adhesion, diapedesis, and tissue injury have reformed our understanding of allergic rhinitis. Because so many redundant mediators have been identified, it is difficult to decide if any single factor can account for the majority of chronic allergic rhinitis complaints or if any single drug will replace the combination of nonsedating antihistamines and topical glucocorticoids or allergy shots that has become the most effective treatment modality. As more is learned about basic processes of atopy, however, it is anticipated that newer drugs with greater specificity and lower potential toxicity will be developed to eliminate this scourge.

ACKNOWLEDGMENT

The writing of this article was supported by US Public Health Service Award AI42403 and US Environmental Protection Agency Award R825814. Although the research described in this article has been funded wholly or in part by the US Environmental Protection Agency through grant number R825814 to James N. Baraniuk, MD, it has not been subjected to the agency's required peer and policy review and therefore does not necessarily reflect the views of the Agency. No official endorsement should be inferred.

REFERENCES AND RECOMMENDED READING

Papers of particular interest, published recently, have been highlighted as:

• Of importance

•• Of major importance

1. Baraniuk JN: Pathogenesis of allergic rhinitis. *J Allergy Clin Immunol* 1997, 99:S763–S772.

2. Druce HM: Allergic and nonallergic rhinitis. In *Allergy Principles and Practice* edn 4. Edited by Middleton E, Jr., Reed CE, Ellis E, *et al.* St. Louis: Mosby; 1993:1433–1453.

3. Togias A: Non-allergic rhinitis. In *Allergic and Non-Allergic Rhinitis: Clinical Aspects.* Edited by Mygind N, Naclerio RM. Philadelphia: W.B. Saunders; 1993:159–166.

4. Andersson M, Greiff L, Svensson C, *et al.*: Allergic and nonallergic rhinitis. In *Asthma and Rhinitis.* Edited by Busse WW, Holgate ST. Boston: Blackwell Scientific Publication; 1995:145–155.

5. Kaliner MA: Allergic rhinitis. In *Allergic and Non-Allergic Rhinitis: Clinical Aspects.* Edited by Mygind N, Naclerio RM. Philadelphia: W.B. Saunders; 1993:152–158.

6. Mygind N, Dahl R, Pedersen S, Thestrup-Pedersen K: *Essential Allergy* edn 2. Oxford: Blackwell Science; 1996:206–208.

7. Raphael GD, Meredith SD, Baraniuk JN, *et al.*: The pathophysiology of rhinitis II: Assessment of the sources of protein in histamine-induced nasal secretions. *Am Rev Respir Dis* 1989, 139:791–800.

8. Baraniuk JN, Clauw JD, Gaumond E: Rhinitis symptoms in chronic fatigue syndrome. *Ann Allergy Asthma Immunol* 1998, 81:359–365.

9. Baraniuk JN, Clauw D, Yuta A, *et al.*: Nasal secretion analysis in allergic rhinitis, cystic fibrosis, and nonallergic fibromyalgia/chronic fatigue syndrome subjects. *Am J Rhinol* 1998, 12:435–440.

10.•• Baraniuk JN, Ali M, Yuta A, *et al.*: Hypertonic saline nasal provocation stimulates nociceptive nerves, substance P release, and glandular mucus exocytosis in normal humans. *Am J Respir Crit Care Med* 1999, 160:655–662.
This article demonstrates that normal human airway nociceptive nerve axon responses cause SP release, which presumably acts on neurokinin-1 receptors on glands to stimulate exocytosis. No vascular leak or permeability was found. This is strikingly different from the "neurogenic inflammation" found in rodent tracheal airways, which had previously led to the conclusion that vascular permeability was the primary endpoint of this reaction.

11. Bonini S, Bonini O, Lambiase A, *et al.*: Vernal keratoconjunctivitis: a model of 5q cytokine gene cluster disease. *Int Arch Allergy Immunol* 1995, 107:95–98.

12. Mareni C, Sessarego M, Montera M, *et al.*: Expression and genomic configuration of GM-CSF, IL-3, M-CSR receptor (C-FMS), early growth response gene-1 (EGR-1) and M-CSF genes in primary myelodysplastic syndromes. *Leuk Lymphoma* 1994, 15:135–141.

13. Frazer KA, Ueda Y, Zhu Y, *et al.*: Computational and biological analysis of 680 kb of DNA sequence from the human 5q31 cytokine gene cluster region. *Genome Research* 1997, 7:495–512.

14. Smirnov DV, Smirnova MG, Korobko VG, Frolova EI: Tandem arrangement of human genes for interleukin-4 and interleukin-13: resemblance in their organization. *Gene* 1995, 155:277–281.

15. Kruskal J, Xiong M, Ferrell R, *et al.*: Linkage and association of adrenergic and dopamine receptor genes in the distal portion of the long arm of chromosome 5 with systemic blood pressure variation. *Hum Mol Genet* 1998, 7:1379–1383.

16. Coombs RRA, Gell PGH: The classification of allergic reactions underlying disease. In *Clinical Aspects of Immunology.* Edited by Gell PGH, Coombs RRA. Oxford: Blackwell Scientific; 1963:317–337.

17. Iliopoulos O, Proud D, Adkinson F Jr, *et al.*: Effects of immunotherapy on the early, late, and rechallenge nasal reaction to provocation with allergen: changes in inflammatory mediators and cells. *J Allergy Clin Immunol* 1991, 87:855–866.

18.•• Cameron L, Hamid Q, Wright E, *et al.*: Local synthesis of epsilon germline gene transcripts, IL-4, and IL-13 in allergic nasal mucosa after ex vivo allergen exposure. *J Allergy Clin Immunol* 2000, 106:46–52.
Local nasal mucosal production of IgE is demonstrated in nasal explants, indicating that IgE plasma cells can differentiate in this tissue ex vivo.

19. Bradding P, Okayama Y, Howarth PH, *et al.*: Heterogeneity of human mast cells based on cytokines content. *J Immunol* 1995, 155:297–307.

20. Bradding P, Mediwake R, Feather IH, *et al.*: TNF-α is localized to nasal mucosal mast cells and is released in acute allergic rhinitis. *Clin Exp Allergy* 1995, 25:406–415.

21. Pawankar RU, Okuda M, Hasegawa S, *et al.*: Interleukin-13 expression in the nasal mucosal of perennial allergic rhinitis. *Am J Respir Crit Care Med* 1995, 152:2059–2067.

22. Juluisson S, Aldenborg F, Enerback L: Protease content of mast cells of nasal mucosa: effects of natural allergen exposure and of local corticosteroid treatment. *Allergy* 1995, 50:15–22.

23. Kawabori Y, Kanai N, Tosho T: Proliferative activity of mast cells in allergic nasal mucosa. *Clin Exp Allergy* 1995, 25:173–178.

24. Simons FE: *Histamine and H1-Antagonists in Allergic Disease.* New York: Marcel Dekker; 1996.

25. Terada N, Kono A, Togawa K: Biochemical properties of eosinophils and their preferential accumulation mechanism in nasal allergy. *J Allergy Clin Immunol* 1994, 94:629–642.

26. Naclerio RM, Baroody FM, Kagey-Sobotka A, Lichtenstein LM: Basophils and eosinophils in allergic rhinitis. *J Allergy Clin Immunol* 1994, 94:1303–1309.

27. Holgate ST, Bradding BM, Sampson AP: Leukotriene antagonists and synthesis inhibitors: new directions in asthma therapy. *J Allergy Clin Immunol* 1996, 98:1–13.

28. Sommerhof CP, Caughey GH, Finkbeiner WE, *et al.*: Mast cell chymase: a potent secretagogue for airway gland serous cells. *J Immunol* 1989, 142:2450–2456.

29. Erjefalt I, Persson CG: Allergen, bradykinin, and capsaicin increase outward but not inward macromolecular permeability of guinea-pig tracheobronchial mucus. *Clin Exp Allergy* 1991, 21:217–224.

30. Iriyoshi N, Takeuchi K, Yuta A, *et al.*: Increased pathology of allergic rhinitis: expression of histamine H1 receptor mRNA in allergic rhinitis. *Clin Exp Allergy* 1996, 26:379–385.

31. Okayama M, Baraniuk JN, Hausfeld JN, *et al.*: Characterization and autoradiographic localization of histamine H1 receptors in human nasal turbinates. *J Allergy Clin Immunol* 1992, 89:1144–1150.

32. Okayama M, Yamauchi K, Sekizawa K, *et al.*: Localization of histamine N-methyltransferase messenger RNA in human nasal mucosa. *J Allergy Clin Immunol* 1995, 95:96–102.

33. Baraniuk JN: Neuropeptide pharmacology. In *Clinical Allergy and Immunology 8: Immunopharmacology of the Respiratory Tract.* Edited by Townley RG, Agarwal DK. New York: Marcel Dekker; 1996:575–603.

34. McDonald DM: Neurogenic inflammation in the respiratory tract: actions of sensory nerve mediators on blood vessels and epithelium of the airway mucosa. *Am Rev Respir Dis* 1987, 136:S65–S72.

35. Stjarne P, Lacroix JS, Anggard A, Lundberg JM: Compartment analysis of vascular effects of neuropeptides and capsaicin in the pig nasal mucosa. *Acta Physiol Scand* 1991, 141:335–342.

36. Svensson C, Andersson M, Greiff L, et al.: Exudative hyperresponsiveness of the airway microcirculation in seasonal allergic rhinitis. *Clin Exp Allergy* 1995, 25:942–950.

37. Joos GF, Germonpre PR, Pauwels RA: Neurogenic inflammation in human airways: it is important? *Thorax* 1995, 50:217–219.

38. Fajac I, Braunstein G, Ickovic MR, et al.: Selective recruitment of eosinophils by substance P after repeated allergen exposure in allergic rhinitis. *Allergy* 1995, 50:970–975.

39.• Proud D, Reynolds CJ, Lichtenstein LM, et al.: Intranasal salmeterol inhibits allergen-induced vascular permeability but not mast cell activation or cellular infiltration. *Clin Exp Allergy* 1998, 28:868–875.
Long-acting β2-adrenergic receptor antagonists had been touted as anti-inflammatory agents in allergic disease. This paper demonstrates that the changes were in the vascular leak component but not other facets of seasonal allergic rhinitis.

40. Mossiman BL, White MV, Hohman RJ, et al.: Substance P, calcitonin-gene related peptide, and vasoactive intestinal peptide increase in nasal secretions after allergen challenge in atopic patients. *J Allergy Clin Immunol* 1993, 92:95–104.

41. Okamoto Y, Shirotori K, Kudo K, et al.: Cytokine expression after the topical administration of substance P to human nasal mucosa: the role of substance P in nasal allergy. *J Immunol* 1993, 151:4391–4398.

42. Rinder J, Lundberg JM: Effects of hCGRP8-37 and the NK1-recptor antagonist SR140.333 on capsaicin-evoked vasodilation in the pig nasal mucosa in vivo. *Acta Physiol Scand* 1996, 156(2):115–122.

43. Baraniuk JN, Silver PB, Kaliner MA, Branes PJ: Effects of ipratropium bromide on bradykinin nasal provocation in humans. *Clin Exp Allergy* 1994, 14:724–729.

44. Baraniuk JN, Kaliner MA, Barnes PJ: Localization of m3 muscarinic receptor mRNA in human nasal mucosa. *Am J Rhinol* 1992, 6:145–148.

45. Mullol J, Baraniuk JN, Logun C, et al.: M1 and M3 muscarinic antagonists inhibit human nasal glandular secretion in vitro. *J Appl Physiol* 1992, 73:2069–2073.

46.•• Costello RW, Jacoby DB, Gleich GJ, Fryer AD: Eosinophils and airway nerves in asthma. *Histol Histopathol* 2000, 15:861–868.
The complex interactions of SP, eosinophil products, and dysfunction of the muscarinic M2 receptors that have been demonstrated in animal models are reviewed.

47. Evans CM, Belmonte KE, Costello RW, et al.: Substance P-induced airway hyperreactivity is mediated by neuronal M(2) receptor dysfunction. *Am J Physiol Lung Cell Mol Physiol* 2000, 279:L477–L486.

48. Altman LC, Ayars GH, Baker C, Luchtel DL: Cytokines and eosinophil derived cationic proteins upregulate intercellular adhesion molecule 1 on human nasal epithelial cells. *J Allergy Clin Immunol* 1993, 92:527–536.

49. Nonaka M, Nonaka R, Jordana M, Dolovich J: GM-CSF, IL-8, IL-1R, TNF-alpha R, and HLA-DR in nasal epithelial cells in allergic rhinitis. *Am J Respir Crit Care Med* 1996, 153:1675–1681.

50. Minshall EM, Cameron L, Lavigne F, et al.: Eotaxin mRNA and protein expression in chronic sinusitis and allergen-induced nasal responses in seasonal allergic rhinitis. *Am J Respir Cell Mol Biol* 1997, 17:683–690.

51. Gosset P, Malaquin F, Delnest Y, et al.: Interleukin 6 and interleukin 1β production is associated with antigen induced late nasal response. *J Allergy Clin Immunol* 1993, 92:878–890.

52. Kenney JS, Baker C, Welch MR, Altman LC: Synthesis of interleukin-1α, interleukin-6, and interleukin-8 by cultured human nasal epithelial cells. *J Allergy Clin Immunol* 1994, 3:1060–1067.

53. Mullol J, Chowdoury BA, White MV, et al.: Endothelin in human nasal mucosa. *Am J Respir Cell Mol Biol* 1993, 8:393–402.

54. Furukawa K, Saleh D, Bayan F, et al.: Coexpression of endothelin 1 and endothelin converting enzyme 1 in patients with chronic rhinitis. *Am J Respir Cell Mol Biol* 1996, 14:248–253.

55. Martin U, Bryden K, Devoy M, Howarth P: Increased levels of exhaled nitric oxide during nasal and oral breathing in subjects with seasonal rhinitis. *J Allergy Clin Immunol* 1996, 7:768–772.

56. Fischer A, Hoffman B: Nitric oxide synthase in neurons and nerve fibres of lower airways and in vagal sensory ganglia of man. *Am J Respir Crit Care Med* 1996, 154:209–216.

57. Masuda S: Quantitative histochemistry of mucus-secreting cells in human nasal mucosa. *Pract Otol (Kyoto)* 1990, 83:1855–1863.

58. Lou YP, Takeyama K, Grattan KM, et al.: Platelet-activating factor induces goblet cell hyperplasia and mucin gene expression in airways. *Am J Respir Crit Care Med* 1998, 157:1927–1934.

59.•• Takeyama K, Dabbagh K, Lee HM, et al.: Epidermal growth factor system regulates mucin production in airways. *Proc Natl Acad Sci U S A* 1999, 96:3081–3086.
This paper demonstrates that cytokines such as epidermal growth factor can modulate the types of mucins and phenotype of exocrine cells in airways.

60.• Sharma P, Dudus L, Nielsen PA, et al.: MUC5B and MUC7 are differentially expressed in mucous and serous cells of submucosal glands in human bronchial airways. *Am J Respir Cell Mol Biol* 1998, 19:30–37.
This paper breaches the mystery surrounding the nature of mucins and their localizations within specific airway exocrine cells.

61. Borchers MT, Carty MP, Leikauf GD: Regulation of human airway mucins by acrolein and inflammatory mediators. *Am J Physiol* 1999, 276:L549–L555.

62. Dabbagh K, Takeyama K, Lee HM, et al.: IL-4 induces mucin gene expression and goblet cell metaplasia in vitro and in vivo. *J Immunol* 1999, 162:6233–6237.

63.•• Wills-Karp M: Immunologic basis of antigen-induced airway hyperresponsiveness. *Annu Rev Immunol* 1999, 17:255–281.
This review covers many mechanisms that may lead to bronchial hyperresponsiveness.

64. Voynow JA, Selby DM, Rose MC: Mucin gene expression (MUC1, MUC2, and MUC5/5AC) in nasal epithelial cells of cystic fibrosis, allergic rhinitis, and normal individuals. *Lung* 1998, 176:345–354.

65. Voynow JA, Young LR, Wang Y, et al.: Neutrophil elastase increases MUC5AC mRNA and protein expression in respiratory epithelial cells. *Am J Physiol* 1999, 276:L835–L843.

66. Yuta A, Baraniuk JN: Therapeutic approaches to airway mucous hypersecretion. In *Airway Mucus: Basic Mechanisms and Clinical Perspectives. Respiratory Pharmacology and Pharmacotherapy series.* Edited by Rogers DF, Lethem MI. Basel: Birkhauser; 1997:365–383.

67. Ziment I: Historic overview of mucoactive drugs. In *Drugs in Bronchial Mucology*. Edited by Braga PC, Allegra L. New York: Raven Press; 1989:1–34.

68. Claman DM, Bousher HA, Lui J, *et al.*: Analysis of induced sputum to examine the effects of prednisone on airway inflammation in asthmatic subjects. *J Allergy Clin Immunol* 1994, 94:861–869.

69. Baroody FM, Cruz AA, Lichtenstein LM, *et al.*: Intranasal beclomethasone inhibits antigen induced nasal hyperresponsiveness to histamine. *J Allergy Clin Immunol* 1992, 90:373–376.

70. White MV: Nasal cholinergic hyperresponsiveness in atopic subjects studied out of season. *J Allergy Clin Immunol* 1993, 92:278–287.

71.• Figueroa JM, Mansilla E, Suburo AM: Innervation of nasal turbinate blood vessels in rhinitic and nonrhinitic children. *Am J Respir Crit Care Med* 1998, 157:1959–1966.
The innervation of human nasal mucosa is displayed in precise photomicrographs.

72. Fang SY, Shen CL: Neuropeptidergic innervation of human nasal mucosa in various pathological conditions. *Proc Natl Sci Counc Repub China B* 1997, 21:8–12.

73. Fang SY, Shen CL: Neuropeptide innervation and neuroendocrine cells in allergic rhinitis and chronic hypertrophic rhinitis. *Clin Exp Allergy* 1998, 28:228–232.

74. Druce HM, Wright RH, Kossoff D, *et al.*: Cholinergic nasal hyperreactivity in atopic subjects. *J Allergy Clin Immunol* 1985, 76:445–452.

75. Kurian, SS, Blank MA, Sheppard MN: Vasoactive intestinal polypeptide (VIP) in vasomotor rhinitis. *Clin Biochem* 1983, 11:425–426.

76. Lucchini RE, Facchini F, Turato G, *et al.*: Increased VIP-positive nerve fibers in the mucous glands of subjects with chronic bronchitis. *Am J Respir Crit Care Med* 1997; 156:1963–1968.

77. Einarsson O, Geba GP, Zhou Z, *et al.*: Interleukin-11 in respiratory inflammation. *Ann NY Acad Sci* 1995, 762:31–40.

78. Jeney EV, Raphael GD, Meredith SD, Kaliner MA: Abnormal cholinergic parasympathetic responsiveness in the nasal mucosa of patients with recurrent sinusitis. *J Allergy Clin Immunol* 1990, 86:10–18.

CHAPTER 5

Allergic Rhinitis

Athena Economides
Michael A. Kaliner

Allergic rhinitis is one of the most common chronic conditions in the United States and the most common immunologic disease. According to some estimates, the symptoms of allergic rhinitis may afflict as many as one in five Americans [1]. Although allergic rhinitis is rarely life threatening, its symptoms can cause extreme discomfort and impairment in the ability to function at work, in school, and in leisure activities. In addition, untreated allergies lead to an increased prevalence of complications, such as sinusitis, asthma, otitis media, craniofacial abnormalities that require orthodontic care, and eustachian tube dysfunction. It is therefore of clinical importance to recognize, understand, and effectively treat this disease.

EPIDEMIOLOGY AND PREVALENCE

Allergic rhinitis is the second most prevalent chronic condition in the United States, outranked only by hypertension [2]. It accounts for 2.5% of physician visits; treatment by immunotherapy accounts for an additional 0.5% [3,4]. According to one estimate, there are more than 40 to 50 million people with allergic disease in the United States; estimates of the prevalence of allergic rhinitis range between 2% and 20% of the population [1]. The disorder is equally common in men and women.

Although allergic rhinitis may develop at any age, approximately 70% of patients develop the disorder before the age of 30 [1]; the incidence is highest between the ages of 15 and 25 years [5]. Additional peaks in incidence of the disease occur in childhood and adolescence [1]. Allergic rhinitis frequently develops by the time a child is 5 to 10 years of age, although it can be identified by 1 year of age. Because immunoglobulin E (IgE) levels are highest during puberty, symptoms are often the most severe during that time.

In some patients, the symptoms of allergic rhinitis are mild and seasonal, whereas others experience severe symptoms almost continually. Approximately 62% of persons with allergic rhinitis are "bothered a great deal" by their symptoms, and 21% are bothered for 41 or more weeks each year. Patients with allergic rhinitis are, on the average, symptomatic for 9 months each year [6]. In a survey conducted to develop and test a clinical trials questionnaire for assessment of quality of life in allergic people, 55% to 88% of adolescents with allergic rhinoconjunctivitis reported feelings of increased irritability, impatience, embarrassment, and anger from their symptoms and appearance [7].

Morbidity associated with allergic rhinitis has significant economic consequences. A survey conducted in 1975 found that Americans experienced 28 million days of restricted activity as a result of allergic rhinitis. They spent six million days bedridden and lost two million school days [8]. A more recent review found that allergic rhinitis accounts for 10 million missed days from work [9]. Total expenditures for antihistamines, decongestants, nasal cromolyn, and nasal corticosteroids in 1988 were approximately $2 billion [10]. In 1995, the direct costs of allergic rhinitis to the American health care system were estimated to be $2.4 billion [11]. In 1998, estimates suggest that the total costs of allergic rhinoconjunctivitis were $6 billion [12].

There is evidence of a genetic predisposition to allergic disorders. The incidence of atopy is roughly one third in children who have one parent or sibling with a history of allergic disease, and a little less than two thirds in children of two such parents [13]. In addition, allergy in twins is more common in identical pairs than in fraternal pairs [14].

PATHOPHYSIOLOGY

Allergic responses are generally considered to be normal protective mechanisms that are activated to an inappropriate degree. Individuals who manifest such atopic responses may develop asthma, eczema (atopic dermatitis), allergic rhinitis, or any combination of these. In rare instances, the allergic response may rapidly escalate to life-threatening anaphylaxis. The suspected genetic component to allergic rhinitis involves an inherited capacity to respond to allergen exposure with increased production of IgE antibodies. These antibodies bind to and sensitize mast cells and basophils, which play pivotal roles in allergic inflammation.

A complex interaction of chemical mediators and inflammatory cells is responsible for the allergic inflammation. Although the clinical manifestations of the allergic response may vary, the allergic reaction consists of a sensitization phase, an immediate-phase response characterized by mast cell degranulation and release of early mediators, and a late-phase response that is characterized by the migration of inflammatory cells from the circulation.

In the human nasal mucosa, the majority of IgE-bearing cells are mast cells [15]. High concentrations of mast cells are found in mucosal linings where external antigens first come into contact with the body. The number of mast cells and eosinophils in the nasal mucosa increases after exposure to an allergen and correlates with the severity of seasonal disease [16]. In fact, eosinophil infiltration is the hallmark of allergic rhinitis and distinguishes allergic inflammation from other inflammatory conditions of the upper respiratory tract.

IgE SENSITIZATION PHASE

The sensitization phase of the allergic response begins when Langerhan's cells act as antigen-presenting cells for allergen fragments to Th0 lymphocytes, which then differentiate into Th2 subtypes. In a process that involves the secretion of interleukin (IL)-4 by Th2 cells, B cells are activated and mature into plasma cells that produce antigen-specific IgE antibodies. The production of IgE antibodies, which recognize these foreign antigens, occurs in nearby lymph tissue. These IgE antibodies bind to receptors on tissue mast cells and circulating basophils. The regulation of IgE production is extremely complex and involves cooperation between B and T lymphocytes as well as the effects of various interleukins and cytokines [17]. Atopic individuals also appear to possess an inherited tendency to express certain amino acid sequences in T-cell receptors that favor the binding to and recognition of specific allergenic antigens [18].

IMMEDIATE PHASE HYPERSENSITIVITY REACTIONS

On subsequent reexposure to the antigen, the allergen molecules bind to the IgE antibodies attached to IgE receptors on the surface of mast cells. This action results in cross-linking of IgE receptors and activation of enzyme cascades in the cell membrane that involves tyrosine kinase, protein kinase C, phospholipase A2, and an influx of calcium ions, resulting in mast cell degranulation. As mast cells degranulate, they release inflammatory mediators, including preformed (histamine) and newly synthesized chemical mediators (serotonin, kinins, leukotrienes, and prostaglandins [13,19]).

Although exocytosis is almost instantaneous, the effects of degranulation occur in several phases. Differences among the many substances released account for the diversity of the effects. The early inflammatory mediators (histamine, kinins, prostaglandins, and leukotrienes) exert their effects in a matter of minutes, and sometimes seconds. Thus, they are responsible for the immediate hypersensitivity reaction. These mediators cause the symptoms of allergic rhinitis that are manifested immediately following exposure to an allergen: itching, sneezing, rhinorrhea, and mild congestion. Early phase allergic reaction occurs in more than 90% of patients with a history of allergic rhinitis and positive skin tests [20•].

Histamine is among the first mediators to be released, and it alone has been shown to cause many of the symptoms seen in allergic rhinitis, inducing nasal itch and sneezing. Histamine, bradykinin, prostaglandins, chymase, and leukotrienes (LTC4, LD4, LTE4) all cause glandular hypersecretion, and therefore rhinorrhea. Histamine also increases nasal airway resistance (congestion), but this effect is also caused both by a neural reflex that causes venous engorgement and increased vascular permeability, causing swelling and inducing serous secretions into the nasal lumen [21]. Similarly, challenges with kinins, prostaglandin D_2, and leukotrienes C4 and D4 have been shown to cause nasal blockage [20•].

LATE-PHASE HYPERSENSITIVITY REACTIONS

Other substances released during mast cell degranulation operate on a different time scale. Cytokines such as tumor necrosis factor, granulocyte macrophage colony-stimulating factor (GM-CSF), and interleukins (specifically, IL-3, IL-4, IL-5, and IL-6) induce the transcription and translation of genes that code for the production of additional inflammatory substances [22]. The process of cytokine and chemokine release from mast cells and lymphocytes takes several hours and contributes to the *late-phase reaction* (LPR). Cutaneous LPR occurs in approximately 50% of allergic patients, approximately 4 to 12 hours after antigen exposure. Nasal LPR has been difficult to demonstrate, but clinically it may be characterized by nasal congestion, irritability, and, to a lesser extent, rhinorrhea and sneezing.

In addition to orchestrating the production of additional inflammatory substances, many cytokines have chemotactic effects. IL4, TNF, and other cytokines produced by mast cells upregulate the expression of adhesion molecules such as ICAM and VCAM, which, via endothelial cell activation, facilitate migration of inflammatory cells through blood vessels to target tissues. Activated eosinophils, polymorphonuclear cells, basophils, and T cells infiltrate the site of the initial insult and escalate the local inflammatory response. This process is referred to as the *cellular recruitment phase* [23].

Allergen challenge studies show that priming is associated with inflammatory cell accumulation at the site of nasal challenge [24]. About half the people with allergic rhinitis experience the priming effect—an increased sensitivity to allergen after repeated daily exposures. For example, a ragweed-sensitive individual requires a larger amount of antigen exposure out of season than at the height of season in order to experience the same symptoms. Nonspecific nasal hyperreactivity or "twitchy nose" is also observed in association with LPR; nonspecific irritants, such as tobacco smoke, strong odors, air pollution, and even climate changes, may exacerbate or prolong symptoms.

Many of the cells recruited to the site of inflammation, including T and B lymphocytes, endothelial cells, macrophages, and platelets, produce substances known as histamine-releasing factors, which cause further histamine to be released, thus renewing the cycle of inflammation [25]. Propagation of the allergic inflammatory response is also accomplished by T cell and mast cell

production of cytokines such as IL-3, IL-5, and GM-CSF, which promote growth, differentiation, and survival of eosinophils. All early-phase mediators (including histamine, LTC4, LD4, LTE4, kinins, kinogenase, and tosyl-L-arginin-methyl-ester [TAME]) are recovered in late phase nasal lavage fluid, except for PGD2, which is released by mast cells but not basophils. This finding suggests a possible role for basophils in LPR [26].

AEROALLERGENS

Most airborne allergens are between 2 and 60 μm in diameter. The allergic components of these particles usually are proteins with molecular weights between 10,000 and 40,000 daltons [27]. Allergens may be found seasonally, as when trees pollinate, or perennially, as with cat exposure. Seasonal allergens include pollens (such as ragweed), molds, and insect parts. Tree pollens generally are released during the early spring, whereas grass pollens usually are released in late spring and early summer. Weed pollens cause the greatest degree of symptomatic illness in the late summer and early fall. In the eastern and midwestern United States, ragweed pollen is most prevalent. Although allergic rhinitis is often called "hay fever" or "rose fever," these terms are inaccurate, as episodes are triggered by pollen allergens (not hay or roses) and are not associated with fever.

Common inhaled perennial allergens include dust, mold, salivary proteins of cats and dogs, and cockroaches. House dust contains many particles, including lint, mites, mite fecal particles, animal dander, insect parts, and fibers. In many geographical areas, two mites, *Dermatophagoides farinae* and *Dermatophagoides pteronyssinus*, are the primary sources of antigenic particles in house dust. They feed on human skin dander (hence the name *Dermatophagoides*, which means eaters of skin). These mites typically live in carpets, bedding, and upholstery, and proliferate in a warm, humid environment, with temperatures of 65°F to 70°F and relative humidity greater than 50%. The fecal particles released by these mites are covered with intestinal enzymes; a protease component of this material is an important allergen. The fecal particles are relatively heavy compared with other airborne allergens and are airborne for only about 30 minutes after being disturbed. Thus, such activities as vacuuming the carpet increase the likelihood of initiating an allergic reaction for about a half an hour. Dust-mite control involves avoidance of *intimate* contact with the dust mite antigen [28••]. Generally this is accomplished by barriers such as allergy-proof encasements for the bedding, as well as weekly washing of the linens in water warmer than 130° and by removal of carpets or other fabric-covered surface areas.

Furry animals, particularly cats, present a serious allergenic threat to susceptible individuals. Allergens from cats are found in either the saliva or the skin; they are much smaller and lighter than dust allergens, and thus may persist in the air for longer periods of time. Essentially, a cat in the household is a constant source of allergenic stimuli. Although there are lower levels of cat allergen in homes without pets (36 to 200 times lower), these lower levels are still sufficient to cause symptoms in some individuals [28••,29]. Cat dander may be considered a ubiquitous allergen found in public places and schools, presumably transferred by clothing [30].

Fungi (molds) are found in both indoor and outdoor environments. Major outdoor allergens include Alternaria, Cladosporium (Hormodendrum), and members of the class Basidiomycetes. Alternaria is a major environmental risk in some arid climates as well as in wet humid areas. The most common molds in basements, bedding, and damp interior areas are Penicillium and Aspergillus. In contrast to pollens, which are more likely to be carried by the wind in dry air and are removed from the air by rain, mold spores are often found in high numbers in moist and humid air. Cockroaches are another significant source of indoor inhaled allergens and should be suspected as a cause of perennial allergies in any patient who lives in an urban environment. Cockroach allergens have been found in high concentrations not only in kitchens but also in bedrooms and family rooms [31].

DIAGNOSIS OF ALLERGIC RHINITIS
History

Taking a careful history from every patient who presents with allergic symptoms is extremely important. Symptoms may include uncontrollable bursts, or paroxysms, of sneezing, itching of the eyes or nose (as well as the palate or pharynx), and nasal congestion, with partial or total obstruction of airflow through the nose and rhinorrhea, often accompanied by postnasal drainage [4]. When the allergic episode is at its worst, patients may experience increased production of tears and soreness of the eyes and a gelatinous conjunctival discharge upon awakening. Patients may complain of irritability, fatigue, sleep-disordered breathing, or depression.

Understanding the triggers for the symptoms is crucial in creating a working diagnosis for the patient. Thus, early phase response triggers are allergens, such as pollens, dander, mites, molds, and cockroaches; however, nasal symptoms can also be triggered by irritants such as tobacco smoke, air pollutants, perfumes, ammonia, changes in temperature relative to humidity or barometric pressure, exercise, emotions (particularly depression), and foods (such as spicy hot food, beer, or wine).

In some cases, the diagnosis may be relatively easy to determine. For example, if a patient experiences symptoms of allergic rhinitis for 2 to 3 weeks at the same time every year, that patient most likely suffers from seasonal rhinitis caused by plant pollens, such as tree pollen or ragweed. Most cases, however, are likely to be more complex, with patients suffering for a longer period of time at variable times of the year and in response to a variety of stimuli. Thus, a patient who vacations during August each year and experiences allergic symptoms may be responding to ragweed pollen or to mold in the vacation home.

In addition to identification of patterns for the symptoms, a personal or family history of atopic disease (allergic rhinitis, asthma, food allergy, and atopic dermatitis) will support the diagnosis of allergic rhinitis. A careful assessment for possible complications or comorbid diseases is also important, particularly when the situation may be complicated by persistence of symptoms beyond the time when clear triggering factors can be implicated. Once the allergic response is initiated, the nasal mucosa may become hyperresponsive due to the effects of the allergic inflammation itself. In such cases, symptoms caused by exposure to tree pollen, for example, persist after the end of the tree pollen "season."

Finally, it is important to note the age of the patient and the length of symptoms; an elderly patient who never had allergies before is unlikely to have allergic rhinitis. A patient with a history of hypertension may have drug-induced rhinitis rather than allergic inflammation. Historical clues that parents may not readily associate with allergies in their children include chronic ear infections, early tonsillo-adenoid surgery, lack of good appetite upon arising (because of postnasal drainage), cradle cap, frequent colds or bronchitis, intolerance to milk or food upon initial introduction to milk or solids, or history of snoring.

Physical findings

While atopic skin manifestations such as dermatitis (eczema) or urticaria may flare up during seasonal allergic episodes, the primary physical findings in allergic rhinitis occur in the nose, eyes, and ears [4]. Nasal examination is best performed with a nasal speculum and a high-power light source. Application of a topical decongestant before examination allows much better visualization of the nasal passages and provides an estimate of the reversibility of mucosal swelling. Attention should be paid to structural deformities that may impede nasal airflow, including a nasal septal deviation, polyps, septal spurs, or hypertrophied turbinates. About 60% of patients have pale, bluish, edematous nasal turbinates, a finding that is classic for allergic rhinitis but not diagnostic. The character of nasal secretions should be noted and is generally thin and clear in allergic rhinitis. Excessive nasal itching may lead to nose rubbing (the "allergic salute") that results in a transverse nasal crease, as well as curvilinear excoriations of the external nasal margin and bleeding of the Kesselbach plexus. Swelling of the nasal membranes and accumulation of clear mucus may block the airway; swelling may also block the sinus ostia, leading to sinusitis. The pneumatic otoscope should be used to examine the ears for the presence of fluid and infections when suspected. Eustachian tube dysfunction may lead to serous otitis media, acute suppurative otitis media, or barotrauma associated with flying or scuba or skin diving. Patients with nasal airway obstruction are likely to breathe through their mouths. Patients who have habitually breathed through the mouth during childhood may have a highly arched, narrow palate, a marked overbite, or dental malocclusion.

A careful eye examination may reveal signs of conjunctivitis, puffiness of the eyelids, Dennie-Morgan lines, or periorbital edema. Venous dilation in the skin under the eyes may cause the appearance of a darkened "black eye," often called "the allergic shiners." These signs are not diagnostic for allergic disease, as they are found in nonallergic rhinitis and sinusitis.

Laboratory diagnostic procedures

The best method for identifying specific allergens associated with allergic rhinitis is skin testing with appropriate positive and negative control substances; however, a positive skin test is only relevant when there is convincing history of symptoms. When the positive skin test to aeroallergens occurs in an asymptomatic person, it may suggest the future development of allergic rhinitis [32•]. A percutaneous skin test is the most commonly performed in vivo test for confirming sensitization to a common aeroallergen. It is preferred to the intradermal test because it is rapid, produces little pain, rarely results in systemic allergic reactions, and has less false-positive reactions. It can be interpreted only when the saline control is negative and the histamine control elicits a wheal and flare in a 15- to 20-minute interval, reproducing the early phase response. Late-phase inflammatory reactions may be elicited hours later with higher concentrations of allergen and in patients with increased sensitivity.

Determining serum IgE levels is generally not useful, as IgE levels are elevated in only 30% to 40% of patients with allergic rhinitis. In addition, serum IgE levels may be elevated in other, nonallergic conditions. Similarly, the peripheral eosinophil count provides little useful information, as it may or may not be elevated in patients with allergic rhinitis. In vitro determination of specific IgE (RAST) usually fail to detect a modest number of skin test–positive individuals (5%–40%); the number ranges depend on the criteria used [24]. This negative rate may be quite important in the evaluation of latex, venoms, or foods. Because of the ease, speed, and accuracy of skin tests, and because of the technical limitations of RASTs,

the latter have limited usefulness in allergic rhinitis. Posterior rhinoscopy is of value if there is suspicion of an anatomic or pathologic abnormality not clearly seen by speculum inspection. When abnormalities in examining the tympanic membrane are detected, impedence audiometry or tympanometry and hearing tests confirm the presence of middle ear fluid and auditory deficit. The main clinical utility of a nasal cytology smear is to differentiate infectious rhinitis (increased numbers of neutrophils and bacteria) from allergic rhinitis (eosinophilia); however, although the presence of eosinophilia suggests allergy, it is not diagnostic, as eosinophilia is also found in the rare syndrome of nonallergic rhinitis with eosinophilia syndrome (NARES).

Differential diagnosis

Whereas seasonal allergic rhinitis is often relatively easy to recognize because of its consistent temporal pattern, perennial rhinitis may be more difficult to recognize. Allergic rhinitis is the most common cause of all rhinitis. Other causes of rhinitis that can be identified with a careful history and physical examination are listed in Table 5-1.

Nonallergic rhinitis with eosinophilia syndrome may cause symptoms that are similar to those of allergic rhinitis; however, NARES is associated with negative skin tests, normal serum IgE levels, abundant eosinophils in the nasal smear, and a tendency to respond clinically to topical corticosteroids.

Vasomotor rhinitis, also called perennial nonallergic rhinitis of unknown cause, is characterized by conges-

---

TABLE 5-1. THE DIFFERENTIAL DIAGNOSIS OF RHINITIS

Allergic inflammation
    Seasonal, perennial, occupational (IgE-driven) rhinitis
Nonallergic inflammation
    Infectious (acute/chronic viral/bacterial, associated
        with immunodeficiency)
    NARES (nonallergic rhinitis with eosinophilia syndrome)
    Vasomotor (noninfectious, nonallergic without eosinophilia)
    Drug-induced or medicamentosa (topical decongestants,
        β-blockers, reserpine, antihypertensives, BCPs,
        a-adrenergic agents, NSAIDs)
    Other (atrophic, gustatory, traumatic/CSF rhinitis)
Systemic diseases with nasal dysfunction
    Endocrine (hypothyroidism, DM, pregnancy, puberty)
    Autoimmune (sarcoid, Wegener's, relapsing polychondritis)
    Ciliary dyskinesia
Anatomical obstruction
    Nasal polyps, Horner's syndrome, foreign body, tumors,
        adenoidal, tonsilar and turbinate hypertrophy, nasal septal
        deviation, concha bullosa, or spurs

tion and rhinorrhea not associated with specific allergens. Symptoms are triggered in response to changes in temperature, barometric pressure or humidity, drafts, irritants, strong smells, ingestion of alcohol, emotional stress, or air pollution. Gustatory rhinitis is rhinorrhea caused by eating spicy foods; it is often accompanied by production of tears and perspiration [33]. Rhinitis medicamentosa may be caused by a rebound effect after withdrawal of topical nasal decongestants. Nasal congestion may also be associated with the administration of some oral medications, including oral contraceptives and antihypertensives (reserpine [Serpasil], methyldopa [Aldomet, Amodopa], propranolol, and hydralazine [Alazine, Apresoline]).

COMPLICATIONS OF ALLERGIC RHINITIS

In addition to the discomfort and impairment of daily living caused by allergic rhinitis, persistence of the symptoms may cause or exacerbate medical conditions that may have significant consequences. Short-term complications include acute sinusitis, eustachian tube dysfunction (which contributes to otitis media [OM]), sleep-disordered breathing, decreased cognitive functioning, and aggravation of underlying asthma. Long-term complications may include chronic sinusitis, sleep apnea, aggravation of nasal polyps, permanent hearing impairment as a result of chronic otitis, craniofacial abnormalities, decreased long-term productivity, and increased propensity to develop asthma (see Table 5-2) [34].

Eustachian tube obstruction due to allergic rhinitis is caused by edema, which prevents fluid from draining from the middle ear. The accumulation of middle ear fluid makes the ear vulnerable to frequent infections. Allergic children appear to be more susceptible to acute

OM and chronic OM with effusion. In a series of 200 unselected pediatric patients with OM with effusion (OME) and tympanostomy tube placement, 24% had allergic rhinitis; among the subset requiring multiple tube insertion, 35% had AR [35]. Chronic serous OM is the most common cause of hearing loss in children today [34]. Further, young children depend on adequate hearing for the development of speech and cognitive function; a history of hearing loss or delayed speech development may be a clue to the presence of chronic serous otitis.

Allergic rhinitis is associated with acute sinusitis [36] and is the most common cause of chronic sinusitis [37]. The manifestations of chronic sinusitis are congestion, purulent nasal discharge with postnasal drip, headache, anosmia, and cough (especially at night). The nasal mucosa may appear inflamed, with a visible purulent discharge and nasal polyp formation. The most frequently occurring pathogens in sinusitis are pneumococci, *Haemophilus influenzae*, and *Moraxella catarrhalis*. A broad-spectrum antibiotic should be used along with decongestants, nasal saline washings, and a topical corticosteroid [38].

Normal nasal functions include air filtration, humidification, and heating. In a normal nose, only 5% of inspired particles that are smaller than 15 μm (such as mold spores) escape nasal filtration and reach the lungs. In an allergic individual who breathes through his or her mouth, the air that reaches the lower airway is not filtered, humidified, or warmed. The exposure to ambient air may contribute to the development of asthma. Increased cough and worsening of asthma symptoms have been reported among seasonal allergic rhinitis patients during pollen seasons. Other physiologic links between asthma and upper airway obstruction are proposed to be via postnasal drainage of inflammatory material; absorption of mediators and chemotactic factors from nasal inflammation into the lower airways; mouth breathing of cold, dry air; activation of nasopharyngeal bronchial reflexes; and diminished beta adrenergic responsiveness [34]. Not only is allergic rhinitis implicated in the worsening of asthma, but recent evidence supports earlier suggestions of allergic rhinitis as a risk factor for the development of asthma [32•,39].

Allergic rhinitis is a common cause of nasal obstruction and is a potentially modifiable risk factor for sleep-disordered breathing. Golbin *et al.* [40] found that 88% of children with perennial allergic rhinitis reported sleep disorders on questionnaires, compared with a 17% frequency in controls. Young *et al.* [41] reported that individuals with chronic nocturnal nasal obstruction were 1.8 times more likely to have moderate to severe sleep-disordered breathing, with episodes of apnea that occurred at least 15 times per hour. Unrecognized and untreated sleep apnea can result in

TABLE 5-2. COMPLICATIONS OF ALLERGIC RHINITIS	
Short-term complications	Long-term complications
Asthma exacerbations	Asthma
Acute sinusitis	Chronic sinusitis
Eustachian tube dysfunction	Acute and chronic otitis media
Serous otitis media with effusion	Hearing and speech impairment
Sleep-disordered breathing	Sleep apnea
Chronic mouth breathing in children	Craniofacial abnormalities
Decreased cognitive functioning	Decrease in long-term productivity
Neuropsychiatric concerns	Allergic irritability syndrome
Anosmia	Anosmia
Ageusia	Ageusia

complications that include not only daytime hypersomnolence, memory loss, depression, and poor cognitive function, but also hypertension, right ventricular hypertrophy, pulmonary hypertension, and right-sided congestive heart failure [42].

Cognitive and neuropsychiatric impairment have received increased attention in recent years, perhaps because they are associated with use of traditional, sedating antihistamines. Marshall and Colon [43] demonstrated seasonal impairment in verbal learning and short-term memory in allergic rhinitis patients during two pollen seasons, compared with test scores obtained outside of the allergy season and to scores of nonatopic controls. These children also suffered from altered moods, scoring lower on a positive-affect scale than their nonatopic controls, or in comparison to themselves when tested outside of their allergic season. The allergic irritability syndrome has been coined to include symptoms of fatigue, malaise, anhedonia, lassitude, irritability, inattention, and performance impairment [34]. Such symptoms usually occur as a complication of severe symptomatic rhinitis and may be perennial, depending on the allergen. Neuropsychiatric impairment due to allergic rhinitis has been reported to result in reduced productivity [34]. Juniper and Guyatt [44] found that 60 of 85 patients with documented allergic rhinoconjunctivitis experienced reduced productivity.

Some craniofacial abnormalities may also be associated with chronic mouth breathing seen in allergic rhinitis or adenoidal hypertrophy. Predominately mouth breathers with allergic rhinitis often have lengthened facial features, including narrower maxillary arch, greater palatal height, and greater anterior facial height [45].

MANAGEMENT OF ALLERGIC RHINITIS

There are three available interventions for allergic rhinitis: avoidance of exposure to triggering allergens, pharmacotherapy for relief of symptoms, and immunotherapy for modification of the immune response. Intervention strategies are frequently evaluated by their measured outcomes. Although a model of outcome evaluations exist for asthma, it is not in place for allergic rhinitis; however, the ideal way to deal with a chronic disease such as allergic rhinitis is to prevent its onset. Primary prevention strategies have been targeted in infancy and early childhood to prevent the onset of allergies and focus on avoidance or environmental control measures. It not only makes intuitive sense that at-risk individuals should attempt to avoid exposure to triggering allergens, but the usefulness of this approach has been confirmed in two longitudinal studies—from the Isle of Wight study [46•] and Japan [47].

If prevention of allergen sensitization is not successful, the next therapeutic aim is to induce remission and prevent persistence of disease through secondary strategies. Preventing the persistence of disease may be accomplished with pharmacologic therapy and immunotherapy, which provide satisfactory relief in the majority of patients. Although there is some evidence that allergen avoidance induces remission of allergic rhinitis [48], immunotherapy is, in fact, the only treatment with consistent long-term improvement and is appropriate for a subpopulation of patients.

What we traditionally think of as "treatment" is actually tertiary disease management, aimed at reducing disease severity and improving outcomes by preventing complications. All three interventions, avoidance, medications, and immunotherapy, are used for disease management. The next section covers each in more detail.

ENVIRONMENTAL CONTROL

The most obvious and effective way to treat symptoms from exposure to an allergenic stimulus is to avoid contact with that stimulus. One assumes that environmental control is affordable to all individuals who need it, but this may not be the case when such interventions are not reimbursable under insurance plans. Also, avoidance may not be effective for the patient who is sensitive to multiple factors in the environment, as elimination of one or a few factors may not suffice. Moreover, it may be virtually impossible to eliminate or completely avoid all offending allergens. For example, during ragweed pollen season, sensitive patients may close their windows, exercise during hours of low pollen counts, and use air filters, but there is no way to avoid all exposure short of relocating to another climate for the duration of that season. Avoidance therapy is also laden with problems. It is tedious, time-consuming, and may require changing living habits. It therefore may not be surprising that compliance is so low [49]. Finally, avoidance cannot control symptoms of nasal hyperresponsiveness, caused by nonallergic triggers such as temperature changes, bright lights, alcohol ingestion, infections, and irritants such as perfumes, automobile exhaust, and tobacco smoke.

Nevertheless, well-controlled studies reinforce the utility of allergen avoidance and reinforce the need to begin allergen avoidance intervention early in life [28••]. The evidence for efficacy is greatest for indoor allergens, such as dust mites, molds, animal dander, and insect parts. Recommendations should include rigorous removal of sources of house dust mites [50], either elimination of furry animals from the house or restriction of their access to the sleeping quarters, dehumidification of the basement, consideration for the use of air filters, use of air conditioning in the car and home, and other considerations based upon the patient's specific sensitivities and living style (see Table 5-3).

NONPHARMACOLOGIC CONTROL

The use of nonmedical treatments for any chronic disease has been an attractive option because of their inherent safety. Vigorous exercise, for example, produces nasal decongestion and may be a useful adjunct in patients with intermittent nasal obstruction caused by nonallergic triggers. This effect is obviously short lived and can be repeated. Saline acts as a mild decongestant, as shown by reduction in nasal blood flow, and may be used as adjunctive therapy improving nasal symptoms. Saline washings improve mucociliary flow and have

been used since ancient times. Saline may be administered by commercially produced buffered spray, bulb syringe, or with the use of a nasal adapter for the Waterpik device (Water Pik Technologies, Inc., Fort Collins, CO), the Grossan adapter (HydroMed Inc., Sherman Oaks, CA).

On the other hand, aromatics, astringents, local hyperthermia, and heated moisturized air have not demonstrated any therapeutic effect for allergic rhinitis in clinical studies [26].

PHARMACOLOGIC APPROACH

As the pathologic events leading to symptoms include allergen inhalation, mast cell activation, mediator release, and cytokine and chemokine generation, there are multiple points at which effective therapy can be interposed. Currently available options for pharmacologic therapy include oral and topical antihistamines, cromolyn sodium, topical corticosteroids, and adjunctive treatments such as decongestants (topical and oral) and nasal Atrovent (Boehringer Ingelheim Pharmaceuticals, Ridgefield, CT). The primary actions of the various approaches to the treatment of allergic rhinitis are summarized on Table 5-4.

Leukotrienes are generated in the nose during allergic reactions and are believed to be important in causing vascular permeability, mucous secretion, and swelling of the nose. Thus, there is a logical basis for use of antileukotriene medications for allergic rhinitis. There is one study suggesting their usefulness, but more evidence is necessary before this class of medications is regularly used for symptoms control.

ANTIHISTAMINES

Antihistamines are histamine H_1-receptor antagonists that prevent histamine from activating the H_1 receptor, thereby preventing histamine-mediated inflammatory effects. Prevention of the effects of histamine reduces nasal itching, rhinorrhea, and sneezing, as well as itching and swelling of the conjunctiva. Antihistamines are not particularly effective in reducing nasal congestion [51]. In general, better results are obtained when antihistamines are taken regularly rather than occasionally because they offer prophylactic benefits—receptor sites can be blocked before histamine is released. Table 5-5 has a summary of common antihistamines.

Traditional antihistamines

Different pharmacologic properties associated with structural variations account for the primary benefits of these antihistamines—some are favored for their antiemetic properties whereas others are more effective as antipruritics. In some cases, their side effects may even be desirable; the sedative properties of diphenhydramine hydrochloride (Benadryl; Warner-Lambert,

---

TABLE 5-3. USUAL STRATEGIES FOR AVOIDANCE OF INDOOR ALLERGENS

Strategies for Dust Avoidance

Encase mattress, box spring, and pillow in mite-proof, impermeable covers

Wash bed sheets and blankets in hot water (at least 130°F) at least once a week

Decrease household humidity (<50%)

Remove all feather pillows and comforters

Minimize dust-collecting surfaces (*eg*, shelves, stuffed animals, books)

Remove Venetian blinds from the bedroom; use washable curtains with shades

Avoid vacuuming when dust-sensitive patients are home; use vacuum cleaners with HEPA filtering devices

Remove carpeting from bedroom or treat carpeting with acaricide

Remove upholstered furniture from the bedroom

Strategies for Animal Allergen Avoidance

Remove pets from home environment

Control reservoirs

   Bar animal entry into bedrooms

   Use air cleaners with HEPA in bedrooms

   Wash animal and animal-contaminated items regularly

Strategies for Mold Allergen Avoidance

Remove mold sources

Clean with fungicides (10% chlorine bleach, Zephiran)

Control humidity (use dehumidifiers, avoid vaporizers or humidifiers)

Strategies for Cockroach Allergen Avoidance

Routine but thorough cleaning (wash, vacuum)

Control sources of food and water (wash dishes, seal food in containers, seal cracks and holes)

Eliminate cockroach populations (bait stations, pesticides)

TABLE 5-4. COMPARISON OF VARIOUS APPROACHES TO THE TREATMENT OF ALLERGIC RHINITIS

	Sneezing	Discharge	Itch	Congestion	Side Effects
Antihistamines					
Traditional (A)	+++	+++	+++	+	+++
Nonsedating (NSA)	+++	+++	+++	+	– to +
Decongestants	–	+	–	+++	++
NSA + decongestants	+++	+++	+++	+++	++
Cromolyn	++	+	+	+	–
Nasal CCS (NCS)	+++	+++	+++	+++	+
NSA +NCS	++++	++++	++++	++++	+
Immunotherapy	+++	+++	+++	+++	+ to ++

TABLE 5-5. ANTIHISTAMINES WITH AND WITHOUT SEDATIVE ACTIVITY

Chemical name	Trade name	Dosage Adult	Children <12 years
Traditional antihistamines			
Ethanolamines			
Diphenhydramine HCl	Benadryl*	25–50 mg tid, qid	5 mg/kg in 3 or 4 divided doses
Alkylamines			
Chlorpheniramine maleate	Chlortrimeton†	4 mg tid, qid	0.4 mg/kg in 3 or 4 divided doses <2 years, 1.25 mg 2–3 times daily
Brompheniramine maleate	Dimetane‡	4 mg tid, qid	0.4 mg/kg in 3 or 4 divided doses
Piperazines			
Hydroxyzine HCl	Atarax§ Vistaril§	10–50 mg tid, qid	2 mg/kg in 4 divided doses
Phenothiazines			
Promethazine HCl	Phenergan¶	12.5–25 mg bid, tid	1 mg/kg divided doses
Piperidines			
Azatadine maleate	Optimine†	1–2 mg bid	
Miscellaneous antihistamines			
Cyproheptadine HCl	Periactin**	4 mg bid–tid, qid	0.25 mg/kg in 3 or 4 divided doses
Clemastine fumarate	Tavist††	2.68 mg bid	
Nonsedating antihistamines			
Fexofenadine	Allegra‡‡	60 mg bid	30 mg bid***
Loratidine	Claritin†	10 mg qd	10 mg qd†††
Cetirizine	Zyrtec§	5–10 mg qd	5–10 mg qd†††
Topical antihistamines			
Azelastine	Astelin§§	274 µg per nostril bid	137 µg per nostril bid‡‡‡

*Warner-Lambert, Morris Plains, NY.
†Schering, Kenilworth, NJ.
‡Robins, Richmond, VA.
§Pfizer, New York, NY.
¶Wyeth-Ayerst, Philadelphia, PA.
** Merck, West Point, PA.
††Novartis Consumer, Summit, NJ.
‡‡Aventis Pharmaceuticals, Parsippany, NJ.
§§Wallace Laboratories, Cranbury, NJ.
***Children 6–12 years old.
†††Children 2–12 years old.
‡‡‡Children 5–11 years old.
Adapted from Kaliner [4].

Morris Plains, NY) are useful in helping patients sleep; however, the side effects of somnolence, dyskinesia, activation of seizure foci, anxiety, confusion, and reduced mental alertness, as well as the anticholinergic effects of dryness, urinary hesitancy, and constipation, restrict the usefulness of these products [52]. Many patients may not be aware of the lingering actions of traditional antihistamines on their cognitive functions [53], and increasing attention has been given to their effects on driving performance [54] as well as occupational injury [55]. With some exceptions, many traditional antihistamines are taken three or four times a day and their side effects may interfere with patient compliance. Many are available over the counter and several of these antihistamines are also available in combination with a decongestant. Because each patient responds differently to each drug, it may be appropriate to try various formulations to find one that adequately relieves the patient's symptoms without producing unacceptable side effects. In some patients, an antihistamine with a relatively weaker sedative effect, such as chlorpheniramine, may be well tolerated. When a new preparation containing an antihistamine with potential sedative activity is tried, the patient should be instructed to take the first dose before bedtime or on a weekend so that school and work performance are not jeopardized. It is important to emphasize to all patients not to drink alcohol while taking a traditional antihistamine.

Nonsedating antihistamines

For the purposes of treating allergic rhinitis, traditional antihistamines, although affordable, have limited usefulness and are no longer recommended as first-line treatment. Nonsedating antihistamines are used widely and have been shown to be safe, effective, and well tolerated [56]. Their once-daily or twice-daily dosage and lack of side effects may improve patient compliance and satisfaction. Nonsedating antihistamines do not cross the blood-brain barrier, and therefore do not cause sedation, which is mediated through central nervous system activity. Moreover, the nonsedating antihistamines are more specific in their actions and do not have anticholinergic or anti-alpha adrenergic activity [53]. Presently available nonsedating antihistamines include fexofenadine (Allegra; Aventis Pharmaceuticals, Parsippany, NJ) and loratadine (Claritin; Schering, Kenilworth, NJ). These drugs are available only by prescription. Cetirizine (Zyrtec; Pfizer, New York, NY) is a selective H_1 antagonist with mild sedative properties (14% somnolence with 10 mg versus 6% with placebo) [57].

Several of the nonsedating antihistamines are available in combination with a decongestant, (Claritin-D, Claritin-D24, and Allegra D). These combination tablets may also reduce nasal congestion. Both Claritin

and Zyrtec are available in pediatric formulations, down to age 2. Topical antihistamines recently became available for nasal use. Azelastine (Astelin; Wallace Laboratories, Cranbury, NJ) is now marketed as a nasal spray and provides a convenient, fast-acting preparation for nasal itching, rhinorrhea, and sneezing. Astelin may be used in children 5 years of age and older, may reduce eye symptoms, seems to affect nasal congestion, and may be associated with a bitter taste and somnolence. Recent data show that Astelin is effective in nonallergic vasomotor rhinitis as well.

Cromolyn sodium (nasal)

The effects of cromolyn are due to its capacity to prevent the release of histamine from mast cells by stabilizing their membranes and decreasing their tendency to release inflammatory mediators in response to allergenic stimuli [58]. In patients with allergic rhinitis, the drug decreases sneezing, itching, and rhinorrhea [59]. Cromolyn must be used prophylactically for optimal effectiveness, as it does not prevent the release of histamine after exposure to the allergenic stimulus. Cromolyn is not useful for as-needed administration. Cromolyn is a moderately effective agent for long-term use in patients with chronic allergic rhinitis and is extremely safe; however, it must be used 3 to 5 times each day for effectiveness. For intranasal use, it is available over the counter.

Nasal corticosteroids

Corticosteroids are effective in treating allergic rhinitis because of their ability to decrease vasodilation, edema, nasal irritability, and inflammation, among many other actions. In addition, these agents diminish the overall response of mucous glands to cholinergic stimulation and the infiltration of inflammatory cells (neutrophils, basophils, and eosinophils) in the late-phase inflammatory response [60]. Corticosteroids also reduce the number of mucosal mast cells and decrease the sensitivity of irritant or sneeze receptors. Thus, nasal corticosteroids are highly effective in reducing the four cardinal symptoms of allergic rhinitis: nasal congestion, rhinorrhea, sneezing, and itchiness [61,62]. The efficacy of nasal corticosteroids for allergic rhinitis has been recognized for many years; they are effective in most patients. The currently available nasal corticosteroids include beclomethasone, budesonide, fluticasone, flunisolide, mometasone, and triamcinolone (Table 5-6). Because they are rapidly metabolized, there is no suppression of the hypothalamic-pituitary-adrenal axis, and therefore, little risk of systemic side effects associated with their use.

Local side effects are also relatively rare. Specifically, there is no evidence that nasal mucosal atrophy occurs, even after 10 years of intranasal use [63]. In addition, there have been no reports of significant incidents of nasal or pharyngeal candidiasis. Local irritation may be less with the aqueous pump and aerosol spray delivery systems, as compared with that resulting from the use of some metered-dose sprays. In general, sprays with a Freon propellant have been reported to sting or cause discomfort from the force of the impact. It is important to instruct the patient not to direct the spray toward the septum, as perforation from trauma, as well as vaso-constriction, can occur.

Nasal corticosteroids are administered once or twice daily, although patients may do well with once-daily or every-other-day administration after symptoms have been controlled. It usually takes 2 to 4 days for the effects of nasal corticosteroids to become noticeable, and local irritation may occur if the mucosa is severely inflamed. For these reasons, it is best to begin treatment before or just after symptoms initially occur and are likely to progress rather than wait until they have become severe.

Although there are data to suggest that topical corticosteroids are more effective than oral antihistamines [22], patients prefer the convenience of oral medications. Moreover, recent data suggest that nasal beclomethasone in recommended doses can affect the growth pattern of young children [64], suggesting some potential for systemic effects. Thus, at this time, it is prudent to suggest that patients use a nonsedating antihistamine in the morning during the allergy season plus the lowest dose of nasal corticosteroid that keeps them comfortable.

Systemic corticosteroids

Systemic or oral corticosteroid therapy is generally inappropriate for patients with allergic rhinitis, except in certain limited circumstances; however, a short course lasting no more than a week is not likely to cause harm and may be helpful in rapidly controlling a severe allergic episode to the point where symptoms may be managed with topical agents or milder oral medications. Systemic injections of corticosteroids for allergic rhinitis are not indicated.

ADJUNCTIVE MEDICAL TREATMENTS FOR ALLERGIC RHINITIS

Decongestants

Decongestants are sympathomimetic agents (alpha-adrenergic agonists) that decrease swelling in the nasal

TABLE 5-6. TOPICAL NASAL CORTICOSTEROIDS

Generic name	Trade name	Dosage (Sprays/Nostril)	
		Adults	Children
Beclomethasone dipropionate	Beconase*	1 puff bid–qid	6–12: 1 puff bid
	Vancenase†		<6: Not recommended
	Beconase AQ*	1–2 sprays bid	6–12: 1–2 sprays bid
	Vancenase AQ†		<6: Not recommended
	Beconase AQ DS*	1–2 sprays qd	6–12: 1–2 sprays qd
	Vancenase AQ DS†		<6: Not recommended
Budesonide	Rhinocort‡	2 sprays bid	<6: not recommended
	Rhinocort AQ‡	1 spray qd	<6: not recommended
Fluticasone	Flonase	2 sprays qd	4–12: 1 spray qd
			<4: Not recommended
Flunisolide	Nasarel§, Nasalide§	2 sprays bid	6–14: 1 spray bid
			<6: Not recommended
Mometasone	Nasonex†	2 sprays qd	3–11: 1–2 sprays qd
			<3: Not recommended
Triamcinolone acetonide	Nasacort¶	2 puffs qd	6–11: 1 spray qd
	Nasacort AQ¶	2 sprays qd	<6: Not recommended
	Tri-Nasal**	2 sprays qd	Not recommended

*Glaxo Wellcome, Research Triangle Park, NC.
†Schering, Kenilworth, NJ.
‡AstraZeneca, Wilmington, DE.
§Dura Pharmaceuticals, San Diego, CA.
¶Aventis Pharmaceuticals, Parsippany, NJ.
**Muro Pharmaceutical, Tewksbury, MA.

mucosa by causing vasoconstriction in the superficial blood vessels [64]. When these blood vessels constrict, they become less leaky. Thus, edema and rhinorrhea may be decreased. Decongestants are more effective when taken in combination with an antihistamine than when taken alone [66].

Topical decongestants

Phenylephrine hydrochloride (Dristan, Neo-Synephrin, etc.) is short acting, whereas oxymetazoline (Afrin, Dristan 12-Hour Spray, etc.) and xylometazoline (Otrivin) have a longer duration of action. The use of topical decongestants avoids the risk of side effects associated with systemic administration of these agents; however, the local side effects are a significant problem. Use of topical decongestants for longer than 3 or 4 days can result in progressively more severe nasal obstruction caused by a rebound effect—the original symptoms worsen after prolonged administration of the drug (rhinitis medicamentosa). Therefore, topical agents should not be used for the long-term treatment of allergic rhinitis.

As will be discussed in the following section, it may be appropriate to use one of these agents in a patient with a completely obstructed nasal airway, permitting the airway to open sufficiently in preparation for use of a topical corticosteroid. Other appropriate uses may be at bedtime to facilitate sleep in a patient with severe exacerbation of symptoms or as part of the medical management of sinusitis. Generally, the use of a topical long-acting decongestant is permitted for 2 to 3 days of any 7-day period.

Oral decongestants

The most commonly prescribed oral decongestant is pseudoephedrine hydrochloride. The potential systemic effects of pseudoephedrine include hypertension, nervousness, irritability, urinary hesitancy, loss of appetite, and insomnia. Some of their stimulatory effects, however, may be tempered by the suppressive or sedative effects of antihistamines when the two are given in combination. Oral decongestants should be used cautiously in patients with heart disease, hypertension, prostate enlargement, or seizure disorders, and should be avoided in patients who are taking a monoamine oxidase (MAO) inhibitor.

Cholinergic stimulation of the nose leads to rhinorrhea and congestion, which can be prevented or treated with topical anticholinergic sprays [67]. Ipratropium (Atrovent Nasal Spray) reduces these symptoms in patients with allergic rhinitis, nonallergic rhinitis, and upper respiratory infections [68].

Ophthalmic medications

For patients who have severe ocular symptoms, including irritation, itching, swelling, and redness associated with allergic rhinitis, topical ophthalmic preparations may be used. Useful combinations of antihistamines and decongestants for the eye include Vascon-A and Naphcon-A (both available over the counter). The following medications are available by prescription for the eyes: the antiallergy products cromolyn (Opticrom [Allergan, Irvine, CA], Crolom), pemirolast (Alamast [Santen, Napa, CA]), lodoxamide (Alomide [Alcon, Fort Worth, TX]), and nedocromil (Alocril [Allergan, Irvine, CA]); the topical antihistamines levocobastine (Livostin) and emedastine (Emadine); the antipruritic compound ketorolac (Acular [Allergan, Irvine, CA]); and the new antiallergy products with antihistamine properties olopatadine (Patanol [Alcon, Fort Worth, TX]), azelastine (Optivar [Muro Pharmaceutical, Tewksbury, MA]), and ketotifen (Zaditor [Novartis Pharmaceuticals, East Hanover, NJ]).

Immunotherapy

Pharmacologic therapy is directed at the symptoms of allergic rhinitis; it does not modify the disease process itself. In some patients, immunotherapy, designed to change the individual patient's immune response to a specific allergen, may be appropriate (Table 5-7) [69]. In general, evaluation, testing, and recommendations for a course of immunotherapy should be performed by a physician with expertise in allergy because of the potential for life-threatening complications. Immunotherapy typically involves once- or twice-weekly subcutaneous injections of the allergens to which the patient is allergic. Initially a dilute solution is used and the concentration is increased gradually until a maintenance dose is reached— the highest level that can be injected without causing significant local reactions. When the maintenance dose is achieved and maintained for 1 to 2 years (with a reduction in symptoms), the interval between injections can usually be increased to 2 to 4 weeks. A course of 3 to 5 years of immunotherapy is usually sufficient to induce a long-lasting remission [70]. Allergens can be combined to minimize the number of injections needed.

TABLE 5-7. INDICATIONS FOR IMMUNOTHERAPY FOR ALLERGIC RHINITIS

Inadequate control by environmental avoidance and pharmacotherapy

Requirement of pharmacotherapy for more than 3–4 months per year

Control with medication, but onset of intolerable side effects (eg, hypertension, insomnia, sedation, irritability)

Progressive severity that requires increasing medications

Aggravation by unavoidable exposure (eg, animal allergy in a veterinarian)

Desire for long-lasting control without medications

The mechanism of action of immunotherapy appears to include stimulation of production of IgG antibodies against the offending allergens. These antibodies enable the patient's immune system to inactivate or neutralize the antigen before it can trigger an allergic episode [71]. The levels of antigen-specific IgA and IgG in nasal secretions rise with treatment; IgE levels rise at first, then fall with continued treatment [72]. Once treatment is started, the expected rise in IgE levels during seasonal exposure to the antigen is blocked. In addition, immunotherapy reduces the late-phase response and the influx of eosinophils [73], and may cause suppression of the allergic response by influencing the type of lymphocyte that controls the immune response [74].

A substantial number of placebo-controlled studies support the efficacy of immunotherapy, and the success rate is generally considered to be approximately 85% to 90% of patients [74]. Additionally, there is good evidence that allergen immunotherapy for allergic rhinitis actually prevents the development of asthma [75,76]. Side effects of immunotherapy, other than local reaction at the injection site, are relatively infrequent; however, the risk of fatal anaphylactic reactions requires that the physician proceed with extreme caution when administering immunotherapy. The concomitant use of pharmacotherapy with immunotherapy keeps patients comfortable during the initial phases of immunotherapy, before it becomes effective. Although pharmacotherapy is excellent for symptomatic control, it does not affect the underlying allergy as does immunotherapy.

APPROACH TO A TYPICAL PATIENT

Education is the first step in treating a patient with a chronic disease. The physician should inform the patient of the etiology and symptoms of allergic rhinitis, as well as explain that the severity of symptoms may vary among individuals, even in the same person, from week to week. The patient's familiarity with the various treatment options and assurance of the physician's concern for his or her long-term health contribute to improved management of allergic rhinitis.

The patient's help should be enlisted in a cooperative effort to control the disease process so that compliance with medication regimens and avoidance of exacerbating factors is improved. Indeed, data on compliance issues paint a grim reality. In a survey of 481 respondents with allergic rhinitis aimed at assessing compliance with environmental control measures, Storms *et al.* [49] reported that only 6% used mattress encasings and 15% washed the bedding in hot water, whereas 25% admitted to no measures. Drug noncompliance rates were very

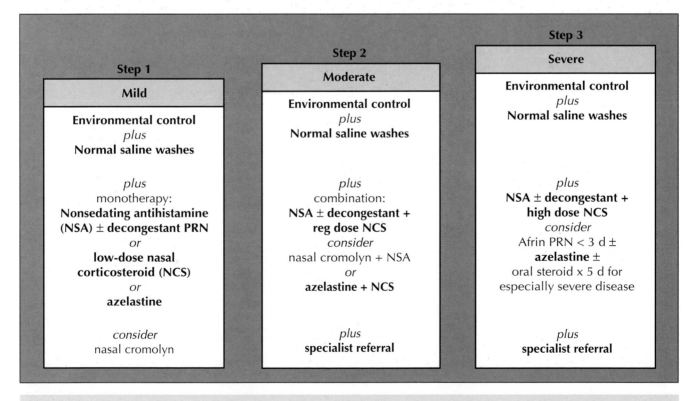

FIGURE 5-1.

Step-wise treatment of allergic rhinitis in adults. (1) Step down treatment once control is achieved; (2) consult a specialist when any complications arise. Highlighted option represents treatment of choice.

high (50%–80%), and patients generally preferred pills rather than inhaled medications [77]. Compliance with immunotherapy regimens in an HMO environment was only 28% for patients with allergic rhinitis alone [78].

Figures 5-1 and 5-2 show algorithms for the stepwise treatment of patients with allergic rhinitis (adults and children, respectively) modified from the recommendations of the Joint Task Force on Practice Parameters in Allergy, Asthma, and Immunology [79] using the step-wise model of the National Institutes of Health (NIH) guidelines for asthma management. Step 1 corresponds to mild disease, such as that seen in seasonal allergic rhinitis. Step 2 corresponds to moderate disease, and may include patients with perennial allergic rhinitis. Step 3 denotes severe, chronic, persistent allergic rhinitis, which may be associated with complications. Environmental control is listed first as a strategy in all steps and for all ages. It is intuitive but not mandatory that a referral to an allergist would facilitate identification of allergens and lead to appropriate instruction in allergen avoidance techniques. Normal saline washes can be quite helpful and are recommended in all steps and all ages.

Occasional exposure to allergen responds well to PRN use of an antihistamine or nasal cromolyn. The treatment strategy for step 1 or mild disease is essentially monotherapy. A nonsedating antihistamine (NSA) alone, or with a timed-release decongestant, can be sufficient. Patients with congestion may benefit from the concomitant use of a decongestant, whereas those whose symptoms include only episodic sneezing, pruritus, and rhinorrhea do not need the additional medication. One can also use a topical nasal antihistamine (Astelin), nasal cromolyn, or a low-dose nasal corticosteroid (NCS). For adults, generally the medications of choice are NSA, Astelin, or NCS. For children, there are NSA choices, Astelin, or low-dose NCS. Because there is no currently available NSA-decongestant combination for children, many physicians use antihistamines and oral decongestants separately for pediatric patients.

Patients whose symptoms last for months or even all year have moderate disease; treatments of choice are listed in Step 2. The key here is combination therapy, eventually stepping down whenever possible to monotherapy or the least medication necessary to control symptoms. For adults, nasal corticosteroids at regular to high doses plus NSA antihistamines with or without decongestants are the combinations of choice. After therapy with an NCS is started and symptoms are controlled, it is appro-

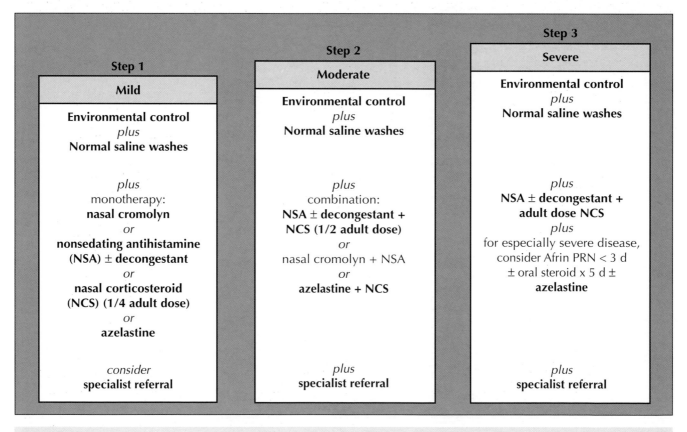

FIGURE 5-2.
Step-wise treatment of allergic rhinitis in children 2 to 11 years old. (1) Step down treatment once control is achieved; (2) consult a specialist when any complications arise. Highlighted option represents treatment of choice.

priate to reduce the medications to the lowest effective dose. NCS may also be combined with topical antihistamines, such as Astelin. For children, combination of low-dose NCS (half the adult dose) with antihistamines should be tried as a reasonable first choice. A combination of cromolyn with antihistamines may also be tried, and one may also consider the occasional use of Afrin.

For patients with more severe symptoms (Step 3), it is probably best to start with a nasal corticosteroid immediately, in addition to an antihistamine and possibly a decongestant. If the patient's nasal passage is completely blocked, a topical decongestant may be used to allow the first few doses of the topical corticosteroid to reach the nasal mucosa. In extreme cases, a short course of oral corticosteroids (30 mg of prednisone per day, tapering off over 5 days) may be necessary.

Within this model, referral to the allergist should be considered for any level of persistent disease in children because early intervention may prevent development of symptoms such as asthma. Both children and adults with moderate or severe disease should be referred to the aller-

gist for a more thorough evaluation of the anatomy and for determining specific triggers. Allergy testing has the dual role of diagnosing IgE-mediated disease and determining the utility of immunotherapy. Immunotherapy is indicated in patients who require more than 3 to 4 months of pharmacotherapy each year or whose symptoms are not satisfactorily controlled with pharmacotherapy. Guidelines have been developed to provide criteria for when a patient should be referred for evaluation of rhinitis and what the referring physician should be provided by the consultant in order to assist in the patient's management (Table 5-8). Other indications for referral to an allergist include severe or chronic complications, persistent or prolonged symptoms, and concurrent diseases that make treatment difficult [80].

There are caveats to the above. Special considerations for pregnant women and the elderly follow the principles of common sense; avoid pseudoephedrine during the first trimester because it has been associated with gastroschisis of the fetus, and consider the optimum treatment of the elderly with other comorbid diseases. Olympic athletes cannot use oral decongestants and may have other limitations because of their sport or Olympic committee regulations. Occupational allergic rhinitis (such as in housekeepers, veterinarians, laboratory technicians) may require allergen immunotherapy earlier rather than later.

CONCLUSIONS

Allergic rhinitis is an extremely common disorder that causes both physical discomfort and inconvenience for many patients. It is characterized by the production of excessive amounts of IgE in response to exposure to specific allergenic antigens; there appears to be a genetic basis for this phenomenon. The binding of specific antigens to IgE antibodies on the surface of mast cells causes these cells to degranulate and release a multitude of immune and inflammatory mediators. Some of these, such as histamine, cause an immediate reaction characterized by sneezing, itching, rhinorrhea, and nasal congestion, the classic symptoms of allergic rhinitis. Other substances cause a late-phase reaction in which additional inflammatory cells are recruited to the site and the inflammatory process is perpetuated.

The first and most important strategy for managing the symptoms of allergic rhinitis is to avoid exposure to the allergens that trigger the response. When that is not sufficient, pharmacologic therapy should be initiated. Antihistamines can be administered on an intermittent or daily basis. Nonsedating antihistamines are preferred and an oral decongestant may be added if nasal congestion is a major symptom. Cromolyn is effective and extremely safe; however, it must be given prophylactically and requires frequent dosage, as many as four or more times daily. Topical nasal corticosteroids are extremely effective

---

TABLE 5-8. INDICATIONS FOR REFERRAL TO AN ALLERGIST

Indications for referral of rhinitis patients to the consultant

When the condition or its treatment is interfering with a patient's performance or causing significant loss of school or work

When the patient's quality of life is significantly affected

When there are complications of rhinitis, such as sinusitis, otitis, hearing loss, asthma, significant snoring, loss of sleep, or bronchitis

When initial treatments have not adequately resolved the symptoms or additional diagnostic approaches are required

When a patient requires systemic corticosteroids

What the consultant should provide to the referring physician

Clarification of allergic or other etiologic basis for the patient's condition

Identification of specific allergens or other triggers for the patient's condition, and education in ways to limit exposure to these triggers

Assistance in developing an effective treatment plan, including allergy avoidance, pharmacotherapy, and immunotherapy

Provision of specialized services, such as preparation of extracts and provision of immunotherapy

Education about the disease state and the therapeutic options

Data from *Kaliner [80]*.

and generally safe. For patients with severe, unresponsive, or prolonged disease, immunotherapy may be appropriate; this decision is best made in consultation with an allergist.

REFERENCES AND RECOMMENDED READING

Recently published papers of particular interest have been highlighted as:
- •   Of interest
- •• Of outstanding interest

1. Evans R: Epidemiology and natural history of asthma, allergic rhinitis, and atopic dermatitis. In *Allergy: Principles and Practice* edn 4. Edited by Middleton E, Reed CE, Ellis EF, *et al*. St. Louis: CV Mosby; 1993:1109–1136.

2. Vital and Health Statistics: Current estimates from the National Health Interview Survey. 1994, Series 10, No. 193.

3. Collins JG, National Center for Health Statistics: Prevalence of Selected Chronic Conditions, United States, 1983–1985. Advance Data from Vital and Health Statistics. No. 155. Hyattsville, MD, Public Health Service, 1988, DHHS publication (PHS) 88-1250.

4. Kaliner MA, Lemanske R: Rhinitis and asthma. *J Am Med Assoc* 1992, 268:2807–2829.

5. Fleming DM, Crombie DA: Prevalence of asthma and hay fever in England and Wales. *Br Med J* 1987, 294:279–283.

6. Naclerio R, Solomon W: Rhinitis and inhalant allergens. *J Am Med Assoc* 1997, 287:1842–1848.

7. Juniper EF, Guyatt GH, Dolovich J: Assessment of quality of life in adolescents with allergic rhinoconjunctivitis. *J Allergy Clin Immunol* 1994, 93:413–421.

8. Young P: Asthma and Allergies: An Optimistic Future. Washington DC: U.S. Department of Health and Human Services; 1980, U.S. Public Health Service, National Institutes of Health publication DIHN 80-388: 4–26.

9. Meltzer EO: An overview of current pharmacotherapy in perennial rhinitis. *J Allergy Clin Immunol* 1995, 96:1097–1110.

10. Meltzer EO: Performance effects of antihistamines. *J Allergy Clin Immunol* 1990, 86:613–619.

11. Baraniuk J, Meltzer E, Spector S: Impact of allergic rhinitis and related airway disorders. *J Resp Dis Suppl* 1996, 17:S11–S23.

12. Ray N, Rinehart C, Thamer M, *et al.*: Cost of allergic rhinoconjunctivitis (AR/AC): estimation by the *Delphi* method. *J Allergy Clin Immunol* 1998, 101:S44.

13. Naclerio RM: Allergic rhinitis. *N Engl J Med* 1991, 325:860–869.

14. Trigg CJ, Davies RJ: Allergic rhinitis. *Arch Dis Child* 1991, 66:565–568.

15. Igarashi Y, Goldrich MS, Kaliner MA, *et al.*: Quantification of inflammatory cells in the nasal mucosa of allergic rhinitis and normal subjects. *J Allergy Clin Immunol* 1995, 95:716–725.

16. Denburg JA, Dolovich J, Harnish D: Basophil mast cell and eosinophil growth and differentiation factors in human allergic disease. *Clin Exp Allergy* 1989, 19:249–254.

17. Barnes PJ: Pathophysiology of allergic inflammation. In *Allergy: Principles and Practice* edn 5. Edited by Middleton E, Reed CE, Ellis EF, *et al*. St. Louis: Mosby; 1998:356–365.

18. Romagnani S: Regulation and disregulation of human IgE synthesis. *Immunol Today* 1990, 11:316–321.

19. Naclerio RM, Baroody FM, Togias AG: The role of leukotrienes in allergic rhinitis: a review. *Am Rev Resp Dis* 1991, 143:S91–S95.

20.• Naclerio R: Clinical manifestations of the release of histamine and other inflammatory mediators. *J Allergy Clin Immunol* 1999, 103 (suppl):382–385.
This is a recent review of the role of chemical mediators to the manifestation of symptoms of early- and late-phase allergic reactions.

21. Kaliner MA: The role of histamine in allergic rhinitis and a guide to management. *Consultant* 1991, 31(suppl):9–12.

22. Saxon A, Diaz-Sanchez D, Zhang K: The allergic response in host defense. In *Clinical Immunology: Principles and Practice*. Edited by Rich RR. St. Louis: Mosby; 1996:847–876.

23. Baraniuk J: Pathogenesis of allergic rhinitis. *J Allergy Clin Immunol* 1997, 99:S763–S772.

24. Ownby DR: Clinical Significance of Immunoglobulin E. In *Allergy: Principles and Practice* edn 5. Edited by Middleton E, Reed CE, Ellis EF, *et al*. St. Louis: CV Mosby; 1998:770–782.

25. Lichtenstein LM: Histamine releasing factors and IgE heterogeneity. *J Allergy Clin Immunol* 1988, 81:814–820.

26. Druce HM: Allergic and nonallergic rhinitis. In *Allergy: Principles and Practice* edn 5. Edited by Middleton E, Reed CE, Ellis EF, *et al*. St. Louis: CV Mosby; 1998:1005–1016.

27. Marsh DG, Norman PS: Antigens that cause atopic disease. In *Immunological Diseases* edn 4. Edited by Samter M. Boston: Little Brown and Co.; 1988:981–1008.

28.•• Tovey E, Marks G: Methods and effectiveness of environmental control. *J Allergy Clin Immunol* 1999, 103:179–191.
A well-rounded and recent overview of the literature on avoidance control.

29. Bollinger ME, Eggleston PA, Flanagan E, Wood RA: Cat antigen in homes with and without cats may induce allergic symptoms. *J Allergy Clin Immunol* 1996, 97:907–914.

30. Berge M, Munir AK, Deborg S: Concentrations of cat (Fel D I), dog (Can f I) and mite (Der f I and Der p I) allergens in the clothing and school environment of Swedish schoolchildren with and without pets. *Pediatr Allergy Immunol* 1998, 9:25–30.

31. Sarpong SB, Wood RA, Eggleston PA: Short term effect of extermination and cleaning on cockroach allergens Bla g 2 in settled dust. *Ann Allergy Asthma Immunol* 1996, 76:257–260.

32.• Settipane RJ, Hagy GW, Settipane GA: Long term risk factors for developing asthma and allergic rhinitis: a 23-year follow-up study of college students. *Allergy Asthma Proc* 1994, 15:21–25.
This is a frequently quoted investigation on the developmental course of allergic respiratory disease. The authors followed a cohort of more than 1000 college students for a total of 23 years, using a prospective and longitudinal design. They document the chronicity of allergic rhinitis and the low risk for spontaneous remission. Also, allergic rhinitis and positive skin tests were identified as significant risk factors for the development of new asthma.

33. Raphael G, Hauptschein-Raphael M, Kaliner M: Gustatory rhinitis: a syndrome of food-induced rhinorrhea. *J Allergy Clin Immunol* 1989, 83:110–115.

34. Settipane RA: Complications of allergic rhinits. *Allergy Asthma Proc* 1999, 20:209–213.

35 Bernstein JM: The role of IgE mediated hypersensitivity in the development of otitis media with effusion. *Otolaryngol Clin North Am* 1992, 25:197–211.

36. Savolainen S: Allergy in patients with acute maxillary sinusitis. *Allergy* 1989, 44:116–122.

37. McNally PA, White MV, Kaliner MA: Sinusitis in an allergist's office: analysis of 200 consecutive cases. *Allergy Asthma Proc* 1997, 18:169–176.

38. Kaliner MA: Recurrent sinusitis: examining medical treatment options. *Am J Rhinol* 1997, 11:123–132.

39. Anderson HR, Pottier AC, Stachan DP: Asthma from birth to age 23: incidence and relation to prior and concurrent atopic disease. *Thorax* 1992, 47:537–542.

40. Golbin A, Bernales R, Lim DT: Perennial allergic rhinitis and sleep disorders [abstract]. 1992, 68:85.

41. Young T, Finn L, Kim H: Nasal obstruction as a risk factor for sleep disordered breathing. *J Allergy Clin Immunol* 1997, 99:S757–S762.

42. Hudgel DW: When to consider surgery for obstructive sleep apnea. *J Resp Dis* 1994, 15: 203–208.

43. Marshall PS, Colon EA: Effect of allergy season on mood and cognitive function. *Ann Allergy* 1993, 71:251–258.

44. Juniper EF, Guyatt GH: Development and testing of a new measure of health status for clinical trials in rhinoconjunctivitis. *Clin Exp Allergy* 1991, 21:77–83.

45. Shapiro G: The role of nasal airway obstruction in sinus disease and facial development. *J Allergy Clin Immunol* 1988, 82:935–40.

46.• Hide DW, Matthews S, Tariq S, Arshad S: Allergen avoidance in infancy and allergy at 4 years of age. *Allergy* 1996, 51:89–93.
This is part of a continuing, prospective, longitudinal study of high-risk infants of atopy in the Isle of Wight, England. A control group of no environmental interventions is compared to a prophylactic group who received either breast milk or hypoallergenic milk formula and extensive dust mite avoidance.

47. Nishioka K, Yasueda H, Saito H: Preventive effect of bedding encasement with microfine fibers on mite sensitization. *J Allergy Clin Immunol* 1998, 101:28–32.

48. Wickman M, Korsgaard J: Transient sensitization to house dust mites: a study on the influence of mite exposure and sex. *Allergy* 1996, 51:511–513.

49. Storms W, Meltzer EO, Nathan RA, Selner JC: Allergic rhinitis: the patients' perspective. *J Allergy Clin Immunol* 1997, 99(suppl):S825–S828.

50. Engler DB, Grant JA: Allergic rhinitis: a practical approach. *Hosp Pract* 1991, 26:105–112.

51. Simons KS, Simons FER: H$_1$-Receptor antagonists: pharamacokinetics and clinical pharmacology. In *Histamine and H$_1$-Receptor Antagonists in Allergic Disease.* Edited by Simons FER. New York: Marcel Dekker; 1996:175–214.

52. Kaliner MA: Clinical use of (H$_1$) antihistamines in elderly patients: considerations in a polypharmaceutic patient population. *Clin Geriatrics* 1997, 5:75–90.

53. Meltzer EO, Welsh MJ: Adverse effects of H$_1$-receptor antagonists in the central nervous system. In *Histamine and H$_1$-Receptor Antagonists in Allergic Disease.* Edited by Simons FER. New York: Marcel Dekker; 1996:357–382.

54. O'Hanlon JF: Antihistamines and driving performance: The Netherlands. *J Resp Dis* 1988, 9 (suppl7A): S12–S7.

55. Gilmore TM, Alexander BH, Mueller BA, *et al.*: Occupational injuries and medication use. *Am J Int Med* 1996, 30:234–239.

56. Kaliner MA: Non-sedating antihistamines: pharmacology, clinical efficacy and adverse effects. *Am Fam Physician* 1992, 45:1337–1342.

57. Honig P, Baraniuk JN: Adverse effects of the H$_1$-receptor antagonists in the cardiovascular system. In *Histamine and H$_1$-Receptor Antagonists in Allergic Disease.* Edited by Simons FER. New York: Marcel Dekker; 1996:383–412.

58. Pelikan Z: The effects of disodium cromoglycate and beclomethasone dipropionate on the late nasal mucosa response to allergen challenge. *Ann Allergy* 1982, 49:200–212.

59. Chandra RK, Heresi G, Woolford G: Double-blind, controlled, crossover trial of 4% intranasal sodium cromoglycate in patients with seasonal allergic rhinitis. *Ann Allergy* 1982, 49:131–134.

60. Pipkorn U, Proud D, Lichtenstein LM, *et al.*: Inhibition of mediator release in allergic rhinitis by pretreatment with topical glucocorticoids. *N Engl J Med* 1987, 316:1506–1510.

61. Orgel HA, Meltzer EO, Kemp JP, *et al.*: Clinical, rhinomanometric, and cytologic evaluation of seasonal allergic rhinitis treated with beclomethasone dipropionate as aqueous nasal spray or pressurized aerosol. *J Allergy Clin Immunol* 1986, 77:858–864.

62. Meltzer EO, Orgel HA, Bush RK, *et al.*: Evaluation of symptom relief, nasal airflow, nasal cytology, and acceptability of two formulations of flunisolide nasal spray in patients with perennial allergic rhinitis. *Ann Allergy* 1990, 64:536–540.

63. Kaliner M, Eggleston PA, Mathews KP: Rhinitis and asthma. *J Am Med Assoc* 1987, 258: 2851–2873.

64. Rachelefsky GS, Chervinsky P, Meltzer EO, *et al.*: An evaluation of the effects of beclomethasone diproprionate aqueous nasal spray (Vancenase AQ) on long-term growth in children. *J Allergy Clin Immunol* 1998, 109:S236.

65. Fraser CM, Potter P, Venter JC: Adrenergic receptors. In *Allergy: Principles and Practice.* Edited by Middleton E, Reed C, Ellis E, *et al.* St. Louis: CV Mosby; 1988:636–647.

66. Falliers CJ, Redding MA: Controlled comparison of a new antihistamine-decongestant combination to its individual components. *Ann Allergy* 1980, 45:75–80.

67. Baraniuk JN, Kaliner MA: Functional activity of upper airway nerves. In *Asthma and Rhinitis.* Edited by Busse W, Holgate S. Boston: Blackwell Scientific; 1994:652–666.

68. Spector S, Dockhorn W, Georgitis J, *et al.*: Intranasal anticholinergic treatment of nasal disorders. *J Allergy Clin Immunol* 1992, 90:1082–1086.

69. Bernstein RA, Nicklas R, Greenberger P, *et al.*: Practice parameter for allergen immunotherapy. *J Allergy Clin Immunol* 1996, 98:1001–1011.

70. Durham SR, Walker SM, Varga E, *et al.*: Long-term clinical efficacy of grass-pollen immunotherapy. *N Engl J Med* 1999, 341:468–475.

71. Van Metre TE, Atkinson NF: Immunotherapy for aeroallergen disease. In *Allergy: Principles and Practice* edn 4. Edited by Middleton E, Reed C, Ellis E, *et al.* St. Louis: CV Mosby; 1993:1489–1510.

72. Gleich JG, Zimmerman BS, Henderson LL, Yunginger JW: Effects of immunotherapy on immunoglobulin E and immunoglobulin G antibodies to ragweed antigens: a six-year prospective study. *J Allergy Clin Immunol* 1982, 70:261–271.

73. Iliopoulos O, Proud D, Adkinson NF Jr, *et al.*: Effects of immunotherapy on the early, late, and rechallenge nasal reaction to provocation with allergen: changes in inflammatory mediators and cells. *J Allergy Clin Immunol* 1991, 87:855–866.

74. Weber RW: Immunotherapy with allergens. *J Amer Med Assoc* 1997, 278:1881–1887.

75. Jacobsen L: Preventative allergy treatment. *Clin Exp Allergy* 1996, 26:80–85.

76. Johnstone DE: Study of the role of antigen dosage in the treatment of pollinosis and pollen asthma. *J Dis Child* 1957, 94:1.

77. Kelloway S, Wyatt RA, Adlis SA: Comparison of patients' compliance with prescribed oral and inhaled asthma medications. *Arch Intern Med* 1994, 154:1349–1352.

78. Donahue JG, Greineder DK, Connor-Lacke L, *et al.*: Utilization and cost of immunotherapy for allergic asthma and rhinitis. *Ann Allergy Asthma Immunol* 1999, 82:339–347.

79. Dykewicz MS, Fineman S: Diagnosis and management of rhinitis: parameter documents of the joint task force on practice parameters in allergy, asthma and immunology. *Ann Allergy Asthma Immunol* 1998, 81:463–518.

80. Kaliner MA: Allergy care in the next millennium: guidelines for the specialty. *J Allergy Clin Immunol* 1997, 99:729–734.

CHAPTER 6

Nonallergic Rhinitis

Russell A. Settipane
Guy A. Settipane

Nonallergic rhinitis represents a broad classification of nasal diseases that share the occurrence of nasal symptoms without an allergic etiology. As many as half the patients presenting to physicians with chronic nasal symptoms (obstruction/congestion, rhinorrhea, and hyperirritability) may have this disorder [1,2•]. Nasal symptoms may be indistinguishable from those in allergic rhinitis; therefore, negative testing for IgE sensitivity to relevant aeroallergens is necessary to confirm this diagnosis. Nonallergic rhinitis may be subclassified on the basis of various characteristics. These include immunologic/cytologic features [3••] (Table 6-1), etiology/systemic disease association (Table 6-2), and frequency of occurrence (Table 6-3). This chapter focuses on frequency of occurrence of chronic rhinitis conditions, excluding acute infectious etiologies, such as viral upper respiratory infections and acute bacterial sinusitis. The epidemiology of nonallergic rhinitis is discussed first, followed by a review of the clinical presentation, diagnosis, pathophysiology, and treatment of individual nonallergic rhinitis syndromes. Discussion focuses on common nonallergic rhinitis syndromes, and only briefly reviews uncommon or rare forms of rhinitis.

EPIDEMIOLOGY OF NONALLERGIC RHINITIS

The frequency of nonallergic rhinitis and the different syndromes that comprise this disorder are gradually becoming better defined (Table 6-4). Mullarkey et al. [2•] determined that 52% of 142 rhinitis patients seen in an allergy clinic could be classified as having nonallergic rhinitis. Togias [4] found that only 17% of 362 rhinitis patients at an academic allergy clinic had nonallergic rhinitis. Rough data from large population surveys indicate the prevalence of chronic sinusitis to be 14.7% [5], chronic rhinitis to be 20.4%, and hay fever to be 9.8% [6]. The European Community Respiratory Health Survey of 1412 subjects selected for participation based on a history suggesting allergic rhinitis reported a 25% frequency of nonallergic rhinitis [7]. Recently, a National Rhinitis Classification Task Force (NRCTF) surveyed 975 patients entering the allergist's office for an evaluation of chronic rhinitis [8]. Forty-three percent of patients were classified as having pure allergic rhinitis, 23% were classified as having pure nonallergic rhinitis, and 34% were classified as having mixed rhinitis (Fig. 6-1). In total, 57% of all patients presenting with chronic rhinitis were classified as having some component of nonallergic rhinitis, either pure or mixed. Further analysis revealed that 44% of patients with allergic rhinitis were also classified as having a component of nonallergic rhinitis. This study, like those that preceded it, may have have produced data skewed toward an overestimation of allergic rhinitis given that subjects were recruited from allergy practices. The true prevalence of nonallergic rhinitis may very well be higher than what this study suggests. This

TABLE 6-1. CLASSIFICATION OF NONALLERGIC RHINITIS BASED ON IMMUNOLOGIC AND NASAL CYTOLOGIC FEATURES

Perennial nonallergic rhinitis (inflammatory)
  Eosinophilic nasal disease (NARES, BENARS)
  Basophilic/metachromatic nasal disease
  Infectious
  Nasal polyps
  Atrophic rhinitis
  Immunologic nasal disease (primary (?): non-IgE–mediated or secondary to systemic immunologic disorders)
Noninflammatory, nonallergic rhinitis
  Metabolic (hormornal)
  Rhinitis medicamentosa
  Reflex-induced rhinitis (bright light and other physical modalities)
  Vasomotor rhinitis
  Rhinitis sicca
  Irritant rhinitis
  Cold air rhinitis
Structurally related rhinitis
  Septal deviation
  Neoplastic and nonneoplastic tumors
  Miscellaneous (choanal atresia/stenosis, trauma, foreign body, malformation, cleft palate, adenoid hypertrophy)

BENARS—blood eosinophilia nonallergic rhinitis syndrome; NARES—nonallergic rhinitis with eosinophils syndrome.
Adapted from *Zeiger* [3••].

TABLE 6-3. CLASSIFICATION OF NONALLERGIC RHINITIS

Common	Infrequent
Vasomotor	Aspirin sensitivity
Chronic sinusitis	Hypothyroidism
Structural (septum, turbinates, valve)	Atrophic
NARES/BENARS	Systemic immunologic disorders
Drug-induced	Cerebral spinal fluid rhinorrhea
Estrogen-related	Other structural disorders
Nasal polyps	Foreign body
Physical/chemical/irritant	Ciliary dyskinesia
	Nasal mastocytosis

BENARS—blood eosinophilia nonallergic rhinitis syndrome; NARES—nonallergic rhinitis with eosinophils syndrome.

TABLE 6-2. CLASSIFICATION OF CHRONIC NONALLERGIC RHINITIS BASED ON ETIOLOGY

Syndromes of suggested etiology
  Chronic infection
    Immunodeficiencies
    Ostiomeatal obstruction
  Metabolic condition
    Acromegaly
    Pregnancy
    Hypothyroidism
  Vasculitides/autoimmune
    Sjögrens syndrome
    Systemic lupus erythematosus
    Relapsing polychondritis
    Churg-Strauss syndrome
  Granulomatous diseases
    Sarcoidosis
    Wegener's granulomatosis
  Drug-induced
    Topical decongestants
    Systemic medications
  Nasal polyps
    Aspirin intolerance
    Chronic sinusitis
    Churg-Strauss syndrome
    Young's syndrome (sinopulmonary disease, azoospermia, nasal polyps)
    Cystic fibrosis
    Kartagener's syndrome (bronchiectasis, chronic sinusitis, nasal polyps)
  Structurally related rhinitis
    Septal deviation
    Turbinate deformation
    Nasal valve dysfunction
    Obstructive adenoid hyperplasia
    Trauma
    Congenital
    Neoplastic
  Atrophic rhinitis
    Excessive surgery
    Ozena
  Rhinitis induced by physical, chemical, or irritant triggers
    Dry air
    Gustatory
    Bright light
    Air pollution
    Occupational
Syndromes of unknown cause
  Vasomotor rhinitis
  Nonallergic rhinitis with eosinophilia (NARES, BENARS)
  Basophilic/metachromatic nasal disease

BENARS—blood eosinophilia nonallergic rhinitis syndrome; NARES—nonallergic rhinitis with eosinophils syndrome.

NRCTF data can be extrapolated to provide an estimate of the prevalence of nonallergic rhinitis in the United States. Assuming that 20% of the United States population has allergic rhinitis [9,10], and based on the above frequencies of rhinitis syndromes, there are an estimated 19 million patients with nonallergic rhinitis in the United States and an additional 26 million with mixed rhinitis.

We looked at the breakdown of nonallergic rhinitis in 78 patients, and found nonallergic rhinitis with eosinophilia syndrome (NARES) in 33% of patients, blood eosinophilia nonallergic rhinitis syndrome (BENARS) in 4%, vasomotor rhinitis in 61%, sinusitis in 16%, and hypothyroidism in 2% (Table 6-5) [11••]. Female sex and increasing age may be risk factors for the development of nonallergic rhinitis. The NRCTF study found that 71% of patients with nonallergic rhinitis were female compared to 55% in the allergic rhinitis group. Togias [4] observed that 70% of patients

diagnosed with nonallergic nasal disease developed their condition in adult life (age > 20 years), whereas approximately 70% of patients diagnosed with allergic rhinitis developed their condition in childhood (age < 20 years). However, a causal relationship between aging and nonallergic rhinitis has not been firmly established.

CLINICAL PRESENTATION, DIAGNOSIS, PATHOPHYSIOLOGY, AND TREATMENT OF INDIVIDUAL NONALLERGIC RHINITIS SYNDROMES

Vasomotor rhinitis

Vasomotor rhinitis refers to a poorly understood syndrome and is a diagnosis of exclusion. The term itself is misleading, because it implies that a cause relating to vascular/neurologic dysfunction has been identified when, in fact, the mechanism has yet to be established.

TABLE 6-4. FREQUENCY OF OCCURRENCE OF ALLERGIC AND NONALLERGIC RHINITIS

Investigator (year)	Number	Allergic (%)	Mixed (%)*	Nonallergic (%)
			Rhinitis type	
Mullarkey (1980)	142	48	Not studied	52
Togias (1990)	362	83	Not studied	17
ECRHS (1999)†	1142	75	Not studied	25
NRCTF (1999)‡	975	43	34	23

*Mixed counted as "allergic" for total analysis except NCRTF.
†European Community Respiratory Health Survey.
‡National Rhinitis Classification Task Force.

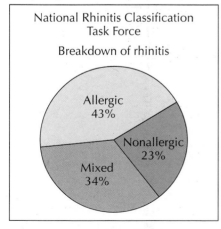

National Rhinitis Classification Task Force

Breakdown of rhinitis

Allergic 43%

Nonallergic 23%

Mixed 34%

FIGURE 6-1.
The National Rhinitis Classification Task Force breakdown of rhinitis: allergic, nonallergic, and mixed.

TABLE 6-5. DIAGNOSIS OF 78 PATIENTS WITH NONALLERGIC RHINITIS

Diagnosis	Patients, n	Patients considered, n	Percentage of patients, %
Vasomotor rhinitis	44	72	61
NARES	25	75	33
Sinusitis (radiographs)*	11	68	16
Possible allergy†	9	76	12
BENARS	3	76	4
Hypothyroidism	1	68	2

BENARS—blood eosinophilia nonallergic rhinitis syndrome;
  NARES—nonallergic rhinitis with eosinophilia syndrome.
* Overlapping of diagnosis present
† Elevated serum IgE levels
Adapted from Settipane et al. [11••].

Mygind [12••] has proposed that the term *vasomotor rhinitis* be replaced by the term *perennial nonallergic rhinitis*, used to describe any nonpurulent rhinitis of unknown cause, regardless of nasal cytology. However, we will use *vasomotor rhinitis* to designate idiopathic, perennial nonallergic rhinitis associated with a lack of identifiable inflammation on nasal cytology, negative allergy skin tests, and normal serum IgE levels.

The symptoms of vasomotor rhinitis tend to be obstructive/congestive rather than secretory/rhinorrhea; sneezing and nasal pruritus are uncommon. In a survey of 678 rhinitis patients [13], nasal blockage was the predominant symptom in the vasomotor rhinitis group, whereas the allergic rhinitis patients suffered from eye irritation, sneezing, and rhinorrhea. Concomitant asthma was more common in the allergic rhinitis group. Togias [4] also found a higher association of asthma with allergic rhinitis compared to those with nonallergic rhinitis. He found nonallergic rhinitis to be associated with fewer sneezes and conjunctival symptoms, but could not differentiate this disorder from perennial allergic rhinitis with regard to rhinorrhea or congestion.

In terms of pathophysiology, little is known except that nonspecific nasal hyperreactivity occurs on exposure to nonimmunologic stimuli, such as changes in temperature or relative humidity, alcohol ingestion, strong odors, and other airborne irritants. Hyperreactivity of the nasal mucosa to methacholine, capsaicin, and histamine has been demonstrated in the laboratory [14–16]. However, the cause of this hyperreactivity remains unexplained. Recent studies have shown an increased number of mast cells, but not goblet cells, in patients with perennial nonallergic rhinitis, whereas no significant difference was found between the number of mast cells in allergic and nonallergic patients [17,18].

Treatment of vasomotor rhinitis can either be nonspecific (directed at the total spectrum of symptoms associated with nonallergic rhinitis) or specific (directed at a single specific symptom). Nonspecific treatment may have an advantage because symptoms of vasomotor rhinitis may often be variable and alternating from obstructive/congestive to secretory/rhinorrhea. Examples of nonspecific treatment include the topical antihistamine azelastine and topical steroids. In clinical trials, azelastine nasal spray has been shown to be nondiscriminatory in regard to the types of nasal symptoms which respond to this topical treatment [19]. Symptoms of vasomotor rhinitis that have been demonstrated to improve in response to azelastine nasal spray include postnasal drip, rhinorrhea, sneezing, and congestion. These clinical trials have also shown a fairly high total response rate. Between 82% and 85% of over 200 subjects with vasomotor rhinitis responded favorably to azelastine nasal spray treatment. Evidence suggests that the mechanism of azelastine's effects may involve anti-inflammatory actions

[20–24]. These include azelastine's ability to reduce the effects of neurokinins like substance P and vasointestinal peptide, to prevent histamine release in vitro and in vivo, to diminish eosinophil activation and the expression of adhesion molecules, to suppress the synthesis of inflammatory cytokines and nitric oxide via an inhibitory effect on NF-κ B, and to reduce vascular permeability [20–23]. Azelastine appears to have the unique combination of anti-inflammatory effects and inhibition of histamine release, calcium transport, and the influx of inflammatory cells into the site of an allergic reaction. Azelastine is effective in vasomotor rhinitis possibly through a combination of all of these activities, especially those involving decreased production of cytokines.

Another form of topical anti-inflammatory treatment is nasal corticosteroids. Topical nasal steroids may also be of nonspecific benefit in vasomotor rhinitis. Because of their anti-inflammatory nature, it has been proposed that nasal steroids may have greater benefit when nasal mucosal inflammation is present. For example, the pharmacologic effects of fluticasone nasal spray in nonallergic rhinitis has been studied. Unilaterally administered fluticasone nasal spray has been shown to have a beneficial effect on nasal inflammatory cells and cytokine profile in both allergic and nonallergic rhinitis patients [25]. The number of CD3, major basin protein (MBP), and tryptase-positive cells were significantly less in both sides of the allergic and nonallergic treated patients, as compared to controls, and interleukin (IL)-4, IL-5 mRNA were downregulated on the treated side. A 2- to 4-week trial of nasal steroid spray therapy is usually worthwhile in that some patients may respond [26,27,28•,29]. Budesonide aerosol preparation, beclomethasone aqueous preparation, and fluticasone aqueous preparation are the only topical corticosteroids that have a Food and Drug Administration indication for the treatment of nonallergic rhinitis.

Although there are no direct comparison studies between azelastine and topical nasal steroids in perennial nonallergic (vasomotor) rhinitis, there is information suggesting that azelastine nasal spray has a more rapid onset of action than intranasal corticosteroids. In dose-ranging trials, azelastine nasal spray resulted in a decrease in symptoms that reached statistical significance within 2 to 3 hours after initial dosing compared to a saline placebo [30,31]. By contrast, a decrease in allergic rhinitis symptoms following fluticasone or budesonide may be seen in 7 to 12 hours [32].

These data suggest that azelastine nasal spray has two significant clinical advantages: it provides rapid onset of action and it does not need to be used for several days to achieve maximum benefit. Azelastine nasal spay is effective on the first day as well as with continual therapy; therefore, daily compliance is not essential for azelastine to be effective.

As mentioned previously, treatment of nonallergic rhinitis may also be specifically tailored to the patient's symptoms. Those patients primarily with obstruction/congestion may be treated with decongestants, as needed, as first-line agents. These agents may be administered topically on a short-term basis, but for long-term use, they should be administered systemically because of the problem of rebound associated with long-term treatment. Those patients with predominantly secretory/rhinorrhea symptoms are best treated with the anticholinergic agent ipatropium bromide nasal spray [33]. This is an effective agent because it is the parasympathetic (cholinergic) nervous system which controls nasal mucosal secretion. Ipatropium bromide is well tolerated because there is little systemic absorption and, therefore, no demonstrable systemic side effects [34•]. Minor infrequent episodes of nasal dryness and epistaxis are the only significant adverse effects reported. Alternatively, classic antihistamines may be used for their drying effect on the nasal mucosa resulting from their parasympathetic activity; however, classic antihistamines may be limited in their usefulness because of frequently associated sedation and tachyphylaxis.

Cost of treatment and clinical implications suggest that oral second generation antihistamines may not be the best approach to the treatment of rhinitis, particularly when a definitive diagnosis has not been established. Oral second generation antihistamines are not indicated for and would not be expected to be effective in nonallergic rhinitis and therefore could be expected to be only partially or intermittently effective in mixed rhinitis. Second-generation oral antihistamines, having essentially no anticholinergic effects, would be even less likely to be effective than first-generation antihistamines.

Another form of therapy from which benefit is sometimes derived for vasomotor rhinitis is topical saline in the form of a spray or irrigation device. Nasal saline may result in reduction of postnasal drip, sneezing, and congestion [34•]. In some cases, using the above therapies in various combinations may produce additive effectiveness.

Experimental treatments for vasomotor rhinitis include topical use of capsaicin intranasally [15]. This is a pungent substance derived from pepper that acts to desensitize sensory neural fibers in the nose, thereby reducing nasal hyperreactivity. Beneficial effects are delayed in onset, with 63% and 69% reduction of nasal blockage and nasal discharge, respectively, after 1 month of therapy. Topical application of 15% to 20% silver nitrate has also been suggested to be effective [35,36]. Surgical approaches to therapy include endoscopic vidian nerve section or electrocoagulation of the anterior ethmoidal nerve [37,38]. In both cases, the parasympathetic supply to the nasal mucosa is divided, resulting in reduced nasal secretions. Although there may be recurrence of symptoms secondary to reinnervation, recent studies report long-term benefits [39]. Sphenopalatine ganglion block has also been reported to relieve symptoms of vasomotor rhinitis; however, the number of blocks required for complete relief ranged from two to four [40]. In cases where congestion is the predominant symptom, turbinectomy is another treatment option. A variety of surgical procedures can be performed for the treatment of hypertrophic inferior turbinates. With radical turbinectomy, there is some concern regarding the extent to which the nasal mucosa returns to a healed and normal functioning state. However, laser turbinectomy has been reported to result in preservation of normal nasal cytology and saccharin time [41].

Chronic sinusitis

Chronic rhinitis symptoms may be associated with or result from chronic infection or inflammation of the paranasal sinuses. The frequency of chronic sinusitis may have been underestimated initially [42]. In 1993, the U.S. National Health Interview Survey placed chronic sinusitis first in rank among the most common chronic diseases, with a prevalence of 14.7% [5].

Chronic sinusitis in adults has recently been defined as a disease of 8 weeks or more of persistent symptoms and signs, or four episodes per year of recurrent acute sinusitis, each lasting for at least 10 days, in association with persistent changes in computed tomography (CT) [43•]. A CT scan of the sinuses should be done 4 weeks after medical therapy without intervening acute infection. In children, the respective figures are 12 weeks of symptoms or more than 6 episodes of sinusitis per year. The symptoms and signs are nasal congestion, discharge, headache, facial pain or pressure, and olfactory disturbance, with fever and halitosis as minor symptoms, and cough and irritability as possible symptoms in children only.

The etiology of chronic sinusitis involves an infectious origin, but the extent to which chronic infection is important in the perpetuation of the disease is unclear. Anaerobes are usually the predominant bacteria in chronic sinusitis, but it is not clear if they are present because of dysfunctional sinus clearance or if they are the primary cause of the condition [44]. It is important to note that bacteria found in culture of the nasal secretions are not representative of those found within the infected sinus cavity. The frequent failure of prolonged and intensive antimicrobial therapy suggests that bacterial infection is not the cause for the persistence of chronic sinusitis. It is more likely that chronic sinusitis represents chronic mucosal inflammation, which is likely to be multifactorial in cause.

The inflammatory nature of chronic sinusitis has been well documented. In the sinus fluid of chronic sinusitis patients undergoing surgery, inflammatory cells are mainly neutrophils, as normally observed in acute sinusitis, but a low percentage of eosinophils, mast cells, and basophils may also be observed [45,46]. High concentrations of histamine, leukotrienes (LT) C_4, D_4, and E_4, and prostaglandin D_2 were found, suggesting mast cell/basophil activation in chronically inflamed sinuses.

The diagnosis of chronic sinusitis in a nonallergic population necessitates a work-up for an underlying cause, as listed in Table 6-6. With proper diagnosis and treatment of the underlying disorder, chronic sinusitis is

optimally controlled. One example is osteomeatal complex obstruction, which when identified and treated first medically and, if unsuccessful, by endoscopic surgery, may successfully reverse chronic sinusitis, at least temporarily. Another example is antibody deficiency syndromes that respond well to intravenous replacement therapy.

There are, however, patients with chronic sinusitis in whom no underlying disorder can be identified. In many of these patients, an underlying inflammatory process is often present and can contribute to inadequate sinus ventilation and drainage. These patients present a therapeutic dilemma because they often respond poorly to therapy. Few data exist on the efficacy of treatment for chronic sinusitis. Intuitively, maintenance of sinus ostial patency is important for proper drainage of retained secretions; therefore, treatment should include a long-term trial of a topical steroid nasal spray in an attempt to reduce tissue inflammation and edema in the region of the osteomeatal complex. Additional therapeutic modalities that may be beneficial include guaifenesin, decongestants, steam inhalation, saline spray or irrigation and,

TABLE 6-6. CONDITIONS THAT MAY UNDERLIE CHRONIC SINUSITIS

Anatomical
Rhinitis
Nasal polyps
Ciliary dyskinesias: Kartagener's syndrome
Cystic fibrosis
Granulomatous disease
Neoplasm
Immunodeficiency

TABLE 6-7. ANTIHYPERTENSIVE DRUGS CAUSING RHINITIS

Trade name	Generic	Symptoms
Aldomet Ester HCL injection*	Methyldopate hydrochloride	Nasal stuffiness
Aldomet oral suspension*	Methyldopa, MSD	Nasal stuffiness
Aldomet tablets*	Methyldopa, MSD	Nasal stuffiness
Apresoline hydrochloride†	Hydralazine hydrochloride USP	Nasal congestion, dyspnea
Apresoline hydrochloride parenteral†	Hydralazine hydrochloride parenteral	Nasal congestion, dyspnea
Cardura‡	Doxazosin	Nasal congestion
Catapres§	Clonidine hydrochloride USP	Dryness of nasal mucosa
Corgard¶	Nadolol, β-blocker	Nasal stuffiness, bronchospasm, cough
Hytrin**	Terazosin	Nasal congestion
Ismelin†	Guanethidine monosulfate	Dyspnea, asthma in susceptible individuals, nasal congestion
Minipress‡	Prazosin hydrochloride	Nasal congestion, dyspnea
Minizide‡	Prazosin hydrochloride, polythiazide	Nasal congestion, dyspnea
Moduretic*	Amiloride HCL-hydrochlorothiazide	1% nasal congestion, 1% dryness
Normodyne††	Brand of labetalol hydrochloride	Nasal stuffiness, wheezing in 1
Trandate‡‡	Labetalol hydrochloride, α- and β-blocker	Nasal stuffiness, dyspnea, bronchospasm
Wytensin§§	Guanabenz acetate	Nasal stuffiness, dyspnea
N/A	Reserpine	Nasal congestion, dyspnea

*Merck and Co, West Point, PA
† Novartis Pharmaceuticals, East Hanover, NJ
‡ Pfizer Inc, New York, NY
§ Boehringer Ingelheim Pharmaceuticals, Ridgefield, CT
¶ Bristol-Myers Squibb, Princeton, NJ
**Abbott Laboratories, Abbott Park, IL
†† Schering, Kenilworth, NJ
‡‡ Glaxo-Wellcome, Research Triangle Park, NC
§§ Wyeth-Ayerst Laboratories, Philadelphia, PA
Adapted from Settipane [58].

for acute flares, intermittent 3-week courses of antibiotics, sometimes combined with systemic glucocorticoids. However, not until a more complete understanding of the pathomechanisms of inflammation in chronic sinusitis is achieved will treatment be more successful.

Anatomical nasal obstruction

Common anatomical causes of nasal obstruction include deviated septum, enlarged turbinates, dysfunctional nasal valve and, in children, adenoid hypertrophy. Anatomical abnormalities account for approximately 5% to 10% of chronic nasal disorders. Obstruction due to tumor is less common and is reviewed under a separate heading. Nasal septal deviation is fairly common, but usually is mild and well tolerated. In cases where the degree of deviation is moderate to severe, particularly when there is concomitant nasal mucosal edema secondary to an underlying rhinitis, symptoms of blockage result and may be complicated by sinusitis, snoring, sleep apnea, and fatigue. Enlarged turbinates and nasal valve disease also are aggravated by concomitant rhinitis. Therefore, whenever there is any question as to the extent of anatomical cause—and before embarking on a surgical procedure to reduce the bulk of turbinates, straighten the septum, or correct a dysfunctional nasal valve—work-up and treatment of associated rhinitis should be pursued. See Table 6-2 for more comprehensive list including less common anatomical causes of rhinitis.

Nonallergic rhinitis with eosinophilia syndrome

Jacobs et al. [47•] presented a series of 52 patients with perennial symptoms of sneezing paroxysms, profuse watery rhinorrhea, and nasal pruritus. Nasal smears showed marked eosinophilia, but allergic disease could not be identified by skin testing or by radioallergosorbent test (RAST). This condition may represent approximately 15% to 33% of adults with nonallergic rhinitis [2•,11••]. This type of nonallergic rhinitis usually occurs as an isolated disorder; however, nonallergic rhinitis with eosinophilia (NARES) may be associated with non-IgE–mediated asthma, aspirin intolerance, and nasal polyps. Blood eosinophilia nonallergic rhinitis syndrome (BENARS) appears to be a subtype of NARES [11••]. BENARS has characteristics similar to NARES, but also includes elevated blood eosinophils (average, 957/mm^3 in three patients). In a study of 78 consecutive patients with nonallergic rhinitis (Table 6-5), NARES was found in 33% and BENARS in 4%. Rare, nonallergic disorders associated with nasal eosinophilia include phaeohyphomycosis of the maxilloethmoid sinus [48] and Churg-Strauss syndrome [49].

Patients with NARES tend to have more intense nasal symptoms than patients with either vasomotor rhinitis or allergic rhinitis [50]. In addition, the presence of anosmia is quite common. The pathology of NARES is marked by eosinophils on nasal cytology, which may range from mild to massive infiltration and is frequently associated with basophilic/metachromatic cell infiltration [3••]. The pathophysiology of NARES is not understood. Eosinophilia may contribute to nasal mucosal dysfunction as a result of toxic substances associated with eosinophils, such as major basic protein and other eosinophil granule-derived proteins. These toxic proteins may damage nasal ciliated epithelium and cause delay in mucociliary clearance [51–56]. In 1992, we reported on 56 nonallergic rhinitis patients and found a significant correlation of nasal eosinophilia with prolonged nasal circulation time (saccharine time) [57]. This delay inhibits mucous flow rate and consequently may be a mechanism resulting in increased propensity toward infection. Recurrent infections are thought to be one cause of nasal polyps. Nasal polyps frequently are associated with nasal eosinophils. Therefore, there is some concern that nasal eosinophilia may be a precursor for nasal polyps or aspirin intolerance syndrome [50]. In cases where aspirin intolerance exists, the aspirin reaction is not the cause of the eosinophilic rhinosinusitis but rather a marker of a severe form of this condition, which is often associated with asthma, sinusitis, and nasal polyps. The presence of nasal eosinophilia in patients with nonallergic rhinitis generally is regarded as a good prognostic indicator for response to treatment with topical steroid therapy. In cases where the eosinophilic infiltration is massive, as is often the case in the aspirin sensitivity syndrome, intermittent-to-frequent use of oral glucocorticoids may be required to control symptomology.

Drug-induced rhinitis

Drugs listed in Tables 6-7 and 6-8 can induce rhinitis in allergic and nonallergic individuals. The term rhinitis medicamentosa is most commonly used to describe the rebound nasal congestion that occurs with overuse of topical decongestants/vasoconstrictor nasal preparations (oxymetazoline, phenylephrine), as well as from abuse of cocaine. Usually, an underlying form of rhinitis has led to this form of self-treatment. Classically, the nasal mucosa is erythematous, congested, granular, with areas of punctate bleeding due to tissue friability. Recent research supports the theory that the rebound swelling is due to interstitial edema rather than to vasodilation [59]. Every patient presenting with the complaint of nasal congestion should be questioned carefully as to the extent of use of decongestant nose sprays and cocaine, especially if the nasal mucosa is erythematous on examination. Treatment of rhinitis medicamentosa requires withdrawal from the topical decongestant as well as treatment of the underlying rhinitis disorder. This is often best accomplished with the use of topical or systemic glucocorticoids, providing there is some component of inflammatory rhinitis present. Many times, patients can be initiated on a topical steroid spray bilaterally and instructed to discontinue the decongestant spray immediately in one nostril and 1 week later in the remaining nostril. If this is ineffective, a 1-week tapering course of oral glucocorticoid, with discontinuation of the decongestant spray on day 2 or 3, usually is effective. Thereafter, the patient should be followed for recurrence and worked up for an underlying cause.

Effect of pregnancy on nonallergic rhinitis

Pregnancy, oral contraceptives, and other estrogens can contribute to rhinitis symptoms. However, the rhinitis that occurs during most pregnancies often has been present before the onset of the pregnancy and often is found to be secondary to common causes unrelated to the pregnancy [60••]. Therefore, the exact extent to which pregnancy is a causal factor is unknown; it may be more of an aggravating factor. During pregnancy, physiologic changes may contribute to increased nasal congestion/obstruction. Among these changes are a massive expansion of circulating blood volume, contributing to an increase in nasal vascular pooling and possible progesterone-induced vascular smooth muscle relaxation. Additionally, pregnancy-associated hormones may have a direct effect on the nasal mucosa, resulting in increased nasal secretion/rhinorrhea secondary to increased nasal mucous gland hyperactivity [61]. Additionally, episodes of bacterial rhinosinusitis have been noted to be more common during pregnancy [62]. A complete discussion of the treatment of rhinitis during pregnancy is beyond the scope of this chapter and is reviewed elsewhere [63••]. It is sufficient to note that the main issue in rhinitis during pregnancy is caution with medication. First-line treatment should include a reliance on the safest forms of treatment, such as steam inhalation, nasal saline sprays, and an avoidance of irritants. Regarding medication, topical medical therapy is preferred to systemic therapy.

Nasal polyps

Nasal polyps occur in approximately 1% of the general population and are not any more frequent in patients with allergic rhinitis [64]. Nasal polyps are associated frequently with aspirin intolerance and the aspirin tetrad syndrome (aspirin intolerance, nasal polyps, sinusitis, and asthma), intrinsic asthma, chronic sinusitis, Young's syndrome, cystic fibrosis, Kartagener's syndrome, Churg-Strauss syndrome, and allergic fungal sinusitis (Table 6-9). Children 16 years or younger with nasal polyps should be evaluated for cystic fibrosis. Nasal polyps are frequently bilateral, multiple, freely movable, pale gray, and arise from the middle meatus of the nose. Polyps in the paranasal sinuses can lead to bone erosion of the sinus walls (Woakes syndrome) [66]. Histologically, they have pseudostratified ciliated columnar epithelium, thickening of the epithelial basement membrane, high stromal eosinophil count, mucin with neutral pH, few glands, and essentially no nerve endings [67]. Cells usually consist of a mixture of lymphocytes, plasma cells, and eosinophils. The majority of nasal polyps are associated with an eosinophilic inflammatory mechanism. However, in polyps from cystic fibrosis patients, neutrophils predominate with insignificant eosinophils [68]. Chemical mediators found in nasal polyps include histamine; serotonin; LTB_4, LTC_4, LTD_4, and LTE_4; IL-5; norepinephrine; kinins; toluene-sulfo-trypsin arginine methyl ester (TAME)-esterase; and possibly prostaglandin D_2 [69,70•]. There is more histamine in nasal polyps than in normal nasal mucosa, and norepinephrine is present in greater concentration in the base of nasal polyps than in

---

TABLE 6-8. ANTIHYPERTENSIVE DRUGS WITH DIURETICS CAUSING RHINITIS

Trade name	Generic	Symptoms
Aldoclor*	Combination of methyldopa and chlorothiazine	Nasal stuffiness
Aldoril*	Methyldopa-hydrochlorothiazide, MSD	Nasal stuffiness
Combipres‡	Clonidine hydrochloride chlorthalidone	Dryness of nasal mucosa
Diutensen-R§	Methylclothiazide and reserpine	Frequent nasal congestion, dyspnea
Enduronyl forte¶	Methylclothiazide and deserpidine	Asthma in asthmatic patients, nasal congestion, dyspnea
Enduronyl tablets¶	Methylclothiazide and deserpidine	Asthma in asthmatic patients, nasal congestion, dyspnea
Rauzide tablets**	Rauwolfia serpentina with bendroflumethazide	Nasal congestion, dyspnea

*Merck and Co, West Point, PA
† Novartis Pharmaceuticals, East Hanover, NJ
‡ Boehringer Ingelheim Pharmaceuticals, Ridgefield, CT
§ Wallace Laboratories, Cranbury, NJ
¶ Abbott Laboratories, Abbott Park, IL
** Bristol-Myers Squibb, Princeton, NJ
Adapted from Settipane [58].

normal nasal mucosa [71]. The concentrations of IgA and IgE and, in some cases, IgG and IgM, are greater in polyp fluid than in serum [72]. At the present time, the pathogenesis of polyp formation is unknown. IgE-mediated disease is not the cause of nasal polyps. In fact, nasal polyps may be associated with a loss of susceptibility to potential additional effects of inhaled allergens [73]. Upper respiratory infections may contribute to the exacerbation of nasal polyps. Despite medical or surgical management, a significant number of nasal polyps are recurrent. Regarding medical therapy, topical corticosteroids alone can frequently control symptoms [74••]. If topical therapy is not effective, systemic corticosteroids should be tried before surgical polypectomy. We routinely use doses of prednisone starting at 60 mg and tapering by 5 mg daily over a 12-day course. Beclomethasone has been approved by the FDA for the prevention of nasal polyp recurrence following surgical removal. Polypectomy does not increase the risk of developing asthma or making asthma worse [75].

Rhinitis induced by physical, chemical, and irritant triggers

Physical triggers of rhinitis symptoms include cold and dry air, ingestion of hot or spicy food, and exposure to bright light. These triggers occur commonly and are most often markers of increased nasal hyperreactivity due to an underlying nasal disorder. However, patients without an underlying disorder, particularly those that work outdoors in cold environments, occasionally present with the chief complaint of excessive nasal symptomatology in response to the above-mentioned stimuli. Some insight into the pathophysiology of this disorder has been gained by experimentally reproducing these conditions in the laboratory. Studies with cold, dry air have demonstrated that both mast cell degranulation and an increased neuronal reflex mechanism are involved [76,77]. The underlying defect appears to be an inability of the nasal mucosa to humidify inhaled air at extreme atmospheric conditions, resulting in an increased osmolality of nasal secretions, which result in nasal epithelial desiccation and detachment and lead to subsequent mast cell degranulation and activation of irritant sensory nerves. Studies with spicy food ingestion have suggested that the pathophysiology involves a purely neurogenic reflex mechanism with the efferent pathway being parasympathetic nerve filters [78•]. This condition is called gustatory rhinitis. Why some patients may have a more responsive reflex mechanism is unknown. Effective treatment for both these conditions is prophylaxis with topical ipratropium bromide prior to cold air exposure or spicy food ingestion.

An increasing array of indoor and outdoor air pollutants are recognized as effecting the nose. Among these are dust, ozone, sulfur dioxide, formaldehyde, volatile organic compounds, wood smoke, and environmental tobacco smoke [79]. The frequency with which these exposures contribute to the development of acute or chronic rhinitis syndromes is unknown, nor has the associated rhinitis been well characterized. Most of these triggers are nasal irritants that cause dryness and reduced nasal airflow, rhinorrhea, and sneezing [79]. Chronic exposure to cigarette smoke results in decreased cilia beat frequency, ineffective movement, and frank deciliation in experimental models [80]. Ciliostasis has been demonstrated in wood workers exposed to wood dust [81]. Neutrophil influx has been shown to occur with ozone exposure and exposure to volatile organic compounds [79,82]. Chronic exposure to formaldehyde vapors may result in nasal histologic abnormalities [83]. Prolonged occupational exposure to nickel, leather or wood dust, chronic formaldehyde, and chlorophenol have been associated with hypertrophic rhinitis, metaplasia, and frank carcinoma [3••].

Occupational rhinitis is defined as the episodic, work-related occurrence of sneezing, rhinorrhea, and nasal obstruction [84•]. Occupational rhinitis can be classified by one of the following reaction types: annoyance, irritant, immunologic, or corrosive (Table 6-10) [85]. Nonallergic rhinitis in the workplace needs to be distinguished from allergic rhinitis secondary to exposure to workplace aeroallergens and from nonoccupational allergic rhinitis aggravated by workplace exposures. The greater the number of symptomatic workers, the more likely it is that the offending agent is nonimmunogenic [87]. Symptoms due to annoyance reactions typically

TABLE 6-9. FREQUENCY OF NASAL POLYPS IN VARIOUS DISEASES

Diagnosis	Frequency, %
Aspirin intolerance	36
Adult asthma	7
Intrinsic asthma	13
Atopic asthma	5
Chronic rhinosinusitis	2
Nonallergic rhinitis	5
Allergic rhinitis	1.5
Childhood asthma/rhinitis	0.1
Cystic fibrosis	20
Churg-Strauss syndrome (asthma, fever, eosinophilia vasculitis, and granuloma)	50
Allergic fungal sinusitis	85
Kartagener's syndrome (bronchiectasis, sinusitis, situs inversus)	?
Young's syndrome (sinopulmonary disease, azoospermia)	?

Adapted from *Settipane [65]*.

TABLE 6-10. OCCUPATIONAL RHINITIS: CAUSATIVE AGENTS IN THE WORKPLACE	
Agent	**Occupational environment**
Annoyance rhinitis	
Perfumes	Beauty salons, department stores
Cooking odors	Restaurants, food manufacturers
Exhaust fumes	Garages, public transportation industry
Detergents	Supermarkets
Cleaning agents	Supermarkets
Room deodorizers	
Flower fragrances	Florist shops, gardening industry
Clothing fragrances	Clothing stores
Cosmetic odors	Cosmetic factories, stores
Tobacco smoke on clothing	
Irritation rhinitis	
Tobacco smoke	
Pollution	
Oxides of nitrogen	Chemical industry
Paint fumes	
Garden sprays	
Toluene, xylene	Petroleum, chemical, paint industries
Capsaicin	Food industry
Formaldehyde	Chemical industry
Sulfur dioxide	
Ozone	
Immunologic rhinitis	
Animal proteins	Animal laboratories, pet stores
Wheat	Food-processing plants
Green tea	
Pyrethrum	Insecticide, gardening industries
Cotton fibers	Cotton mills
Reactive dyes	
Toluene diisocyanate	Auto body spray painting
Bacillus subtilis	Detergent factories
Trypsin	
Papain	Meat-processing plants
Latex	Health care industry
Platinum salts	
Colophony	Metal, electronics industries
Acid anhydrides	Adhesive industry
Plicatic acid	Cedar sawmills
Corrosive rhinitis	
Ammonia	Tanneries; dye, bronzing industries
Chloride	Pulp, paper industry; swimming pool maintenance
Hydrochloric acid	Bleach, battery manufacturing
Vinyl chloride	
Organophosphide compounds	Pesticide industry
Acrylamide	Resins, plastics manufacturing
Cyanide, nitriles	Steel, plastics, herbicide industries
Organic sulfur-containing compounds	

Adapted from *Bardana* [85] and *Chan-Yeung and Lam* [86].

result from exposure to strong odors in patients with heightened olfactory awareness. Symptoms due to irritant reactions result from exposure to one or more known respiratory irritants at levels exceeding threshold limits. Symptoms due to corrosive reactions result from exposure to high concentrations of irritating and soluble chemical gases, causing significant nasal inflammation, often manifesting as mucosal burns, frank ulceration, and at times associated inflammation of the skin, mouth, and eyes. Environmental control is the mainstay of therapy, and is achieved by removing the causal agent, improving ventilation, wearing protective masks, or changing job duties or work site. Recommended medical therapy includes nasal saline lavage to remove accumulated particulate.

Infrequent causes of rhinitis symptoms

The remaining nonallergic rhinitis syndromes occur rarely and warrant only brief discussion. Atrophic rhinitis in industrialized countries is usually only seen as a rare complication of radical nasal tissue removal by surgery aimed to relieve obstruction [88•,89]. In undeveloped countries, symptoms of epistaxis, severe crusting, and stuffiness are associated with a foul or fetid odor and *Klebsiella* colonization. Presumably, greater use of antibiotics has reduced the occurrence of this syndrome in developed countries. Atrophic rhinitis is resistant to treatment. The standard modality is antibiotic treatment of bacterial overgrowth and aggressive nasal saline irrigations. One suggested form of saline therapy is the use of a dental Waterpik (Water Pik Technologies, Inc., Fort Collins, CO) device with the attachment of a nasal irrigator nozzle. An alternative form of therapy is the implantation of bone chips, which reportedly reduces the symptom of nasal stuffiness.

Basophilic/metachromatic cell nasal disease or nasal mastocytosis is a subcategory of nonallergic rhinitis that, like NARES, is a histologic diagnosis [90•, 91]. Mast-cell infiltration (frequently > 2000/mm^3) without nasal eosinophilia is the hallmark of this syndrome. Nasal symptoms are secretion/rhinorrhea and congestion/blockage without significant sneezing/pruritus. Physical examination reveals an especially pale mucous. Unlike NARES, patients with this condition do not develop aspirin sensitivity, nasal polyps, asthma, or sinusitis. The cause of this condition is unknown. Because it is an inflammatory condition, treatment with topical anti-inflammatories should be tried; some patients benefit from intranasal cromolyn or intranasal corticosteroids, whereas others may require oral corticosteroids.

We have already discussed common structural causes of rhinitis symptoms, but rare causes of obstruction/congestion also deserve mention. The differential diagnosis includes tumors and neoplasms, such as chordoma, chemodectoma, neurofibroma, angiofibroma, inverting papilloma, squamous cell carcinoma, sarcoma, and encephaloceles or meningocele.

A rare cause of rhinorrhea is cerebral spinal fluid (CSF) leak, most commonly occurring as a result of trauma, but also occurring either spontaneously, or as a complication of surgery [92•]. Although traumatic CSF leaks usually present within 48 hours of trauma, delayed onset can be seen. However, 95% of cases present within 3 months. Because CSF contains sugar and nasal mucus does not, testing for the presence of glucose is helpful in making the diagnosis. Quantitative glucose measurements accurately identify the fluid as CSF if it contains > 30 mg/100 mL glucose. A more specific test for CSF rhinorrhea is β2 transferrin, which has come into common use in recent years [93]. In addition, thin coronal CT, radionuclide cisternography, and magnetic resonance cisternography can help to localize the site of CSF leakage [94].

Foreign bodies in the nose may present as unilateral nasal blockage and purulent nasal discharge. This may be seen not only in children with objects such as pebbles, erasers, buttons, peas, and beans, but also in hospitalized adults with nasal tubes in place.

Systemic autoimmune/vasculitis diseases, such as Churg-Strauss vasculitis, systemic lupus erythematosus, relapsing polychondritis, and Sjögrens syndrome, can also result in rhinitis [49,95–97]. Granulomatous diseases such as sarcoidosis and, more commonly, Wegner's, can produce nasal manifestations in a large proportion of affected patients [98,99].

Rhinitis sicca can result from Sjögrens syndrome. It also may occur as a normal part of aging. Treatment with the liberal use of nasal saline sprays is appropriate.

CONCLUSIONS

Nonallergic rhinitis is a common disease entity that occurs in about 45 million Americans. These patients have negative allergy skin tests and normal serum IgE. Symptoms are similar to allergic rhinitis but usually are not associated with sneezing episodes and conjunctival complaints. Nonallergic rhinitis is more frequently found in adults (> 20 years of age) than in children. Common types of nonallergic rhinitis include vasomotor, chronic sinusitis, NARES/BENARS, drug-induced, pregnancy, nasal polyps, and physical/chemical/irritant triggers. Infrequent causes include hypothyroidism, acromegaly, systemic immunologic disorders, atrophic mucosa, CSF rhinorrhea, ciliary dyskinesia, and nasal mastocytosis. The most common subtype of nonallergic rhinitis, vasomotor rhinitis, represents almost two thirds of all cases of nonallergic rhinitis. The pathophysiology of vasomotor rhinitis appears to involve proinflammatory chemical mediators in some cases. Treatment should be based on a differential diagnosis that includes skin testing for allergens. When skin testing cannot be obtained, vasomotor rhinitis is often treated empirically with oral antihistamines; however, this tradition is not supported by current clinical data.

Oral antihistamines have not been shown to be effective for nonallergic rhinitis and would be expected to be only partially or intermittently effective for mixed rhinitis. If empirical treatment is chosen, treatment options should be limited to those agents demonstrated to be effective in both allergic and nonallergic disease, either azelastine nasal spray or intranasal corticosteroids. Topical medications are preferred to systemic medications for long-term control of symptoms, and treatment should address all symptoms whether allergic or nonallergic. Alternatively, treatment of nonallergic rhinitis could be targeted to a specific symptom such as decongestants for congestion and anticholinergic agents for rhinorrhea. Nasal saline washing is sometimes worthwhile. The frequency of these causes ranges from vasomotor rhinitis (61%) to hypothyroidism (2%). Treatment of nonallergic rhinitis should be individualized according to patient symptoms and should include antihistamines, decongestants, anticholinergic agents, a trial of nasal steroids, and nasal lavage (saline washing). Experimental medical treatment includes capsaicin and silver nitrate applications. Experimental surgical treatment includes vidian nerve section, electrocoagulation of anterior ethmoidal nerve, sphenopalatine ganglion block, and turbinectomy.

REFERENCES AND RECOMMENDED READING

Recently published papers of particular interest have been highlighted as:
•   Of interest
•• Of outstanding interest

1. Dykewicz MS, Fineman S: Diagnosis and management of rhinitis: complete guidelines of the joint task force on practice parameters in allergy, asthma, and immunology. *Ann Allergy Asthma Immunol* 1998, 81(5):478–518.

2.• Mullarkey MF, Hill JS, Webb DR: Allergic and nonallergic rhinitis: their characterization with attention to the meaning of nasal eosinophilia. *J Allergy Clin Immunol* 1980, 65:122–126.
This is one of the few studies to provide data on the prevalence of nonallergic rhinitis.

3.•• Zeiger RS: Differential diagnosis and classification of rhinosinusitis. In *Nasal Manifestations of Systemic Diseases*. Edited by Schatz M, Zeiger RS, Settipane GA. Providence, RI: OceanSide Publications; 1991:3–20.
This paper provides an excellent review of rhinitis secondary to underlying systemic disease.

4. Togias A: Age relationships and clinical features of nonallergic rhinitis. *J Allergy Clin Immunol* 1990, 85:182.

5. Benson V, Marono MA: Current estimates from the National Health Interview Survey, 1993, National Center for Health Statistics. *Vital Health Stat* 1993, 10:182.

6. Turkeltaub PC, Gergen PJ: The prevalence of allergic and nonallergic respiratory symptoms in the US population: data from the second national health and nutrition examination survey 1976–1980 (NHANES II). *J Allergy Clin Immunol* 1988, 81:305.

7. Leynaert B, Bousquet J, Neukirch C, *et al.*: Perennial rhinitis: an independent risk factor for asthma in nonatopic subjects. Results from the European Community Respiratory Health Survey. *J Allergy Clin Immunol* 1999, 104:301–304.

8. Data presented at the National Allergy Advisory Council Meeting (NRCTF): The broad spectrum of rhinitis: etiology, diagnosis, and advances in treatment. St. Thomas, U.S. Virgin Islands, October 16, 1999.

9. Hagy GW, Settipane GA: Prognosis of positive allergy skin tests in an asymptomatic population. *J Allergy* 1971, 48:200–211.

10. Nathan RA, Meltzer EO, Selner JC, *et al.*: Prevalence of allergic rhinitis in the United States. *J Allergy Clin Immunol* 1997, 99:808–814.

11.•• Settipane GA, Klein DE: Nonallergic rhinitis: dermography of eosinophils in nasal smear, blood total eosinophil counts and IgE levels. *NER Allergy Proc* 1985, 6:363–366.
This article provides insight into the prevalence of various nonallergic rhinitis subtypes.

12.•• Mygind N: Definition, classification, terminology. In *Allergic and Nonallergic Rhinitis: Clinical Aspects.* Copenhagen: Munksgaard; 1993:11–14.
Definition, classification, and terminology for nonallergic rhinitis is proposed in this paper.

13. Lindberg S, Malm L: Comparison of allergic rhinitis and vasomotor rhinitis patients on the basis of a computer questionnaire. *Allergy* 1993, 48:602–607.

14. Borum P: Nasal methacholine challenge. *J Allergy Clin Immunol* 1979, 63:253–257.

15. Stjärne P, Lundblad L, Änggard A, *et al.*: Local capsaicin treatment of the nasal mucosa reduces symptoms in patients with nonallergic nasal hyperreactivity. *Am J Rhinol* 1991, 5:145–151.

16. Togias A, Proud D, Kagey-Sobotka A, *et al.*: Cold dry air (CDA) and histamine (HIST) induce more potent responses in perennial rhinitis compared to normal individuals. *J Allergy Clin Immunol* 1991, 87:148.

17. Berger G, Marom Z, Ophir D: Goblet cell density of the inferior turbinates in patients with perennial allergic and nonallergic rhinitis. *Am J Rhinol* 1997, 11:233–236.

18. Berger G, Goldberg A, Ophir D: The inferior turbinate mast cell population of patients with perennial allergic and nonallergic rhinitis. *Am J Rhinol* 1997, 11:63–66.

19. Banov C, La Force C, Lieberman P: Double-blind trial of astelin nasal spray in treatment of vasomotor rhinitis. *Ann Allergy Asthma Immunol* 84:138, 2000.

20. Shinoda M, Watanabe N, Suko T, *et al.*: Effects of substance P (SP) and vasoactive intestinal peptide (VIP) in nasal secretions. *Am J Rhinol* 1997, 11:237–241.

21. Takao A, Shimoda T, Matsuse H, *et al.*: Inhibitory effects of azelastine hydrochloride in alcohol-induced asthma. *Ann Allergy Asthma Immunol* 1999, 82:390–394.

22. Ciprandi G, Prozanto C, Passalacqua G, *et al.*: Topical azelastine reduces eosinophilic activation and intracellular adhesion molecule-1 expression on nasal epithelial cells: an anti-allergic activity. *J Allergy Clin Immunol* 1996, 981:1088–1096.

23. Yoneda K, Yamamoto T, Ueta E, Osaki T: Suppression by azelastine hydrochloride of NF-κ B activation involved in generation of cytokines and nitric oxide. *Jpn J Pharmacol* 1997, 73:145–153.

24. Tamaoki J, Yamawaki I, Tagaya E, *et al.*: Effect of azelastine on platelet-activating factor-induced microvascular leakage in rat airways. *Am J Physiol* 1999, 276:L351–357.

25. Kondo H, Nachtigal D, Frenkiel S, *et al.*: Effect of steroids on nasal inflammatory cells and cytokine profile. *Laryngoscope* 1999, 109:91–97.

26. Malm L, Wihl J: Intranasal beclomethasone dipropionate in vasomotor rhinitis. *Acta Allergol* 1976, 31:245–253.

27. Wight RG, Jones AS, Beckingham E, *et al.*: A double-blind comparison of intranasal budesonide 400 micrograms and 800 micrograms in perennial rhinitis. *Clin Otolaryngol* 1992, 17:354–358.

28.• Small P, Black M, Frenkiel S: Effects of treatment with beclomethasone dipropionate in subpopulations of perennial rhinitis patients. *J Allergy Clin Immunol* 1982, 70:178–182.
This reference, as well as the four preceding references, demonstrate the effect of intranasal corticosteroid therapy for patients with perennial nonallergic rhinitis.

29. Blom HM, Godhthelp T, Fokkens WJ, *et al.*: The effect of nasal steroid aqueous spray on nasal complaint scores and cellular infiltrates in the nasal mucosa of patients with nonallergic, noninfectious perennial rhinitis. *J Allergy Clin Immunol* 1997, 100:739–747.

30. Weiler JM, Meltzer EO, Benson PM, *et al.*: A dose-ranging study of the efficacy and safety of astelin nasal spray in the treatment of seasonal allergic rhinitis with an acute model. *J Allergy Clin Immunol* 1994, 94:972–980.

31. Meltzer EO, Weiler JM, Dockhorn RJ, *et al.*: Azelastine nasal spray in the management of seasonal allergic rhinitis. *Ann Allergy* 1994, 72:354–359.

32. Day JH, Briscoe MP, Rafeiro E, *et al.*: Onset of action of intranasal budesonide (Rhinocort Aqua) in seasonal allergic rhinitis studied in a controlled exposure model. *J Allergy Clin Immunol* 2000, 105:489–494.

33.• Grossman J, Banov C, Boggs P, *et al.*: Use of ipratropium bromide in chronic treatment of nonallergic perennial rhinitis, alone and in combination with other perennial rhinitis combinations. *J Allergy Clin Immunol* 1995, 95:1123–1127.
This paper demonstrates that added effectiveness may be obtained by combining ipratropium bromide and corticosteroid nasal spray therapy.

34.• Bronsky EA, Druce H, Findlay SR, Hampel FC: A clinical trial of ipratropium bromide nasal spray in patients with perennial nonallergic rhinitis. *J Allergy Clin Immunol* 1995, 95:1117–1122.
This is one of the primary references demonstrating the effectiveness of ipratropium bromide for treatment of perennial nonallergic rhinitis.

35. Bhargava KB, Shirali GN, Abhyankar US, Gadre KC: Treatment of allergic and vasomotor rhinitis by the local application of different concentrations of silver nitrate. *J Laryngol Otol* 1992, 106:699–701.

36. Samarrae SM: Treatment of vasomotor rhinitis by the local application of silver nitrate. *J Laryngol Otol* 1991, 105:285–287.

37. Guindy A: Endoscopic transseptal vidian neurectomy. *Arch Otolaryngol Head Neck Surg* 1994, 120:1347–1351

38. Dong Z: Anterior ethmoidal electrocoagulation in the treatment of vasomotor rhinitis. *Chung Hua Erh Pi Yen Hou Ko Tsa Chih* 1991, 26:358–359.

39. Fernandes CM: Bilateral transnasal vidian neurectomy in the management of chronic rhinitis. *J Laryngol Otol* 1994, 108:569–573.

40. Prasanna A, Murthy PS: Vasomotor rhinitis and sphenopalatine ganglion block. *J Pain Symptom Manage* 1997, 13:332–338.

41. Mladina R, Risavi R, Subaric M: CO_2 laser anterior turbinectomy in the treatment of nonallergic vasomotor rhinopathia. A prospective study upon 78 patients. *Rhinology* 1991, 29:267–271.

42. NIAID Task Force Report: Asthma and the other allergic diseases: National Institutes of Health publication 79-387. Washington, DC: US Department of Health, Education and Welfare; 1979:23–31.

43.• Lund VJ, Kennedy DW: Quantification for staging sinusitis. *Ann Otol Rhinol Laryngol* 1995, 104(suppl):17–21.
This paper proposes definitions for chronic sinusitis in adult and pediatric populations.

44. Gwaltney JM Jr: Microbiology of sinusitis. In *Sinusitis*. Edited by Druce HM. New York: Marcel Dekker; 1994:41–56.

45. Stierna P, Carlsoo B: Histopathological observations in chronic maxillary sinusitis. *Acta Otolaryngol (Stockh)* 1990, 110:450–458.

46. Georgitis JW, Matthews BL, Stone B: Chronic sinusitis: characterization of cellular influx and inflammatory mediators in sinus lavage fluid. *Int Arch Allergy Immunol* 1995, 106:416–421.

47.• Jacobs RL, Freedman PM, Boswell RN: Nonallergic rhinitis with nasal eosinophilia (NARES syndrome). *J Allergy Clin Immunol* 1981, 67:253–262.
This is a landmark article first describing and characterizing NARES.

48. Sobol SM, Love RG, Stutman HR, Pysher TJ: Phaeohyphomycosis of the maxilloethmoid sinus caused by *Drechslera spicifera*: a new fungal pathogen. *Laryngoscope* 1984, 94:620–627.

49. Olsen KD, Neel HB, DeRemee RA, Weiland LH: Nasal manifestations of allergic granulomatosis and angiitis (Churg-Strauss syndrome). *Otolaryngol Head Neck Surg* 1980, 88:85–89.

50. Moneret-Vautrin DA, Hsieh V, Wayoff M, *et al.*: Nonallergic rhinitis with eosinophilia syndrome a precursor of the triad: nasal polyposis, intrinsic asthma, and intolerance to aspirin. *Ann Allergy* 1990, 64:513–518.

51. Bousquet J, Chanez P, Lacoste JY, *et al.*: Eosinophilic inflammation in asthma. *N Engl J Med* 1990, 323:1033–1039.

52. Hastie AT, Loegering DA, Gleich GJ, Kueppers F: The effect of purified human eosinophil major basic protein on mammalian ciliary activity. *Am Rev Respir Dis* 1987, 135:848–853.

53. Flavahan NA, Slifman NR, Gleich GJ, Vanhoutte PM: Human eosinophil major basic protein causes hyperreactivity of respiratory smooth muscle. *Am Rev Respir Dis* 1988, 138:685–688.

54. Venge P, Dahl R, Fredens K, Peteerson CGB: Epithelial injury by human eosinophil. *Am Rev Respir Dis* 1988, 138:S54–S57.

55. Spector SL, English G, Jones L: Clinical and nasal biopsy response to treatment of perennial rhinitis. *J Allergy Clin Immunol* 1980, 66:129–137.

56. Ayars GH, Altman LC, McManus MM, *et al.*: Injurious effect of the eosinophil peroxide-hydrogen peroxide-halide system and major basic protein on human nasal epithelium in vitro. *Am Rev Respir Dis* 1989, 140:125–131.

57. Davidson AE, Miller SD, Settipane RJ, *et al.*: Delayed nasal mucociliary clearance in patients with nonallergic rhinitis and nasal eosinophilia. *Allergy Proc* 1992, 13:81–84.

58. Settipane GA: Nasal manifestations of systemic diseases. In *Rhinitis*, edn 2. Providence, RI: OceanSide Publications; 1991:197–208.

59. Graf P, Hallen H, Juto-Je: The pathophysiology and treatment of rhinitis medicamentosa. *Clin Otolaryngol* 1995, 20:224–229.

60.•• Incaudo GA, Schatz M: Rhinosinusitis associated with endocrine conditions: hypothyroidism and pregnancy. In *Nasal Manifestations of Systemic Diseases*. Edited by Schatz M, Zeiger RS, Settipane GA. Providence, RI: OceanSide Publications; 1991:53–62.
This reference provides an excellent review of rhinosinusitis associated with endocrine conditions and pregnancy.

61. Toppozada H, Michaels L, Toppazada M, *et al.*: The human respiratory nasal mucosa in pregnancy. *J Larynol Otol* 1982, 96:613–626.

62. Sorri M, Bortikanen-Sorri AL, Kanja J: Rhinitis during pregnancy. *Rhinology* 1980, 18:83–86.

63.•• Schatz M, Hoffman CP, Zeiger RS, *et al.*: Course and management of asthma and allergic diseases during pregnancy. In *Allergy Principles and Practice* edn 4, vol 2. Edited by Middleton E, Reed CE, Ellis EF, *et al.* St. Louis: Mosby; 1997:1301–1342.
This is a thorough review of rhinitis in pregnancy.

64. Connell J: Nasal hypersensitivity in comprehensive immunology. In *Cellular, Molecular and Clinical Aspects of Allergic Disorders* vol 6. Edited by Gupta S, Good RA. New York: Plenum; 1979:397.

65. Settipane GA: Nasal polyps. In *Rhinitis* edn 2. Providence, RI: OceanSide Publications; 1991:173–184.

66. Wentges RT, Woakes E: The history of an eponym. *J Laryngol Otol* 1972, 86:501.

67. Oppenheimer EH, Rosenstein BJ: Differential pathology of nasal polyps in cystic fibrosis and atopy. *Lab Invest* 1979, 40:445–449.

68. Rowe-Jones JM, Shembekar M, Trendell-Smith N, *et al.*: Polypoidal rhinosinusitis in cystic fibrosis: a clinical and histopathological study. *Clin Otolaryngol* 1997, 22:167–171.

69. Salari H, Borgeat P, Steffenrud S, *et al.*: Immunological and nonimmunological release of leukotrienes and histamine from human nasal polyps. *Clin Exp Immunol* 1986, 63:711–717.

70.• Bachert C, Wagenmann M, Hauser U, *et al.*: IL-5 synthesis is upregulated in human nasal polyp tissue. *J Allergy Clin Immunol* 1997, 99:837–842.
Interleukin-5 may represent a main target for therapy of nasal polyposis. Nasal polyposis may, in turn, serve as a good model for investigating and treating other eosinophilic diseases, such as asthma.

71. Bumsted RM, El-Ackad T, Smith JM, Brody MJ: Histamine, norepinephrine, and serotonin content of nasal polyps. *Laryngoscope* 1979, 89:832–843.

72. Chandra RK, Abrol BM: Immunopathology of nasal polypi. *J Laryngol Otol* 1974, 88:1019–1024.

73. Keith PK, Conway M, Evans S, *et al.*: Nasal polyps: effects of seasonal allergy exposure. *J Allergy Clin Immunol* 1994, 93:567–574.

74.•• Lindholdt T, Rundcrantz H, Bende M, *et al.*: Glucocorticoid treatment for nasal polyps: the use of topical budesonide powder, intramuscular betamethasone, and surgical treatment. *Arch Otolaryngol Head Neck Surg* 1997, 123:595–600.
The literature on medical therapy for nasal polyps is limited. This study shows that most patients do well with medical treatment. Surgery was required in very few patients.

75. Downing ET, Braman S, Settipane GA: Bronchial reactivity in patients with nasal polyps before and after polypectomy. *J Allergy Clin Immunol* 1982, 69:102.

76. Proud D, Bailey GS, Naclerio RM, *et al.*: Tryptase and histamine as markers to evaluate mast cell activation during the responses to nasal challenge with allergen, cold, dry air and hyperosmolar solutions. *J Allergy Clin Immunol* 1992, 89:1098–1110.

77. Togias AG, Naclerio RM, Proud D, *et al.*: Nasal challenge with cold, dry air results in the production of inflammatory mediators: possible mast cell involvement. *J Clin Invest* 1985, 76:1375–1381.

78.• Raphael GD, Hauptschein-Raphael M, Kaliner MA: Gustatory rhinitis. *Am J Rhinol* 1989, 3:145–149.
The diagnosis of gustatory rhinitis is described and characterized.

79. Bascom R: Air pollution. In *Allergic and Nonallergic Rhinitis*. Edited by Mygind N, Naclerio RM. Copenhagen: Munksgaard; 1993:32–45.

80. Coggins CRE, Fouilet XLM, Lam R, *et al.*: Cigarette smoke–induced pathology of the rat respiratory tract: a comparison of the effects of the particulates and vapour phases. *Toxicology* 1980, 16:83.

81. Black A, Eans JC, Hadfiled EH, *et al.*: Impairment of nasal mucociliary clearance in woodworkers in the furniture industry. *Br J Ind Med* 1974, 31:10.

82. Graham D, Henderson F, House D: Neutrophil influx measured in nasal lavages of humans exposed to ozone. *Arch Environ Health* 1988, 43:228–233.

83. Olsen JH, Jensen SP, Hink M, *et al.*: Occupational formaldehyde exposure and increased nasal cancer risk in man. *Int J Cancer* 1984, 34:639–644.

84.• Slavin RG: Occupational rhinitis. *Immunol Allergy Clin North Am* 1992, 12:769.
Occupational rhinitis is probably underrecognized. This reference serves to classify this disorder and provides a comprehensively different diagnosis.

85. Bardana EJ Jr: Occupational asthma and related respiratory disorders. *Dis Mon* 1995, 41:141–200.

86. Chan-Yeung M, Lam S: Occupational asthma. *Am Rev Respir Dis* 1986, 133:689–690.

87. Bernstein DI: Clinical assessment and management of occupational asthma. In *Asthma in the Workplace.* Edited by Bernstein IL, Chan-Yeung M, Malo JL. New York: Marcel Dekker; 1993:103–123.

88.• Han-Sen C: The oxena problem: clinical analysis of atrophic rhinitis in 100 cases. *Acta Otolaryngol* 1982, 93:461.
This reference provides insight into the diagnosis of atrophic rhinitis by reviewing 100 cases.

89. Holopainen E: Nasal mucous membrane in atrophic rhinitis with reference to symptom-free nasal mucosa. *Acta Otolaryngol (Stockh)* 1967, 227(suppl):26–47.

90.• Connell JT: Nasal mastocytosis. *J Allergy* 1969, 43:182.
This is a landmark reference describing and characterizing nasal mastocytosis.

91. McKenna EL: Nasal mastocytosis. *Laryngoscope* 1974, 84:112–125.

92.• Zlab MK, Moore GF, Daly DT, Yonkers AJ: Cerebrospinal fluid rhinorrhea: a review of the literature. *Ear Nose Throat J* 1992, 71:314–317.
This article provides a literature review of CSF rhinorrhea.

93. Skedros DG, Cass SP, Hirsch BE, Kelly RH: β-2 transferrin assay in clinical management of cerebral spinal fluid and perilymphatic fluid leaks. *J Otolaryngol* 1993, 22:341–344.

94. Sillers MJ, Morgan CE, Gammal T: Magnetic resonance cisternography and thin coronal computerized tomography in the evaluation of cerebrospinal fluid rhinorrhea. *Am J Rhin* 1997, 11:387–392.

95. Reiter D, Myers AR: Asymptomatic septal perforations in systemic lupus erythematosus. *Ann Otol Rhinol Laryngol* 1980, 89:78–80.

96. Hughes RAC, Berry CL, Seifert M, Lessof MH: Relapsing polychondritis: three cases with a clinicopathological study and literature review. *Q J Med* 1972, 41:363–380.

97. Henkin RI, Talal N, Larson AL, Mattern CFT: Abnormalities of taste and smell in Sjögrens syndrome. *Ann Intern Med* 1972, 76:375–383.

98. Wilson R, Lund V, Sweatman M, *et al.*: Upper respiratory tract involvement in sarcoidosis and its management. *Eur Respir J* 1988, 1:269–272.

99. Fauci AS, Haynes BF, Katz P, Wolff SM: Wegener's granulomatosis: prospective clinical and therapeutic experience with 85 patients for 21 years. *Ann Intern Med* 1983, 98:76–85.

CHAPTER 7

Viral Rhinitis

Deborah A. Gentile
David P. Skoner

Viral rhinitis is a common, morbid, and costly malady, often complicated by otitis media, sinusitis, and asthma. Earlier research implicated roles for cytopathology, cellular infiltration, and inflammatory mediators such as bradykinin in disease pathogenesis, but these factors are now recognized as late events with specific and limited contributions to disease expression. Current therapies are relatively ineffective and aimed at reducing symptoms rather than moderating underlying mechanisms. Nasal elevations of proinflammatory cytokines track symptom expression during viral rhinitis, and it is hypothesized that these chemicals orchestrate a common response to infection with many different viruses that cause rhinitis. Also, recent evidence supports a role for neurogenic inflammation in the development of complications. Future studies should dissect the role of proinflammatory cytokines and neuropeptides in the expression of symptoms, signs, pathophysiologies, and complications of viral rhinitis.

INTRODUCTION

Viral rhinitis is extremely common in children and adults. For most segments of the population, this condition is self-limited and associated with relatively short periods of morbidity. However, in infants, the elderly, and the immunocompromised, infection with some of the causal viruses is associated with a significant excess mortality. Also, viral rhinitis is well established as a predisposition to other diseases involving the lungs, paranasal sinuses, and middle ears (1–3). These complications are characterized by a more prolonged time course than that of the precipitating virus infection and are often refractory to conventional medical treatment. Medications of questionable efficacy sold for the relief of symptoms and signs of viral rhinitis represent a major component of the over-the-counter drug market, and prescription medications for treating associated complications including sinusitis, otitis media, and pneumonia represent a significant financial burden to society. These costs are compounded by the decreased economic productivity resulting from the large number of days lost to industry and education.

PATHOGENESIS OF VIRAL RHINITIS

Viruses that cause rhinitis include rhinovirus (RV), adenovirus, influenza virus (FLU), parainfluenza virus, coxsackie virus, and respiratory syncytial virus (RSV). Comparative studies of experimental infection of adult humans with RSV, FLU, RV, and cox-sackie A virus show that all of these viruses provoke a similar local symptom-sign presentation (with varying degrees of systemic involvement), nasal secretory response, pattern of complications (with varying frequencies), and panel of elaborated inflammatory mediators (IMs) and cytokines [4,5]. Differences that exist among viruses primarily reflect the types of cells that are infected (tissue tropism) and thus the degree to which the infection is localized. For example, whereas RVs are generally confined to the upper airways by their sensitivity to temperature, RSV can be disseminated to the lung and middle ear by way of the contiguous mucosa, and FLU can infect leukocytes with viremic dissemination. These observations suggest that the pathogenesis of the local, cold-like signs, symptoms, and complications is common to the different etiological agents and most likely represents the consequences of a generalized host response to viral infection of the nasal mucosa.

The most prominent signs and symptoms of viral rhinitis include rhinorrhea, sneezing, nasal obstruction, sore throat, cough, malaise, fever, and sweats [6]. In some studies, the development of pulmonary hyperreactivity was reported [3], and complications involving the paranasal sinuses are common [1]. Also reported are otological complications, including eustachian tube obstruction, middle ear underpressures, and otitis media [7]. Most studies failed to culture virus from the site of the complication (sinus, lung, or middle ear), and the development of complications has been associated with the extension of the inflammatory response as opposed to in situ viral infection.

The pathogenesis of symptoms and signs of illness and pathophysiologies and complications of viral rhinitis have been studied using epidemiological surveys, animal models, and adults experimentally infected with different respiratory viruses. Importantly, similar patterns and magnitudes of the pathophysiologic and symptomatic responses to infection were documented for experimental and natural viral rhinitis [6]. A distinct advantage offered by the experimental model over nat-

ural infection is its high degree of control over several factors: the health of the subjects; the dose and nature of the infecting agent; the precise temporal sequence of infection, symptom, sign and pathophysiology presentation; cytokines; and IMs.

Early studies of the host response to viral rhinitis focused on the humoral system. High homotypic serum neutralizing IgG antibody titers have been associated with protection from infection and lessened signs and symptoms [8]. Similarly, high nasal IgA antibody titers have been significantly correlated with decreased duration of viral shedding. There is also evidence that the cellular immune response may play a role in the pathogenesis of viral rhinitis. Phenotypic and functional changes in circulating immune/inflammatory parameters have been documented during experimental viral upper respiratory infections (URIs) [9].

The role of IMs has been the focus of recent studies of viral URI pathogenesis. The similarity between the clinical manifestations of allergic rhinitis and the common cold has prompted repeated attempts to establish a role for histamine and other IMs in the pathogenesis of viral rhinitis. Three generalized methods have been used to provide evidence for a role of IMs and cytokines in the pathogenesis of viral rhinitis: 1) documentation of a time-dependent increase in the concentration of the IM/cytokine (in nasal secretion, blood, or urine) during the period of infection that parallels symptoms; 2) provocation of signs, symptoms, and mucosal inflammation by topical application of the IM/cytokine; and 3) moderation of the inflammatory process or symptom expression by inhibitors of these IMs/cytokines.

Elevated nasal secretion levels during natural or experimental viral rhinitis have been observed for bradykinin, leukotrienes (LTs), interferon-α, interferon-β, interferon-γ, interleukin (IL)–1, IL-6, IL-8, IL-11, and tumor necrosis factor (TNF) [10–12,13••]. These elevations were directly correlated with symptom expression for IL-1, IL-6, and bradykinin. Direct application to the nasal mucosal of histamine, bradykinin,

TABLE 7-1. EFFECTS OF TOPICAL ADMINISTRATION OF SELECTED INFLAMMATORY MEDIATORS AND CYTOKINES

Mediator/cytokine	Rhinorrhea	Sneezing	Congestion
Histamine	X	X	X
Bradykinin	X		X
Leukotrienes	X		X
IL-6	X		
IL-8			X

IL—interleukin.

LTs, IL-8, and IL-6 in noninfected humans reproduced certain symptoms of the common cold (Table 7-1) [14–16]. However, efficacy trials using synthesis or action inhibitors have largely been disappointing. Most were underpowered, poorly designed, or used inhibitors with questionable potency or target tissue delivery [17], and none examined the possible interactions between cytokines and other mediators.

ROLE OF INFLAMMATORY MEDIATORS

Histamine, a classic mediator of allergic rhinitis, is stored in granules of tissue mast cells and circulating basophils and is released immediately upon cellular contact with a variety of stimuli. Local histamine in nasal secretions [4] and urinary histamine metabolites can be detected during viral rhinitis [18]. Mucosally applied histamine triggers a full spectrum of rhinitis symptoms and is the only mediator studied that provokes sneezing [14]. Of interest, antihistamine treatment during viral rhinitis consistently depresses symptoms and signs of sneezing and rhinorrhea but has little effect on other aspects of disease expression [17].

Bradykinin is a potent mediator of inflammation and is synthesized locally from precursors delivered with other serum proteins by transudation. Application of bradykinin to the nasal mucosa provokes rhinorrhea, congestion, facial pain, and sore throat [14]. Kinins were found in the nasal secretions recovered from subjects with experimental and natural viral rhinitis [10]. The concentration and time course of the production of kinins are correlated with symptom severity. However, steroid therapy significantly reduced kinins in nasal lavage fluids but had no effect on symptoms, and bradykinin antagonists did not affect signs and symptoms in a number of experimental RV studies [19].

Leukotrienes are potent mediators generated by different cell types that participate in inflammatory reactions. The sulfidopeptide LTs increase the permeability of post-capillary venules and facilitate plasma leakage, edema formation, and cellular diapedesis. LBT4 is one of the most potent chemoattractants for neutrophils and, to a lesser degree, eosinophils. Both the sulfidopeptide LTs and LTB4 are potent enhancers of mucus secretion. According to data on a 5-lipoxygenase knockout mouse model, LTs are critically involved in many, but not all, causes of inflammation. Combined with the results reported for mast cell–deficient mice, chemotactic LTs released by mast cells can be shown to be important in neutrophil recruitment during the early acute inflammatory response to insult. Elevated levels of LTs were observed in nasal secretions of children infected with RSV, parainfluenza virus, and FLU and in experimentally infected adults [11]. Moreover, LTs applied directly to the nasal mucosa in noninfected individuals reproduced symptoms of nasal congestion and rhinorrhea [20]. Both 5-lipoxygenase enzyme inhibitors and LTD4 antagonists have efficacy in treating nasal congestion in allergic rhinitis. No trials of LT blockers or inhibitors have been conducted in viral rhinitis, but corticosteroids, which downregulate LT synthesis in vitro but not in vivo, had a demonstrable effect on cough.

Recent evidence also implicates a role for nitric oxide (NO) in the pathogenesis of viral rhinitis. Increased concentrations of nasal NO have been reported during viral rhintis in vivo. Moreover, NO inhibited RV-induced cytokine production and viral replication in a human respiratory epithelial cell line. However, recent studies have failed to find an association between NO and the signs, symptoms, and complications during experimental viral rhinitis [21].

ROLE OF NEUROGENIC INFLAMMATION

Mediators of neurogenic inflammation may also play a role in the pathogenesis of viral rhinitis. It is hypothesized that virus infection provokes the release from epithelial cells of IL-11 and endothelins (ETs), which conjointly and synergistically activate nociceptive nerves leading to local mucosal axon responses and the subsequent release of inflammatory neuropeptides. These peptides, in turn, cause neurogenic inflammation which is expressed as nasal irritation, sneezing (nociceptive nerve activation), engorgement of venous sinusoids (mucosal swelling with decreased nasal patency), increased vascular permeability (major source of rhinorrhea fluid), glandular exocytosis, low-grade inflammatory cell infiltration, and reflex obstruction of the eustachian tube and sinus ostia. Several lines of evidence support a role for neurogenic inflammation in the pathogenesis and expression of viral rhinitis. These include the following observations: 1) parasympathetic reflexes mediate the glandular exocytosis and mucous hypersecretion; 2) hyperresponsiveness of the nasal mucosa to histamine and cold dry air was reported during RV and FLU infections; 3) viral infection in humans causes release of IL-11, a "neurokine" that increases the sensitivity of nociceptive neurons to activation, increases neural responses to painful stimuli, and provokes bronchial hyperresponsiveness; and 4) ETs are synthesized and secreted by nasal epithelial and glandular cells in response to virus infection [22–24]. In other inflammatory diseases such as asthma and rhinitis, ETs and IL-11 are released, stimulate nociceptive neurons, and recruit parasympathetic reflexes. Also, in allergen challenge studies, the release of substance P, calcitonin gene–related peptide, and vasoactive intestinal peptide is associated with itch, nasal blockage, and rhinorrhea, showing that these nociceptive neuropeptides can be measured in nasal secretions and that their concentrations are related to specific symptoms [25].

ROLE OF CYTOKINES

Recent studies have focused on elucidating the role of cytokines in the pathogenesis of viral rhinitis. The cytokine network provides a complex and highly interactive mechanism for regulation and amplification of the immune system and inflammatory response. During an inflammatory event, proinflammatory cytokines are typically upregulated in a cascading fashion. On the continuum of proinflammatory and immune system–stimulating chemicals, TNF-α and IL-1 hold central roles. TNF-α is the first cytokine to be upregulated in response to an inflammatory stimulus, with levels peaking within several hours. IL-1 is the second cytokine to be upregulated, with levels peaking within 24 to 48 hours. TNF-α and IL-1 then trigger the sequential upregulation of other cytokines, including IL-6, IL-8, and IL-10. Interestingly, results from recent studies suggest that the severity of URI-induced illness and the development of complications are orchestrated by the sequential elaboration of these various proinflammatory cytokines [12,13••, 26••].

TNF-α and IL-1 also play roles in regulating T-helper type 1 (T_H1) and type 2 (T_H2) immune responses. T-helper lymphocytes can be divided into several subsets including T_H1 and T_H2 cells, which are involved in cellular and humoral immunity, respectively. T_H2 lymphocytes and their cytokines, including IL-4, have been implicated in the pathogenesis of viral URI-induced illness and complications. Increases in local and systemic IL-4 mRNA and protein levels were observed during viral URIs. Several studies reported associations between IL-4 elevations, severity of viral rhinitis, and incidence of virally induced complications [27]. In animal models, overexpression of IL-4 was shown to delay RSV clearance, and treatment with anti–IL-4 was shown to decrease the severity of RSV-induced illness [28].

Tumor necrosis factor-α is produced primarily by activated macrophages, induces synthesis of acute phase reactants by the liver, induces fever, and causes the relaxation of vascular smooth muscle. TNF-α can also activate endothelial cells to upregulate other cytokines and adhesion molecule expression, thus enhancing vascular permeability, cellular adhesion, and procoagulant activity. TNF-α is a proinflammatory cytokine with pleiotropic expression consistent with a primary role in the pathogenesis of virally induced rhinitis. In several studies, release of TNF-α was increased from epithelial cells and monocytes following in vitro infection with respiratory viruses [29]. Other studies reported elevated levels of TNF-α protein in nasal lavage samples recovered from otherwise healthy infants during primary

RSV infection and from adults following experimental infection with a variety of respiratory viruses [30]. Several studies reported that TNF-α production was biphasic with peaks occurring 6 hours and 2 to 3 days following infection with respiratory viruses. Another study reported a positive association between local elevations of TNF-α protein and severity of virally induced rhinitis [31], and preliminary studies conducted in our laboratory related elevated TNF-α to the expression of otological complications during FLU infection (Gentile and Skoner, unpublished data, 2000). These data are consistent with the hypothesis that TNF-α contributes to the pathogenesis of viral rhinitis.

Interleukin-1 is produced by epithelial cells, mononuclear phagocytes, and fibroblasts and shares many of the same activities as TNF-α. The IL-1 family has three members: IL-1α, IL-1β, and an endogenous IL-1 receptor antagonist (IL-1ra). IL-1 has been implicated in the activation of T lymphocytes. Blocking the action of IL-1 has many diverse effects that include inhibiting neutrophil accumulation in lung tissue of animal models. As with TNF-α, release of IL-1 was increased from nasal epithelial cells following in vitro virus infection [32]. One recent study reported a small increase in IL-1α, a modest increase in IL-1β, and an impressive increase in IL-1ra in nasal lavages obtained from adults with experimental RV infection [33••]. Maximal induction of IL-1α and IL-1β was noted at 48 hours, whereas maximal induction of IL-1ra occurred between 48 and 72 hours. These times corresponded to the peak periods for symptomatology and symptom resolution, respectively. These data support the hypotheses that IL-1 contributes to the pathogenesis of viral rhinitis and that IL-1ra plays an important role in disease resolution.

IL-1 and TNF-α interact with other cytokines to modulate inflammation. IL-6 is produced by a wide spectrum of cells in response to a number of stimuli, including IL-1–induced activation of transcription factors. IL-6 mediates many biological functions that are relevant to virus infection. These include its abilities to act as an endogenous pyrogen, stimulate the acute phase response, stimulate T lymphocytes, induce the terminal differentiation of B lymphocytes, and stimulate immunoglobulin production. IL-6 is a potent regulator of pulmonary inflammation and an important component of biologic homeostasis. Dysregulation is implicated in a wide array of inflammatory and viral disorders. Increases in local IL-6 production were reported during URIs caused by RV, FLU, and RSV and coincide with peaks in symptomatology and pathophysiology [12,13••,30]. Moreover, IL-6 causes significant increases in nasal secretions after topical application [16].

Interleukin-8 is a neutrophil-chemotactic cytokine whose production by monocytes, fibroblasts, endothelial cells, epithelial cells, and neutrophils is induced by

IL-1 and TNF-α. In addition to its activity as a potent neutrophil chemoattractant, IL-8 activates neutrophil degranulation and respiratory burst, T lymphocyte chemotaxis, and release of histamine and LTs from basophils. IL-8 has been identified in a number of inflammatory conditions (including nasal allergic responses) at plasma concentrations of up to 1.2 μg/ml, which fall within the range at which neutrophils are stimulated in vitro. IL-8 has been detected in nasal secretions of volunteers infected with RV, FLU, and RSV [13••,26••,34]. Moreover, IL-8 causes marked increases in nasal airway resistance and tissue neutrophilia after topical application and has been associated with disease severity during experimental RV infection [15,34].

Interleukin-10 is produced by T lymphocytes, blood monocytes, and tissue macrophages and is considered to be an intrinsic antiinflammatory and immunosuppressive cytokine. IL-10 inhibits cytokine production by T lymphocytes, mononuclear phagocytes, and natural killer cells. Expression of IL-10 by antigen-presenting cells may have a role in lessening inflammation by inhibiting the synthesis of proinflammatory cytokines such as IL-1, IL-6, IL-8, and TNF-α. This role for IL-10 is supported by its ability to induce T-cell tolerance to antigen. Indeed, lack of macrophage IL-10 production has been purported to underlie the chronic airway inflammation characteristic of asthma [35]. Increases in local IL-10 production were reported during experimental viral rhinitis, and maximal IL-10 levels typically coincide with the onset of resolution of viral URI–induced symptomatology and pathophysiology [36].

Several recently developed tools are available for dissecting the role of various proinflammatory cytokines in the pathogenesis of viral rhinitis and its complications. One such tool is the use of animal models of cytokine knockout and blockade. In mice deficient for IL-6 or in those treated with IL-1ra, symptoms of FLU-induced illness were partially reduced [37]. Moreover, mortality was reduced in those animals treated with IL-1ra. Another recently developed tool is cytokine genotyping. Recent studies demonstrated associations between specific cytokine genotypes associated with high production of TNF-α or IL-1β and increased susceptibility to several infectious diseases [38••]. These results suggest that certain cytokines are necessary for the development of symptomatology during viral rhinitis and that specific cytokine polymorphisms may be associated with increased susceptibility to viral rhinitis and its complications.

In summary, cytokines promote the initiation, amplification, and persistence of inflammation by their direct cellular effects and by their role in inducing synthesis or release of other inflammatory chemicals in a cascading fashion. A common pathway in viral rhinitis may be the early release of nonspecific, host-alert cytokines, including TNF-α and IL-1. These have both local effects (eg, depress protein synthesis and upregulate major histocompatibility complex presentation) and systemic effects (eg, pyrogenic and stem cell maturation) that are expressed as the more general symptoms and signs of illness (eg, fever and malaise). They also upregulate integrin and selectin expression and thereby mediate the local recruitment of inflammatory cells, which in turn promotes the release or synthesis of IMs (eg, histamine, bradykinin, eicosanoids, and other cytokines). Some of those IMs initiate neurogenic inflammation and increased vascular permeability (rhinorrhea) and cause sneezing, cough, and nasal congestion. In a cascading and networking fashion, TNF-α and IL-1 also regulate the production of other pro- or anti-inflammatory cytokines via transcription factor activation in an autocrine or paracrine manner. Additionally, there is strong evidence for cross-talk between IMs, especially those products of the lipoxygenase pathway and the cytokines. In spite of the data demonstrating an association between cytokines and symptoms of viral rhinitis, the role of these mediators in pathogenesis will not be clear until specific inhibitors are available for use in clinical trials.

PREVENTION AND TREATMENT

The pharmacologic agents currently available for the treatment and/or prevention of viral rhinitis are summarized in Table 7-2. For certain pathogens, viral rhinitis and its complications can be prevented by effective

TABLE 7-2. PHARMACOLOGIC AGENTS CURRENTLY MARKETED FOR THE TREATMENT/PROPHYLAXIS OF VIRUSES CAUSING RHINITIS

Active immunization
  Influenza vaccine
Passive immunization
  Anti-RSV monoclonal antibody
Antiviral agents
  Ribavirin (RSV)
  Amantadine, rimantadine, zanamivir, oseltamivir (influenza)
Symptomatic treatment
  Antihistamines
  Decongestants
  Anticholinergics
  Combination products
Other
  Zinc

RSV—respiratory syncytial virus.

immunization against the precipitating virus or by effective antiviral prophylaxis or treatment. For example, populations at risk for severe FLU- or RSV-induced lower respiratory illness can be actively immunized with a FLU vaccine or passively immunized with an anti-RSV monoclonal antibody [39,40]. Moreover, several antiviral agents are available for prophylaxis or treatment [41]. These include ribavirin for RSV and amantadine, rimantadine, zanamivir, and oseltamivir for FLU. Antiviral agents for RV, such as pleconaril, are currently under development and testing. However, at present, the use of immunization or antiviral agents is not applicable to the majority of episodes viral rhinitis for several reasons: 1) the large number of viruses that cause viral URIs; 2) the high degree of antigenic variability exhibited by most of these viruses; 3) the limited arsenal, high specificity, and significant side-effects of available antivirals; and 4) concerns regarding selection of resistant virus strains during extended antiviral prophylaxis [42].

Symptomatic therapy remains the mainstay of treatment. The first-generation antihistamines have been used for many years for the treatment of rhinorrhea and sneezing associated with viral rhinitis. Oral antihistamines have no effect on nasal congestion. First-generation antihistamines are lipophilic molecules, which can easily cross the blood-brain barrier and induce pharmacologic actions in the central nervous system. Representative

TABLE 7-3. ADVERSE EFFECTS OF ANTIHISTAMINES

Central nervous system*
  Stimulation
  Neuropsychiatric
  Peripheral
  Depressive (includes sedation and cognitive impairment)
Cardiac†
  Prolongation of QT interval
  Ventricular arhythmias
Anticholinergic*
  Dry mouth and eyes
  Urinary retention
  Impotence
  Worsening of glaucoma
Others
  Weight gain
  Rashes
  Photosensitivity
  Hypersensitivity reactions
  Blood disorders
  Hepatic dysfunction

*Less common with second-generation agents.
†Associated with astemizole and terfenadine only.

first-generation antihistamines include diphenhydramine, tripolidine, chlorpheniramine, brompheniramine, and hydroxyzine and are available in oral formulations; many are sold over the counter. Several large studies of experimental viral rhinitis have confirmed that these agents are efficacious for the treatment of viral-induced rhinorrhea and sneezing [17,43]. However, their use is limited by their adverse effect profile [44,45••]. Their major limitation is sedation; other limitations are summarized in Table 7-3.

Second-generation antihistamines are lipophobic, have a large molecular size, and possess an electrostatic charge. Because of their physiochemical properties, they generally do not cross the blood-brain barrier, and therefore exhibit negligible central nervous system effects. Second-generation antihistamines are also grouped into different classes based on their chemical structure. Currently marketed second-generation antihistamines include three oral medications (loratadine, cetirizine, and fexofenadine) and one intranasal (azelastine). All of these medications require a prescription. None of these medications are approved by the Food and Drug Administration (FDA) for the treatment or prevention of viral rhinitis. Second-generation antihistamines administered as treatment for viral rhinitis had small effects on sneezing and rhinorrhea [46]. In general, second-generation antihistamines are less effective than first-generation agents at relieving virally induced rhinorrhea. This is most likely due to the relative lack of anticholinergic and antimuscarinic effects of second-generation antihistamines. Prophylactic use of second-generation antihistamines has not been tested. Interestingly, second-generation antihistamines have been shown to downregulate expression of intercellular adhesion molecule (ICAM), the RV receptor, in vitro [47]. It is conceivable that prophylactic use of second-generation antihistamines may prevent or limit infection and thereby reduce complications via downregulation of ICAM expression. In support of in vivo clinical relevance of that effect, the results of a recent study showed that children with recurrent otitis media who were placed on a second-generation antihistamine had a lower incidence of viral URIs than children placed on placebo [48]. One of the primary advantages of second-generation antihistamines is that they are nonsedating, or significantly hyposedating. They also have a long duration of action and are amenable to once- or twice-daily dosing. Limitations of second-generation antihistamines are summarized in Table 7-3 [44,45••].

Both topical and oral adrenergic agents are effective for the treatment of nasal congestion associated with viral rhinitis. Oral decongestants include pseudoephedrine, phenylpropanolamine, and phenylephrine. Topical decongestants include phenylephrine, oxymetazoline, naphthazoline, tetrahydrozoline, and zylometazoline. Prolonged use of the topical adrenergic agents should be avoided to prevent the development of rhinitis medicamentosa, an apparent rebound effect when the drug is discontinued. The primary adverse effects of decongestants are summarized in Table 7-4 [44,45••]. Efficacy against symptoms of viral rhinitis, including nasal congestion, rhinorrhea, and sneezing, may be improved by the combination of an antihistamine with a decongestant.

Ipratropium bromide is effective for the treatment of rhinorrhea associated with viral rhinitis. This agent exerts its effect by blockade of cholinergic stimulation of glandular secretions. It is available as a topical nasal spray, requires a prescription, and is FDA approved for the treatment of viral rhinitis. In large studies of subjects with naturally acquired viral URIs, ipratropium produced a 22% to 31% decrease in rhinorrhea compared to placebo [49]. The most common adverse effects include nasal irritation and bleeding.

Numerous studies have examined the efficacy of zinc for the treatment of viral rhinitis. Despite the in vitro effect of zinc on viral replication, there has been no detectable effect of zinc on virus replication in vivo. The effect of zinc on symptoms of viral rhinitis has been inconsistent. Some studies reported dramatic decreases in the duration and severity of symptoms, while other studies have shown no effect [50•]. The most common adverse effect is unpleasant taste.

CONCLUSIONS

The majority of current treatments for viral rhinitis were "borrowed" from other nasal inflammatory diseases (eg, allergy). The rational development of specific therapies for viral rhinitis is complicated by our incomplete understanding of disease pathogenesis, the similar expression of illness for different viruses, and the relatively late presentation of identifiable symptoms and signs. Future studies should contribute to a better understanding of the inflammatory responses to viral URIs and clarify the roles of the targeted proinflammatory cytokines and neurogenic inflammation in disease expression. This knowledge will lay the foundation for rationally targeted therapies directed at the host inflammatory or immune responses that have the potential to alter the course of a viral URI, suppress disease expression and limit complications, including otitis media, sinusitis and airway hyperreactivity.

REFERENCES AND RECOMMENDED READING

Papers of particular interest, published recently, have been highlighted as:

• Of importance

•• Of major importance

1. Gwaltney JM Jr, Phillips CD, Miller RD, Riker DK: Computed tomographic study of the common cold. N Engl J Med 1994, 330:25–30.

2. Henderson FW, Collier AM, Sanyai MA, et al.: A longitudinal study of respiratory viruses and bacteria in the etiology of acute otitis media with effusion. N Engl J Med 1982, 306:1377–83.

3. Lemanske RF Jr, Dick EC, Swenson CA, et al.: Rhinovirus upper respiratory infection increases airway hyperreactivity and late asthmatic reactions. J Clin Invest 1989, 83:1–10.

4. Igarashi Y, Skoner DP, Doyle WJ, et al.: Analysis of nasal secretions during phases of experimental rhinovirus upper respiratory tract infection. J Allergy Clin Immunol 1993, 92:722–731.

5. Doyle WJ, Skoner DP, White MV, et al.: Pattern of nasal secretions during experimental influenza virus infection. Rhinology 1996, 34:2–8.

6. Turner RB, Witek TJ, Riker DK: Comparison of symptom severity in natural and experimentally induced colds. Am J Rhinol 1996, 10(3):167–172.

7. Doyle WJ, Skoner DP, Hayden F, et al.: Nasal and otologic effects of experimental influenza A virus infection. Ann Otol Rhinol Laryngol 1994,103:59–69.

8. Alper C, Doyle W, Skoner D, et al.: Prechallenge antibodies moderate disease expression in adults experimentally exposed to rhinovirus strain Hanks. Clin Infect Dis 1998, 27:119–128.

9. Skoner DP, Whiteside TL, Wilson JW, et al.: Effect of rhinovirus 39 (RV-39) infection on immune parameters in allergic and non-allergic subjects. J Allergy Clin Immunol 1993, 92:732–743.

10. Naclerio RM, Proud D, Lichtenstein LM, et al.: Kinins are generated during experimental rhinovirus colds. J Infect Dis 1988, 157:133–142.

11. Gentile DA, Patel A, Doyle WJ, et al.: Elevations of local leukotriene C4 levels during experimental viral upper respiratory infections. Am J Respir Crit Car Med 2000, 161:A179.

12. Gentile D, Doyle W, Whiteside T, et al.: Increased IL-6 levels in nasal lavage samples following experimental influenza A virus infection. Clin Diagn Lab Immunol 1998, 5:604–608.

13.•• Skoner DP, Gentile DA, Patel A, Doyle WJ: Evidence for cytokine mediation of symptoms in adults experimentally infected with influenza A virus. J Infect Dis 1999, 180:10–14.
This study demonstrates an association between viral replication, local IL-6 production, and symptom expression during experimental infection of adults with influenza A virus. These results suggest that IL-6 may have a role in mediating symptoms and signs of infection during influenza A infection.

TABLE 7-4. ADVERSE EFFECTS OF DECONGESTANTS

Central nervous system
  Stimulation
  Headache
Cardiac
  Tachycardia
  Palpitations
  Arrhythmias
  Hypertension
Others
  Nausea
  Vomiting
  Urinary retention

14. Doyle WJ, Boehm S, Skoner DP: Physiologic responses to intranasal dose-response challenges with histamine, methacholine, bradykinin and prostaglandin in adult volunteers with and without nasal allergy. *J Allergy Clin Immunol* 1990, 86:924–935.

15. Douglass JA, Dhami D, Gurr CE, et al.: Influence of interleukin-8 challenge in the nasal mucosa in atopic and nonatopic subjects. *Am J Respir Crit Care Med* 1994, 150:1108–1113.

16. Gentile DA, Yokitis J, Angelini BL, et al.: Effect of intranasal challenge with IL-6 on airway symptomatology and physiology in allergic and non-allergic subjects. *Ann Allergy Asthma Immunol* 2000, 84:130.

17. Doyle WJ, McBride TP, Skoner DP, et al.: A double-blind placebo-controlled clinical trial of the effect of chlorpheniramine on the response of the nasal airway, ME and eustachian tube to provocative rhinovirus challenge. *J Pediatr Inf Dis* 1988, 7:229–238.

18. Skoner DP, Fireman PF, Doyle WJ: Urine histamine metabolite elevations during experimental colds. *J Allergy Clin Immunology* 1997, 99:S419.

19. Higgins PG, Barrow GI, Tyrrell DA: A study of the efficacy of the bradykinin antagonist, NPC 567, in rhinovirus infections in human volunteers. *Antiviral Res* 1990, 14(6):339–344.

20. Bisgaard H, Olsson P, Bende M: Effect of leukotriene D4 on nasal mucosal blood flow, nasal airway resistance and nasal secretion in humans. *Clin Allergy* 1986, 16:289–297.

21. Kaul P, Singh I, Turner R: Effect of nitric oxide on rhinovirus replication and virus-induced IL-8 elaboration. *Am J Respir Crit Care Med* 1999, 159:1193–1198.

22. Yuta A, Doyle WJ, Gaumond E, et al.: Rhinovirus infection induces mucus hypersecretion. *Am J Physiol* 1998, 274:L1017–L1023.

23. Einarsson O, Geba GP, Zhu Z, et al.: Interleukin-11: stimulation in vivo and in vitro by respiratory viruses and induction of airway hyperresponsiveness. *J Clin Invest* 1996, 97:915–924.

24. Mullol J, Chowdoury BA, White MV, et al.: Endothelin in human nasal mucosa. *Am J Respir Cell Mol Biol* 1993, 8:393–402.

25. Mosimann BL, White MV, Hohman RJ, et al.: Substance P, calcitonin-gene related peptide, and vasoactive intestinal peptide increase in nasal secretions after allergen challenge in atopic patients. *J Allergy Clin Immunol* 1993, 92:95–104.

26.•• Hayden FG, Fritz R, Lobo MC, et al.: Local and systemic cytokine responses during experimental human influenza A virus infection: relation to symptom formation and host defense. *J Clin Invest* 1998, 101:643–649.
This study examines serial levels of cytokines in nasal lavage fluid, serum, and plasma in adults experimentally infected with influenza A virus. The results support a role for IL-6 and interferon-α in the development of symptoms and host defense during influenza infection.

27. Pitkaranta A, Nokso-Koivisto J, Jantti V, et al.: Lowered yields of virus-induced interferon production in leukocyte cultures and risk of recurrent respiratory infections in children. *J Clin Virol* 1999, 14:199–205.

28. Tang YW, Graham BS: Anti-IL-4 treatment at immunization modulates cytokine expression, reduces illness, and increases cytotoxic T lymphocyte activity in mice challenged with respiratory syncytial virus. *J Clin Invest* 1994, 94:1953–1958.

29. Raza M, Essery S, Weir D, et al.: Infection with respiratory syncytial virus and water-soluble components of cigarette smoke alter production of TNF-α and nitric oxide by human blood monocytes. *FEMS Immunol Med Microbiol* 1999, 24:387–394.

30. Matsuda K, Tsutsumi H, Okamoto Y, Chiba C: Development of IL-6 and TNF-α activity in nasopharyngeal secretions of infants and children during infection with respiratory syncytial virus. *Clin Diag Lab Immunol* 1995, 2:322–324.

31. Hornsleth A, Klug B, Nir M, et al.: Severity of respiratory syncytial virus disease related to type and genotype of virus and to cytokine values in nasopharyngeal secretions. *Pediatr Infect Dis J* 1998, 17:1114–1121.

32. Subauste MC, Jacoby DB, Richards SM, Proud D: Infection of a human respiratory epithelial line with rhinovirus: induction of cytokine release and modulation of susceptibility to infection by cytokine exposure. *J Clin Invest* 1995, 96:549–557.

33.•• Yoon HJ, Zhu Z, Gwaltney JM, Elias JA: Rhinovirus regulation of IL-1 receptor antagonist in vivo and in vitro: a potential mechanism of symptom resolution. *J Immunol* 1999, 162:7461–7469.
This study examines the mechanism of disease resolution during rhinovirus infection. The results suggest that IL-1ra may play an important role in the resolution of rhinovirus infection.

34. Turner RB, Weingand KWQ, Yeh CH, Leedy DW: Association between interleukin-8 concentration in nasal secretions and severity of symptoms of experimental rhinovirus colds. *Clin Exp Allergy* 1995, 25:46–49.

35. Borish L, Aarons A, Rumbyrt J, et al.: Interleukin-10 regulation in normal subjects and patients with asthma. *J Allergy Clin Immunol* 1996, 97:1288–1296.

36. Gentile DA, Patel A, Ollila C, et al.: Diminished IL-10 production in subjects with allergy after infection with influenza A virus. *J Allergy Clin Immunol* 1999, 103:1045–1048.

37. Swiergiel AH, Smagin GN, Johnson LJ, Dunn AJ: The role of cytokines in the behavioral responses to endotoxin and influenza virus infection in mice: effects of acute and chronic administration of the interleukin-1 receptor antagonist (IL-1ra). *Brain Res* 1997, 776:96–104.

38.•• Mira J, Cariou A, Grall F, Delclaux C: Association of TNF2, a TNF-α promoter polymorphism, with septic shock and susceptibility to mortality. *JAMA* 1999, 282:561–568.
This study reports a higher frequency of TNF2, a polymorphism associated with high production of TNF-α, in individuals with septic shock compared with the general population. This study also shows increased concentrations of TNF-α in subjects with this polymorphism. It is conceivable that this polymorphism is associated with increased susceptibility to viral rhinitis and its complications.

39. Sawyer LA: Antibodies for the prevention and treatment of viral diseases. *Antiviral Res* 2000, 47(2):57–77.

40. Deguchi Y, Takusugi Y: Efficacy of influenza vaccine in the elderly: reduction in risks of mortality and morbidity during an influenza A (H3N2) epidemic for the elderly in nursing homes. *Int J Clin Lab Res* 2000, 30(1):1–4.

41. Doyle WJ, Skoner DP, Alper CM, et al.: Effect of rimantadine treatment on clinical manifestations and otologic complications in adults experimentally infected with influenza A (H1N1) virus. *J Infect Dis* 1998, 177:1260–1265.

42. Hayden FG, Hay AJ: Emergence and transmission of influenza A viruses resistant to amantadine and rimantadine. *Curr Top Microbiol Immunol* 1992, 176:119–1130.

43. Gwaltney JM Jr, Park J, Paul RA, et al.: Randomized controlled trial of clemastine fumarate for treatment of experimental rhinovirus colds. *Clin Infect Dis* 1996, 22:656–662.

44. Gentile DA, Friday G, Skoner DP: Management of rhinitis: antihistamines and decongestants. In *Immunology and Allergy Clinics of North America*. Edited by Vassallo J. Philadelphia:W.B. Saunders Company; 2000:355–368.

45.•• Dykewicz MS, Fineman S, Skoner DP, et al.: Diagnosis and management of rhinitis: parameter documents of the joint task force on practice parameters for allergy, asthma and immunology. *Ann Allergy Asthma Immunol* 1998, 36:2992–3000.
This document contains complete guidelines for diagnosis and management of rhinitis developed by the Joint Task Force on Practice Parameters in Allergy, Asthma and Immunology. It includes a review of clinical characterizations and diagnosis of different forms of rhinitis, recommendations on evaluation, and parameters on management, including pharmacologic therapy. Guidelines are also presented on special considerations in patient subsets (children, the elderly, and pregnant women).

46.   Berkowitz RB, Tinkelman DG: Evaluation of oral terfenadine for treatment of the common cold. *Ann Allergy* 1991, 67:593–597.

47.   Paolieri F, Battifora M, Riccio AM, *et al.*: Terfenadine and fexofenadine reduce in vitro ICAM-1 expression on human continuous cell lines. *Ann Allergy Asthma Immunol* 1998, 81:610–607.

48.   Garabedian EN: Effect of loratadine syrup in the treatment of otitis media with effusion (OME): a randomized, double blind, placebo controlled trial. *J Allergy Clin Immunol* 1999, 103:S255.

49.   Dockhorn R: A double-blind, placebo-controlled study of the safety and efficacy of ipratropium bromide nasal spray versus placebo in patients with the common cold. *J Allergy Clin Immunol* 1992, 90:1076–1082.

50.• Prasad AS, Fitzgerald JT, Bao B, *et al.*: Duration of symptoms and plasma cytokine levels in patients with the common cold treated with zinc acetate: a randomized, double-blind, placebo-controlled trial. *Ann Intern Med* 2000, 133:245–252.
This randomized, double-blind, placebo-controlled trial examines the efficacy of zinc in reducing the duration of symptoms of the common cold. Administration of zinc was associated with reduced duration and severity of cold symptoms, especially cough.

CHAPTER 8

Differential Diagnosis of Chronic Rhinitis at Various Ages

John W. Georgitis

The prevalence and differential diagnosis of rhinitis changes as we progress from birth to senescence. The heavy burden of allergic rhinitis is often overlooked in infants and disregarded in childhood and adolescence. In women, especially in pregnancy, hormonal changes can significantly affect nasal mucosal hyperreactivity and worsen ongoing syndromes. Various types of inflammatory and noninflammatory nonallergic rhinitides become more prevalent in the fifth decade and beyond. The burgeoning elderly population with irritant, atrophic, and medication-related rhinitis will constitute a greater proportion of our practices as the general population ages.

INTRODUCTION

Rhinitis is one of the most common chronic disorders worldwide, affecting all age groups from infancy to the elderly [1–3]. Allergens are the major cause of symptoms; however, other conditions should be considered when evaluating patients with chronic nasal complaints, especially coexisting disorders such as asthma, sinusitis, and atopic dermatitis [4••]. Chronic rhinitis symptoms are often associated with dentofacial abnormalities, otitis, and behavior difficulties in children. Chronic rhinitis also affects cognitive function [5–7,8••] and quality of life.

Based on the age group, certain factors and conditions alter the differential diagnosis for the patient with nasal complaints such as atopic dermatitis in infants, asthma in young adults and adolescents, or atropic rhinitis in the elderly [9,10]. Food-induced rhinitis symptoms are now appreciated as causative agents in some individuals. Occupational exposure to allergens and irritants also play an important role for working adults and students [11]. Lastly, because all practitioners face an aging population, the role of medications used to treat other chronic conditions must be considered in the elderly patient with rhinitis symptoms.

In the United States, the prevalence of rhinitis ranges from 4% to 40%. In Japan the cumulative prevalence in first-graders is 17.6%, which did not change from 1981 to 1995 [2,12,13]. In Italy, studies of adults 20 to 44 years of age showed that the prevalence of allergic rhinitis, or hay fever, was 16.7%, with no differences related to sex or age [14]. In England, 16.9% of individuals aged more than 14 years reported the symptom of "nasal obstruction every day for more than 14 days" [15]. In this survey, 19.8% of respondents noted having "runny nose," 7.1% reported "bouts of sneezing," and 19.6% noted "hay fever." Rhinosinusitis—defined by at least two out of the three symptoms of congestion, rhinorrhea, and sneezing for more than 1 hour per day for at least 2 weeks—was noted by 13.7%, and 8.6% stated that they had perennial symptoms. Thus, a significant proportion of the population has chronic nasal symptoms.

The environment plays an important role in the development of chronic rhinitis symptoms [16]. The location of one's home and work is extremely significant, as are exposure to tobacco smoke, air pollution, animal dander, and humidity conditions [17–19]. In a Swiss study of childhood allergies, children living on farms had lower rates of sneezing compared with their peers who did not live on farms. The allergen type and exposure are also important factors. For example, sensitivity to olea, a minor allergen, requires higher pollen concentrations than does sensitivity to grass pollens [20].

Parents and family genetics play an important role in the development of allergic conditions. There is an association of birth month, social class, and birth order with the development of rhinitis [21,22]. In contrast, maternal smoking is associated with wheezing but not rhinitis symptoms. In Japanese familial studies, parental allergy (rhinitis, asthma, or eczema) was associated with a 15% prevalence with a relative risk ratio of 2.4 [23]; however, there was no specific association with the allergic condition in the offspring and that in the parent.

The cost of rhinitis is significant. The cost for patients with a primary diagnosis of allergic rhinoconjunctivitis is 1.9 billion US dollars per year (1996 estimate); there is an additional 4.0 billion dollars in cost when allergic rhinitis is a secondary diagnosis [24]. When allergic rhinitis is comorbid with anxiety or depression, the average outpatient health care expenditures are $207 and $363 per year per patient, respectively [25].

This chapter discusses patient groups arbitrarily divided by age: infants are aged less than 3 years, children are aged 3 to 12 years, adolescents are aged 12 to 21 years, adults are aged 21 to 55 years, and the elderly are aged more than 55 years. This chapter also discusses hormone-associated rhinitis conditions.

Several diagnostic studies are used to evaluate the patient with rhinitis. Most important are patient history (specific nasal symptoms; location, severity, frequency, and seasonality of symptoms; associated airway conditions; quality-of-life assessments; and home, work, and school environment) and physical examination [26]. Allergen skin testing (prick, intradermal, and patch) remains the classic study for the rhinitis patients; in selected individuals, serologic studies for allergen-specific IgE (radioallergoabsorbent testing [RAST]) may be needed. Other diagnostic studies include simple nasal smear of the nasal secretions (looking for eosinophils and other cellular components), serum IgE titer, and quantitative immunoglobulins. Imaging studies of the upper airway and contiguous structures may be indicated. Other useful diagnostic studies used for the complex or complicated rhinitis patient are nasal peak flow, rhinomanometry, acoustic rhinometry, olfactory threshold, and measures of mucociliary function.

INFANTS

Infants are unique because of their nasal function and size. In an Italian study of young children, 35% had allergic rhinitis by the first year of life, with an additional 5% by age 2 to 5 years. Infants are obligate nasal breathers and are often referred to as "rug rats" because of their tendency to crawl on floors and carpets, which results in close proximity to the carpet allergens. Infants have functional sinus cavities at birth, so development of sinusitis is possible despite the young age. Lastly, foods are often implicated as causative agents for rhinitis symptoms, especially if there is a concomitant skin disorder such as atopic dermatitis.

The differential diagnosis in infants includes allergic rhinitis due to common allergens such as house dust mite, cockroach, molds, animal dander, and food. In older infants, seasonal allergens may be considered (ie, grasses, tree pollens, and weed pollen). Gastroesophageal reflux disease (GERD) should be considered, even in the absence of a significant history of vomiting. Frequent rhinitis complaints in infants may be due to infection by viral or bacterial agents. Anatomical abnormalities—such as tracheoesophageal fistula, laryngotracheomalacia, deviated septum, and choanal atresia or narrowing—should be considered. Swallowing dysfunction may exist in which liquids reflux into the posterior nasopharynx. Cystic fibrosis with early nasal polyp development and immunodeficiency of the antibody production lines should also be considered.

Diagnostic studies for infants are limited. They include skin testing and simple imaging studies such as a lateral neck radiograph or Waters' view of the paranasal sinuses. Skin testing can be done, but allergen selection is limited by the small size of the patient. A carefully selected panel of eight to 16 allergens can generally identify infants with allergic rhinitis. In selected cases, RAST for foods or perennial allergens may be useful. In this situation, the allergens selected are important and should be the common foods: cow's milk, egg protein, wheat, peanut, soybean, tree nuts, house dust mite, cockroach, or animal danders [27]. In cases where one does not suspect an allergic condition and wishes not to proceed with skin testing, a serum IgE level will be helpful before embarking on skin testing to "rule out" atopy. In addition, a simple nasal smear for eosinophils or neutrophils may help in differentiating allergic from infectious rhinitis. The nasal infiltrate can also contain eosinophils and mast cells in allergic children [28]. Nasal cultures are not warranted and may be misleading because of natural bacterial agents present in the nasal cavity and normal nasal flora. The exception is gonococcal purulent rhinitis.

CHILDREN AND ADOLESCENTS

Children and adolescents comprise one of the major groups affected by allergic rhinitis, and most nasal complaints are due to allergen exposure. However, infectious rhinitis, especially sinusitis and otitis, is still prominent. Viral infections (eg, common rhinoviruses) often lead to rhinitis symptoms as well. Children with allergic rhinitis consistently report lower quality of life than do their nonallergic peers [5]. Their rhinitis leads to embarrassment, frustration with decreased cognitive function, slower psychomotor speed, and decreased verbal learning and memory during the allergy season.

Seasonal allergic and perennial allergic rhinitis are the major diagnoses [29]. Environmental allergens are important, but seasonal allergens now play a more important role. Other conditions to consider include sinusitis, GERD, infectious rhinitis, and, much less commonly, nonallergic rhinitis. Anatomic causes for rhinitis include tonsillar or adenoidal hypertrophy with airway obstruction or narrowing, septal deviation, nasal polyps, and foreign body in the nasal passage. Systemic disorders to consider are cystic fibrosis, midline granuloma, and Wegener's granulomatosis.

The prevalence of allergic rhinitis in British children by age 16 years was 12% in 1958, increasing to 23% in 1970. In children aged 18 years in the United States, the prevalence was 15% to 18% in 1962 to 1965, increasing to 26% in 1976 to 1980 [30]. In a study of Tucson infants, Wright *et al.* [31] reported that 42% of their subjects had physician-diagnosed allergic rhinitis by age 6 years. In contrast, the prevalence of allergic rhinitis by age 7 years is 3.3% in Finland [32]. In desert conditions, a higher sensitization rate was present in children aged 6 to 17 years, compared with adults and the children were sensitized to multiple allergens [33]. The sensitization rate was 77.3% to pollens (*Chenopodium*, Bermuda grass, and prosopis tree), 62.3% to dust mite and cockroach, and 14.7% to molds [34]. Children with atopic dermatitis often develop allergic rhinitis over time. In a study of 94 children with dermatitis, 45% had developed allergic rhinitis by age 7 years [35]. This is a "classic" transition from one allergic target organ to another.

Skin testing, predominantly using the prick method, remains the most fruitful diagnostic study in children and adolescents. A nasal smear for eosinophils may be useful for the skin test–negative individual with significant nasal complaints [36]. Imaging studies, especially a limited coronal sinus CT, should be considered because

of the possibility of concomitant sinusitis. For complex cases, flexible rhinoscopy can be performed to assess the patency of the nasal passage, septal anatomy, and adenoid tissue size.

ADULTS

Adults comprise the largest group with seasonal or perennial allergic rhinitis. Most people report the onset of symptoms before the age of 30 years [37]. In a study in Minnesota, allergic rhinitis was diagnosed before age 25 years in 59% of asthmatic patients, whereas it was diagnosed in less than 15% of patients after age of 40 years [38••]. In a frequently cited study of Brown University students, the incidence of allergic rhinitis at school enrollment was 175 (24%) of 738 students. When examined at age 40 years, an additional 131 (18%) had developed allergic rhinitis [39]. In a Danish study of adults surveyed 8 years apart, there was increased prevalence with time of rhinitis symptoms to seasonal pollens (odds ratio [OR] = 1.6; 95% CI, 1.4 to 1.9), furry animals (OR = 1.6; 95% CI, 1.3 to 2.0), and house dust (OR = 1.3; 95% CI, 1.1 to 1.6). This was independent of sex and age [40].

Seasonal and perennial allergic rhinitis are the major diagnoses [2,41–44]. Other possible conditions include nonallergic rhinitis (often associated with nasal eosinophilia), vasomotor rhinitis, and gustatory rhinitis (food-induced). The infectious conditions include acute and recurrent sinusitis, allergic fungal sinusitis, and eosinophilic mucin sinusitis when there is fungal infection in nonatopic subjects. Other conditions of the nasal tissues include nasal polyposis and rhinitis medicamentosa. Anatomical considerations to consider are nasal neoplastic processes, septal deviations or spurs, and adenoidal hypertrophy. Hypothyroidism, severe GERD, hormonal factors, and systemic disorders such as rheumatoid diseases (eg, systemic lupus erythematosus), and Wegener's granulomatosis are often associated with chronic rhinitis symptoms. Interestingly, 70% of patients with chronic fatigue syndrome or fibromyalgia report having nasal symptoms. Drug-induced rhinitis must also be considered because this age group begins to require chronic medications for other disorders.

Diagnostic studies for adults include classical skin prick testing. Intradermal testing may be needed in patients with classical symptoms but negative prick skin tests. Occupational environmental allergens should be reviewed in detail. RAST and serum IgE tests are helpful but not commonly performed. Imaging studies with sinus CT and barium swallow or pH probe for acid reflux may be indicated for complex or unresponsive cases. Lastly, flexible rhinoscopy in the outpatient setting helps for anatomic or serious conditions such as nasal neoplasms.

THE ELDERLY

With the aging "baby boomer" population, it is estimated that 52 million Americans, 17% of the US population, will be aged 65 or older by 2020. In a recent survey of allergy-immunology specialists, one of every five patients being evaluated is aged more than 55 years, and 6% are aged more than 70 years [45]. Individuals aged in their 80s represent the fastest growing population in the United States. This population presents unique problems.

Fortunately, allergic rhinitis is still a very uncommon rhinitis condition for the elderly. However, skin test reactivity decreases with age and symptoms tend to be milder [46]. The incidence of nonallergic rhinitis as a diagnosis rises with age. In addition, the elderly have changing nasal physiologic function. It is common to see drier nasal mucosa in individuals with a sicca type of condition. They frequently complain of severe congestion without significant turbinate edema and have negative skin tests. Therefore, the diagnosis of "atropic rhinitis" should be entertained in this population but not in the other age groups.

Elderly patients often take multiple and varied daily medications, especially for chronic cardiac and gastrointestinal disorders (*ie*, "polypharmacy" therapy) [47••]. Rhinitis due to medications is a condition for some patients on long-term β-blockers, diuretic therapy for treatment of cardiovascular conditions, and antireflux agents. Rhinitis medicamentosa may be present in patients using chronic nasal sympathomimetics for relief of nasal congestion. This population has financial constraints and socioeconomic issues unique to their age. Often, they are on fixed incomes and use expensive long-term medications for nonnasal conditions. They may also have cognitive dysfunction that affects their ability to remember to use daily medications correctly. Chronic nasal congestion may lead to overuse of topical nasal sympathomimetics, with the development of rhinitis medicamentosa, or oral α-adrenergic agonists, with hypertension or sleep irregularities.

HORMONE-RELATED RHINITIS

Cyclic changes in hormones present a different challenge for the appropriate diagnosis of rhinitis in women. Allergic rhinitis affects approximately one third of women of childbearing age. However, cyclic changes in rhinitis intensity may be related to the changes in relative concentrations of the complex mix of hormones during the menstrual cycle. In nasal provocation experiments, allergic patients on oral contraceptive having grass challenges had less nasal congestion at day 14 of the menstrual cycle but more sneezing at the end of the cycle. Thus, the hormone levels affect nasal reactivity in complex ways [48].

Therefore, for women of childbearing age or who are pregnant, nasal complaints may stem from these mucosal changes of hormonal rhinitis. These hormonal variations worsen or exacerbate active perennial or seasonal allergic rhinitis symptoms as well.

Rhinitis of pregnancy has been attributed to increasing concentrations of female hormones during pregnancy and the need for swollen mucosae with mucous hypersecretion for protection of the vagina and cervix [49••]. Symptoms range from sneezing and itching to severe nasal congestion with profuse rhinorrhea similar to vasomotor rhinitis. Physicians are severely limited in diagnosing and treating rhinitis during pregnancy because of the potential risks to the fetus and mother that are associated with medications. Nasal saline sprays and lavage, topical oxymetazoline, oral pseudoephedrine, and chlorpheniramine are the most widely recommended medications. These choices are not optimal because there are legitimate risks when taking a first-generation, sedating antihistamine such as chlorpheniramine and driving or using other equipment. Allergy testing is generally deferred because of the remote (1:1000) risk of anaphylaxis during testing. Allergy shots may be continued; some allergists maintain the same dose throughout the pregnancy or cut the dose in half. If pregnancy and rhinitis are complicated by asthma, then shots may have to be discontinued because of the risk of inducing acute asthmatic reactions.

CONCLUSIONS

Special nasal conditions that mimic allergic rhinitis may be present in each age group. However, seasonal and perennial allergic rhinitis remain the most common diagnoses for the patient with chronic nasal complaints.

REFERENCES AND RECOMMENDED READING

Papers of particular interest, published recently, have been highlighted as:

- • Of importance
- •• Of major importance

1.　Rachelefsky GS: National guidelines needed to manage rhinitis and prevent complications. *Ann Allergy Asthma Immunol* 1999, 82:296–305.

2.　The American Academy of Allergy, Asthma & Immunology: The Allergy Report. Milwaukee: American Academy of Allergy, Asthma & Immunology; 2000. [http://www.theallergyreport.org/]

3.　Dykewicz MS, Fineman S: Executive Summary of Joint Task Force Practice Parameters on Diagnosis and Management of Rhinitis. *Ann Allergy Asthma Immunol* 1998, 81:463–468.

4.•• Fireman P: Rhinitis and asthma connection: management of coexisting upper airway allergic diseases and asthma. *Allergy Asthma Proc* 2000, 21:45–54.
This article reviews the association of upper and lower airway diseases at various ages and details their significance.

5. Marshall PS, O'Hara C, Steinberg P: Effects of seasonal allergic rhinitis on selected cognitive abilities. *Ann Allergy Asthma Immunol* 2000, 84:403–410.

6. Blaiss MS: Quality of life in allergic rhinitis. *Ann Allergy Asthma Immunol* 1999, 83:449–454.

7. Settipane RA: Complications of allergic rhinitis. *Allergy Asthma Proc* 1999, 20:209–213.

8.•• Blaiss MS: Cognitive, social and economic costs of allergic rhinitis. *Allergy Asthma Proc* 2000, 21:7–13.
The cognitive costs of allergic rhinitis, particularly to school children, are outlined.

9. Hadley JA: Evaluation and management of allergic rhinitis. *Med Clin North Am* 1999, 83:13–25.

10. Dykewicz MS, Fineman S, Skoner DP, *et al.*: Diagnosis and management of rhinitis: complete guidelines of the Joint Task Force on Practice Parameters in Allergy, Asthma and Immunology. *Ann Allergy Asthma Immunol* 1998, 81:478–518.

11. Benninger MS: The impact of cigarette smoking and environmental tobacco smoke on nasal and sinus disease: a review of the literature. *Am J Rhinol* 1999, 13:435–438.

12. Schoenwetter WF: Allergic rhinitis: epidemiology and natural history. *Allergy Asthma Proc* 2000, 21:1–6.

13. Matsumoto I, Odajima H, Nishima S, *et al.*: Change in prevalence of allergic diseases in primary school children in Fukuoka City for the last fifteen years. *Jpn J Allergol* 1999, 48:435–442.

14. Campello C, Ferrari M, Poli A, *et al.*: Prevalence of asthma and asthma-like symptoms in an adult population sample from Verona. *Monaldi Arch Chest Dis* 1998, 53:505–509.

15. Jones NS, Smith PA, Carney AS, Davis A: The prevalence of allergic rhinitis and nasal symptoms in Nottingham. *Clin Otolaryngol* 1998, 23:547–554.

16. Braun-Fahrlander C, Gassner M, Grize L, *et al.*: Prevalence of hay fever and allergic sensitization in farmers' children and their peers living in the same rural community. *Clin Exp Allergy* 1999, 29:28–34.

17. Leino T, Tammilehto L, Hytonen M, *et al.*: Occupational skin and respiratory diseases among hairdressers. *Scand J Work Environ Health* 1998, 24:398–406.

18. Hauschuldt P, Molhave L, Kjaergaard SK: Reactions of healthy persons and persons suffering from allergic rhinitis when exposed to office dust. *Scand J Work Environ Health* 1999, 25:442–449.

19. Keles N, Ilicali C, Deger K: The effects of different levels of air pollution on atopy and symptoms of allergic rhinitis. *Am J Rhinol* 1999, 13:185–190.

20. Florido JF, Delgado PG, de San Pedro BS, *et al.*: High levels of Olea europaea pollen and relation with clinical findings. *Internat Arch Allergy Immunol* 1999, 119:133–137.

21. Vovolis V, Grigoreas C, Galatas I, Vourdas D: Is month of birth a risk factor for subsequent development of pollen allergy in adults. *Allergy Asthma Proc* 1999, 20:15–22.

22. Lewis SA, Britton JR: Consistent effects of high socioeconomic status and low birth order, and the modifying effect of maternal smoking on the risk of allergic disease during childhood. *Respir Med* 1998, 92:1237–1244.

23. Matsuoka S, Nakagawa R, Nakayama H, *et al.*: Prevalence of specific allergic diseases in school children as related to parental atopy. *Peds International* 1999, 41:46–51.

24. Ray NF, Baraniuk JN, Thamer M, *et al.*: Direct expenditures for the treatment of allergic rhinoconjunctivitis in 1996 including the contributions of related airway illnesses. *J Allergy Clin Immunol* 1999, 103:401–407.

25. Cuffel B, Wamboldt M, Borish L, *et al.*: Economic consequences of comorbid depression, anxiety and allergic rhinitis. *Psychosomatics* 1999, 40:491–496.

26. Lund V: Allergic rhinitis—making the correct diagnosis. *Clin Exp Allergy* 1998, 28:25–28.

27. Cantani A: The growing genetic links and the early onset of atopic diseases in children stress the unique role of the atopic march: a meta-analysis. *J Investig Allergol Clin Immunol* 1999, 9:314–320.

28. Vinke JG, KleinJan A, Severijnen LW, *et al.*: Differences in nasal cellular infiltrates between allergic children and age-matched controls. *Eur Resp J* 1999, 13:797–803.

29. Fireman P: Therapeutic approach to allergic rhinitis: treating the child. *J Allergy Clin Immunol* 2000, 105:S616–S621.

30. Sly RM: Changing prevalence of allergic rhinitis and asthma. *Ann Allergy Asthma Immunol* 1999, 82:233–248.

31. Wright A, Holberg CJ, Martinez FD, *et al.*: Epidemiology of physician-diagnosed allergic rhinitis in childhood. *Pediatrics* 1994, 94:895–901.

32. Xu B, Jarvelin MR, Pekkanen J: Prenatal factors and occurrence of rhinitis and eczema among offspring. *Allergy* 1999, 54:829–836.

33. Katz Y, Verleger H, Barr J, *et al.*: Indoor survey of moulds and prevalence of mould atopy in Israel. *Clin Exp Allergy* 1999, 29:186–192.

34. Dowaisan A, Al-Ali S, Khan M, *et al.*: Sensitization to aeroallergens among patients with allergic rhinitis in a desert environment. *Ann Allergy Asthma Immunol* 2000, 84:433–438.

35. Gustafsson D, Sjorberg O, Foucard T: Development of allergies and asthma in infants and young children with atopic dermatitis—a prospective follow-up to 7 years of age. *Allergy* 2000, 55:240–245.

36. Okano M, Nishizaki M, Kawarai Y, *et al.*: Prevalence and prediction of allergic rhinitis using questionnaire and nasal smear examination in school children. *Acta Otolaryngol Suppl* 1999, 540:58–63.

37. Corren J: Allergic rhinitis: treating the adult. *J Allergy Clin Immunol* 2000, 105:S610–615.

38.•• Yawn BP, Yunginger JW, Wollan PC, *et al.*: Allergic rhinitis in Rochester, Minnesota residents with asthma: frequency and impact on health care charges. *J Allergy Clin Immunol* 1999, 103:54–59.
This article outlines the consequences and interactions of allergic rhinitis at the health care interface.

39. Greisner WA, Settipane RJ, Settipane GA: Natural history of hay fever: a 23-year follow-up of college students. *Allergy Asthma Proc* 1998, 19:271–275.

40. Linneberg A, Nielsen NH, Madsen F, *et al.*: Increasing prevalence of allergic rhinitis in an adult Danish population. Allergy 1999, 54:1194–1198.

41. Wu LY, Steidle GM, Meador MA, *et al.*: Effect of tree and grass pollens and fungal spores on spring allergic rhinitis: a comparative study. *Ann Asthma Allergy Immunol* 1999, 83:137–143.

42. Shiomori T, Yoshida S, Miyamoto H, Makishima K: Relationship of nasal carriage of Staphylococcus aureus to pathogenesis of perennial allergic rhinitis. *J Allergy Clin Immunol* 2000, 105:449–454.

43. Gurkan F, Ece A, Haspolat K, Dikici B: Parental history of migraine and bronchial asthma in children. *Allergol Immunopathol* 2000, 28:15–17.

44. Baraniuk JN, Clauw D, Yuta A, *et al.*: Nasal secretion analysis in allergic rhinitis, cystic fibrosis, and nonallergic fibromyalgia/chronic fatigue syndrome subjects. *Am J Rhinol* 1998, 12:435–440.

45.   Lang DM, Visintainer PF, Howland WC, *et al.*: Survey of the
       extent and nature of care for adults and older adults by aller-
       gy/immunology practitioners. *Ann Asthma Allergy Immunol*
       2000, 85:106–110.

46.   Simola M, Holopainene E, Malmberg H: Changes in skin and
       nasal sensitivity to allergens and the course of rhinitis; a long
       term follow-up study. *Ann Asthma Allergy Immunol* 1999,
       82:152–156.

47.•• Montanaro A: Allergic disease management in the elderly: a
       wakeup call for the allergy community. *Ann Asthma Allergy
       Immunol* 2000, 85:85–86.
       *The growing elderly population presents unique rhinitis and sinusitis
       problems for allergists and primary care providers alike.*

48.   Stubner UP, Gruber D, Berger UE, *et al.*: The influence of
       female sex hormones on nasal reactivity in seasonal allergic
       rhinitis. *Allergy* 1999, 54:865–871.

49.•• Mazzotta P, Lorbstein R, Koren G: Treating allergic rhinitis in
       pregancy: safety considerations. *Drug Safety* 1999,
       20:361–375.
       *This important review describes the risks of allergy therapies in
       pregnancy.*

CHAPTER 9

Pediatric Rhinitis

William E. Berger

Epidemiologic and pathophysiologic evidence indicate that allergic rhinitis, whether seasonal or perennial, is one piece of a larger atopic clinical picture that often occurs concomitantly with asthma. Allergic rhinitis usually develops during childhood and has a prevalence of up to 40% in the pediatric population. Careful attention to food allergies and the presence of household allergens during infancy and early childhood may limit potential sensitization. Optimal management of allergic rhinitis with antihistamines and topical corticosteroids may improve quality of life and curtail the development of serious sequelae.

INTRODUCTION

Allergic rhinitis is the most common chronic condition in the pediatric population, affecting 20% to 40% of children [1]. Of the 40 million people in the United States estimated to suffer from this IgE-mediated nasal disorder, approximately 6 million are children [2]. Allergic rhinitis usually develops before 20 years of age, with a mean onset between 8 and 11 years [3].

The personal and societal impact of allergic rhinitis is staggering. Overall estimates of the direct and indirect costs of allergic rhinitis in the United States in 1996 were $5.3 billion [4••]. In children, more than 2 million absentee school days can be attributed to allergic rhinitis each year. The disorder impairs cognitive functioning, which can be further impaired by the use of first-generation antihistamines [4••]. Children with allergic rhinitis also are more likely to exhibit shyness, depression, anxiety, and fearfulness than other children, and their inability to sleep soundly may have deleterious effects on both school performance and self-esteem [5••].

The morbidity of allergic rhinitis can be substantial, considering that half the patients experience symptoms for more than 4 months each year and 20% are symptomatic for at least 9 months of the year [4••]. In addition to the characteristic nasal inflammation that may be accompanied by a constellation of symptoms including rhinorrhea, nasal congestion, pruritus, postnasal drip, and sneezing, many allergic rhinitis patients experience headache and fatigue. Chronic nasal obstruction can cause severe complications in children, and the excessive mouth breathing results in facial abnormalities such as retrognathic maxilla and mandible, increased facial length, high arched palate, and dental malocclusions [6•]. Allergic rhinitis is associated with conjunctivitis, loss of olfaction and taste, sleep apnea, an increased frequency of asthma, and two conditions, otitis media and sinusitis, that result from the respective obstruction of the eustachian tube and sinus ostia [6•].

CHARACTERISTICS OF ALLERGIC RHINITIS

In addition to serving as a conduit for air, the nose processes air by humidifying, warming, and filtering it. It also provides olfaction, vocal resonation, and initial microbial defense mechanisms [6•]. Allergic rhinitis is an IgE-mediated reaction provoked by either seasonal or perennial airborne allergens. Although seasonal allergens vary with geographic location, the most common seasonal allergens in temperate climates are pollens and molds. Generally, tree pollens produce symptoms in the spring, grass pollens trigger rhinitis in the early summer, and ragweed pollen is problematic in the late summer. Approximately 75% of allergic rhinitis patients are sensitive to ragweed pollen (hay fever), 40% are sensitive to grass pollen, and 9% are sensitive to tree pollen [7••]. Perennial allergens commonly include dust mites, molds, cockroaches, and animal saliva and dander continually present in the indoor environment. Depending upon the provoking allergen(s), patients may be symptomatic throughout the year, exclusively during certain seasons, perennially with seasonal exacerbations, or sporadically after encountering specific allergens.

Allergic rhinitis is a prototype of IgE-mediated disease, manifesting as a biphasic response to both seasonal and perennial allergens. The immediate or early phase reaction occurs within minutes of exposure to an aeroallergen, beginning with sneezing followed by an increase in nasal secretions [6•,8,9]. After 5 minutes, reduced airflow develops as a result of mucosal swelling. These acute symptoms abate within 1 hour [9]. The recurrence of symptoms 4 to 8 hours later is referred to as the late-phase reaction.

Continued exposure to allergens leads to chronic inflammatory changes within the nasal mucosa, producing an effect more profound than acute nasal symptoms. The consequences are hyperirritability of the turbinates, characterized by enhanced sensitivity to all exacerbants of rhinitis (aeroallergens and irritants), and priming, where the dose of allergen required to produce symptoms is greatly diminished [6•,8]. Chronic inflammation of the upper airways is also associated with pathophysiologic changes in the epithelial lining, manifesting as epithelial cell proliferation following prolonged allergen exposure [8].

The clinical changes in the early- and late-phase reactions are choreographed by the release of numerous mediators and the influx of inflammatory cells. Upon re-exposure of an atopic patient to inhaled allergens, the cross-linking of specific IgE molecules on the surface of nasal mast cells triggers the release of chemical mediators, including histamine, leukotrienes, prostaglandins,

tryptase, and kinins (Table 9-1) [9,10]. These chemical mediators cause physiologic changes in the upper airway that manifest as acute symptoms: congestion resulting from mucosal permeability, vasodilation, and edema; increased mucous secretion; and rhinorrhea, pruritus, and sneezing resulting from disturbances in the autonomic nervous control of nasal function that lead to cholinergic predominance [2,4••,8–12]. Many of these symptoms are mediated by the binding of histamine to H_1 receptors located on mast cells, mucous-secreting cells, subepithelial blood vessels, and nerve endings [11]. The release of chemotactic factors and the increased number of adhesion molecules on the vascular endothelium, which bind circulating cells called to the site by the chemotactic agents, together trigger an influx of inflammatory cells into the nasal mucosa and submucosa [6•,8,11]. Within 3 hours of allergen challenge, there is a rich infiltration of eosinophils, neutrophils, basophils, and T-helper cells, eliciting the late-phase reaction [4••,13].

The T-helper cells serve as a source of cytokines that amplify and regulate local immune responses, although they also may induce the hypothalamus to promote fatigue, malaise, irritability, and cognitive impairment [4••]. Of the two classes of T-helper cells that have been identified (T_H1 cells that affect cell-mediated immunity and T_H2 cells that control humoral, or antibody, responses), the predominant lymphocytes present in allergic mucosal inflammation are the T_H2 cells [8,11]. Biopsy and bronchial lavage studies demonstrate that T-cells from atopic individuals are biased toward secreting cytokines from T_H2 cells, while nonatopic individuals secrete more cytokines from T_H1 cells [14•]. The effects of the T_H2 cytokines, including IL-4 and IL-5, are counteracted by the T_H1 cytokines, which induce a protective proinflammatory response [14•].

PREVALENCE AND NATURAL HISTORY OF ATOPY

The natural history of atopic disease frequently begins with atopic dermatitis and food allergy in infancy and early childhood and progresses to allergic rhinitis and/or atopic asthma [4••,15]. The overall incidence of allergic rhinitis increases from 10% in childhood to 30% during adolescence, reaching its height between the ages of 12 and 15 [16,17]. The mean age of onset of seasonal allergic rhinitis (10.6 years) is slightly older than that for perennial allergic rhinitis (9.1 years) [3]. Symptoms tend to worsen for the first two or three seasons, after which time disease severity usually stabilizes, generally improving in middle age. In approximately 20% of cases, symptoms disappear during childhood [7••]. In this respect, allergic rhinitis differs significantly from asthma, since the incidence of asthma is highest during the first years of life and most affected children experience their first asthmatic episode before 3 years of age [7••]. Nevertheless, both asthma and allergic rhinitis are atopic responses of the airways to airborne allergens and their incidences have continued to rise despite improved management.

Recent epidemiologic studies indicate that the prevalence of allergic disease in general is increasing in children and adolescents. For example, a study of 18-year-old Swedish military conscripts showed that the prevalence of allergic rhinitis rose from 4.4% in 1971 to 8.4% in 1981 [18]. In the same time period, the prevalence of asthma increased from 1.9% to 2.8%. Similarly, in the 20-year period beginning in 1971, the prevalence of allergic rhinitis and asthma tripled in Finnish adolescents, allergic rhinitis increasing from 5.0% to 14.9%, and asthma increasing from 1.0% to 2.8% [19]. In the United States, the prevalence of asthma in 6- to 11-year-olds rose from 4.8% in 1974 to 7.6% in 1988 [20].

Mounting evidence indicates that the conditions under which an allergen is encountered in infancy may have lifelong effects on atopy [21]. There appears to be a critical period during early infancy when an individual genetically predisposed to atopy is at greater risk of sensitization upon exposure to food or aeroallergens [4••,21]. Risk factors for developing allergic rhinitis include early exposure to perennial aeroallergens and a family history of atopy [21]. Compared to a 13% frequency of developing atopic disease when neither parent is atopic, children with one atopic parent develop allergies with a frequency of 29% and tend to be symptomatic later in life; children with two atopic parents develop allergies with a frequency of 47% and tend to be symptomatic in childhood. The risk of atopy increases to nearly 72% when both parents have the same atopic manifestation [5••,7••].

A SPECTRUM OF AIRWAY DISORDERS

The link between disorders of the upper and lower airways has long been recognized; numerous studies document the frequent comorbidity of allergic rhinitis, asthma, and sinusitis. Supporting evidence has been drawn from epidemiologic and pathophysiologic data, as well as from the simple observations that asthma and allergic rhinitis share a genetic predisposition for atopy, a continuous respiratory mucosa, and a common inflammatory etiology mediated by the same molecular and cellular constituents.

Epidemiologic surveys indicate that allergic rhinitis is far more common among asthma patients than the general population. Between 60% and 78% of patients with asthma have coexisting allergic rhinitis, compared to a general prevalence of 20% for allergic rhinitis [22–24]. Conversely, between 19% and 38% of patients with allergic rhinitis have coexisting asthma, compared to a prevalence of 3% to 5% for asthma in the general population [22–24]. In a recent study, rhinitis was found to be present in 92.5% of teenage asthmatics; rhinitis began either simultaneously with or before the asthma in 72% [25]. The prevalence of rhinitis also was significantly higher in atopic (98.9%) than in nonatopic (78.4%) individuals. Although the temporal relationship between the onset of rhinitis and asthma has been independently confirmed in other studies conducted in children and adults, the results of a prospective longitudinal study of 694 college freshmen is considered more definitive. Among this population that had no evidence of asthma in 1961, students who reported having symptoms of rhinitis were 3 times more likely (10.5%) to develop asthma during the ensuing 23 years than individuals without rhinitis (3.6%) [26].

Other evidence that suggests a link between upper and lower airway disorders is the occurrence of

TABLE 9-1. CHEMICAL MEDIATORS OF ALLERGIC RHINITIS

Mediator	Pathophysiology	Clinical correlates
Histamine	Vascular permeability	Nasal congestion
	Vasodilatation	Nasal congestion
	Irritated nerve endings	
	Glandular secretion	Sneezing, rhinorrhea
Leukotrienes	Vascular permeability	Nasal congestion
	Vasodilatation	Nasal congestion
	Glandular secretion	Rhinorrhea
Kinins	Vascular permeability	Nasal congestion
	Vasodilatation	Nasal congestion
Chemotactic agents	Influx of inflammatory cells, late phase reaction, nasal hyperresponsiveness	Prolongation and magnification of all symptoms

bronchial hyperreactivity after nasal provocation in rhinitis patients with no evidence of asthma and the beneficial effects of rhinitis therapy on asthma in patients with coexistent disease. Although patients with rhinitis have a greater likelihood of having comorbid asthma, and rhinitis is considered a risk factor for asthma, it has not been possible to predict which rhinitis patients are at greatest risk for developing asthma. Several studies have examined whether enhanced bronchial hyperreactivity after nasal provocation by allergen or methacholine is a harbinger of asthma in rhinitis patients, but the results are still inconclusive [27–29]. However, the beneficial effects of treatment for rhinitis on asthma patient outcomes is unequivocal.

In patients with concomitant disease, topical intranasal corticosteroids, including beclomethasone dipropionate and flunisolide, have been shown to reduce the symptoms of both seasonal allergic rhinitis and asthma as well as hyperresponsiveness of the lower airways [30,31]. Similar beneficial effects of intranasal beclomethasone have been demonstrated for perennial allergic rhinitis and asthma, including a reduction in exercise-induced bronchospasm, even in studies that showed less than 2% drug deposition in the chest [23]. A dramatic improvement in bronchial responsiveness after treatment with intranasal beclomethasone also has been demonstrated in rhinitis patients who do not have asthma, which is all the more poignant since oral inhalation of beclomethasone had no effect [32]. Similar effects on bronchial hyperreactivity have been obtained with second-generation antihistamines [23]. Additionally, both medical and surgical treatment of sinusitis have proven beneficial to asthma outcomes in the pediatric population [33].

Three broad categories of mechanisms have been proposed to account for the link between upper and lower airway disease: 1) neural reflex mechanisms; 2) loss of nasal air conditioning functions; and 3) dissemination mechanisms [23,34]. A nasobronchial reflex mechanism has been suggested, based on the ability of nonspecific nasal irritation (from silica particles, allergen, or histamine) to cause a rapid reflex bronchoconstriction that can be inhibited by atropine [23,34]. A second possible mechanism is the direct result of nasal blockage, a common symptom of rhinitis that often causes a shift from the normal pattern of nasal breathing to mouth breathing. When this occurs, the air that reaches the lower airway is inadequately warmed, filtered, and humidified, potentially leading to a reduction in osmolality similar to that thought to trigger exercise-induced asthma. A third possibility is seeding of the lungs with postnasally drained fluid containing inflammatory mediators and cells. While evidence for the latter mechanism is inconclusive, there is little data to support the notion that systemic communication could account for this mechanism

[34]. It is likely that all three mechanisms contribute to the alterations in lung function present in patients with comorbid asthma and rhinitis.

RECOGNIZING ALLERGIC RHINITIS IN CHILDREN

Diagnosing allergic rhinitis in the pediatric population presents unique challenges. Because children often lack the ability to verbalize their symptoms, the disorder frequently remains undiagnosed and untreated, increasing the potential for developing serious sequelae and detracting from the child's quality of life. It is therefore important that the physician recognize the signs that herald allergic rhinitis. These include the "allergic shiner," a darkening of the lower eyelid due to suborbital edema, the "allergic crease" or Dennie-Morgan's line, a transverse skin line above the tip and below the bridge of the nose caused by constant rubbing, and the "allergic salute," the upward rubbing of the nose with the palm of the hand performed to reduce the itching and open the nasal passages [4••,5••,35•]. Parents also may be aware of the child's nasal voice, constant mouth breathing and chapped lips, frequent snoring, coughing due to postnasal drainage, paroxysmal sneezing, and chronic gaping of the mouth [35•]. In addition to these localized signs, children with allergic rhinitis may exhibit systemic symptoms such as weakness, malaise, irritability, and poor appetite. They may not look well or feel well because of lack of sleep, providing additional clues to the presence of allergic rhinitis.

The diagnostic clues evident upon physical examination do not necessarily indicate an underlying allergic etiology (Table 9-2). Allergy testing is necessary to establish a definitive diagnosis of allergic rhinitis. Inhalant allergens are the most common triggers of allergic rhinitis in children as well as in adults. Seasonal allergens usually do not surface because at least two seasons of exposure are required to elicit sensitization [5••]. Food is a significant source of allergic reaction before 2 or 3 years of age. Perennial inhalant allergens also can trigger allergic responses after several weeks or months of daily exposure in the very young child [5••]. Skin tests for both food allergens and perennial inhalant allergens can be performed in children less than 2 years of age, if clinically indicated, with the proviso that a positive allergy test causes a smaller wheal-and-flare response than in older children and adults due to lower levels of specific IgE [4••,5••,36]. While nasal cytology testing may be helpful, nasal allergen challenge in children is reserved for research purposes only. The levels of nasal eosinophils and basophilic cells (basophilic leukocytes or mast cells) correlate highly with each other in children between 4 months and 7 years of age, with high levels of both suggesting aeroallergen sensitization [4••].

MANAGEMENT OF ALLERGIC RHINITIS

A tripartite approach to the management of allergic rhinitis incorporates environmental control, immunotherapy, and pharmacologic treatment. Although several new drugs are available for children, the first two elements of this management approach are particularly important in children because of their focus on prevention.

Environmental control

Logic dictates that reducing or eliminating the presence of the offending allergen is the first course of treatment. However, in atopic children, families should be instructed about the importance of this step during early infancy and childhood when sensitization first occurs [4••]. As a secondary prevention, the early institution of effective allergen avoidance measures may reduce IgE production and abolish allergic sensitization. For example, early exposure to perennial allergens in the home carries the greatest risk of sensitization, especially in children with a strong family history of atopy. Should sensitization occur, removal of the allergen would require several steps, depending on the offending allergen (Table 9-3).

Immunotherapy

The 1998 World Health Organization position paper on allergen immunotherapy stipulates three clinical indications for immunotherapy in children: 1) IgE-mediated rhinoconjunctivitis; 2) allergic asthma; and 3) severe anaphylactic reactions to *Hymenoptera* stings [37]. Given the existence of any of these indications, there are differing schools of thought regarding immunotherapy in children. Because immunotherapy carries an inherent risk of anaphylaxis, the more conservative approach dictates that immunotherapy is appropriate when complete avoidance of the offending allergen either is not possible or is not successful and pharmacologic treatment has failed.

Another line of reasoning, however, is aimed at changing the potential clinical course of allergic rhinitis in an effort to prevent the development of multiple sensitizations or asthma. In addition, since the morbidity and mortality of rhinitis and asthma continue to rise despite improved pharmacologic management, measures that prevent the initiation and progression of inflammation in the airways may be beneficial. Evidence from preliminary studies indicates that immunotherapy may either trigger a switch from predominantly T_H2 cytokine production to protective T_H1 cytokine production or may induce a state of unresponsiveness to allergen [14•,38•]. The nature of

---

TABLE 9-2. IMPORTANT ELEMENTS OF PATIENT HISTORY

Age of onset
Chronologic variations in symptoms
Exacerbating factors
  Allergens
  Irritants
  Ingestants
Nature of symptoms
  Sneezing
  Congestion
  Postnasal drip
  Pruritus
  Rhinorrhea
Environmental exposure
  Home
  Pets
  Feathers
  Air conditioning, heating
Activities
Medications used to treat rhinitis and patient's response to them
  Topical
  Oral
Family history of atopy
Personal manifestations of atopy
  Asthma
  Atopic dermatitis
  Allergic conjunctivitis

TABLE 9-3. ALLERGEN AVOIDANCE MEASURES

House dust mites

Enclose mattress, box spring, and pillows in allergen-proof casings
Wash bed linen weekly in hot water (130°F)
Reduce indoor humidity to 50%
Vigorously clean inside, consider using benzyl benzoate or tannic acid to cleanse
Remove carpeting from floors
Replace feather duvets and pillows with synthetic products

Pollens and outdoor molds

Avoid fresh-cut grass; do not mow lawn
Stay inside with windows closed
Use air conditioning on indoor cycle
Reduce outdoor exposure during periods of high pollen counts in season
Shower after outdoor activity to remove pollen and avoid contaminating bedding

Pets

Remove pet from home whenever possible
Consider making the pet an outdoor animal
Cat allergen can be reduced by frequent (biweekly) bathing of cat
Use HEPA filter

this switch is the subject of ongoing research. Some studies have demonstrated the efficacy of immunotherapy in preventing the development of asthma in rhinitis patients, and others have shown the usefulness of specific immunotherapy in preventing the development of new sensitivities in children with asthma [38•,39]. New routes of immunization, such as sublingual immunotherapy, are also being examined in children.

Patient compliance is of the utmost importance because therapy must continue for 3 to 5 years to establish long-range effects. Before embarking on a course of immunotherapy, an assessment of the caretaker's and child's attitudes toward this mode of treatment is crucial. Immunotherapy should only be initiated in those children for whom high-quality allergen extracts are available, the clinical efficacy and safety of which have been documented in clinical studies.

Pharmacotherapy

When avoidance and supportive measures are inadequate for controlling rhinitis symptoms, pharmacotherapeutic management is required. Antihistamines, which act as competitive antagonists of histamine at the H_1 receptor, continue to be the mainstay of treatment for allergic rhinitis [4••]. Oral antihistamines effectively reduce symptoms of rhinorrhea, pruritus, and sneezing, as well as the conjunctivitis that frequently accompanies rhinitis. They have a rapid onset of action, although most have little objective effect on congestion or postnasal drainage.

The second-generation antihistamines are more specific and do not cross the blood/brain barrier, resulting in minimal anticholinergic activity and less drowsiness than the first-generation antihistamines. Many second-generation antihistamines, including cetirizine and loratadine, also possess additional anti-inflammatory activities (eg, blocking histamine and leukotriene release, reducing inflammatory cell influx) and are available in combination with decongestants, providing additional symptom relief (Table 9-4) [40•]. Additionally, both cetirizine and loratadine plus pseudoephedrine were shown in separate studies to improve rhinitis and asthma symptoms in patients with comorbid disease, although this has only been examined in adults [41].

The absence of sedative effects is critical for children, since rhinitis itself can impair cognition. In a study comparing the first-generation antihistamine diphenhydramine with the nonsedating second-generation antihistamine loratadine and placebo in school-aged children, cognition in all the atopic children was considerably poorer than in their nonatopic peers [42]. Children with rhinitis who were treated with loratadine or placebo performed considerably better than those treated with diphenhydramine, indicating that while rhinitis impairs cognition, these effects are not reversed by nonsedating antihistamines and they are exacerbated by sedating antihistamines.

Topical antihistamines are potentially useful alternatives in children. Azelastine was recently approved for

TABLE 9-4. SECOND-GENERATION ANTIHISTAMINES FOR ALLERGIC RHINITIS

Trade name	Chemical name	Age	Dosage
Oral			
Allegra Tablets (Aventis Pharmaceuticals, Parsippany, NJ)	Fexofenadine	≥12 years 6–11 years	60 mg po bid or 180 mg po qd 30 mg po bid
Allegra-D Tablets (Aventis Pharmaceuticals, Parsippany, NJ)	Fexofenadine 60 mg/pseudoephedrine 120 mg	>12 years	60 mg po bid
Claritin Tablets/Syrup (Schering, Kenilworth, NJ)	Loratadine	≥6 years 2–5 years	10 mg po qd 5 mg po qd
Claritin-D Tablets (Schering, Kenilworth, NJ)	Loratadine 5 mg/pseudoephedrine sulfate 120 mg	≥12 years	5 mg po bid
Claritin-D 24-Hour Tablets (Schering, Kenilworth, NJ)	Loratadine 10 mg/pseudoephedrine 240 mg	>12 years	10 mg po bid
Zyrtec Tablets (Pfizer, New York, NY)	Cetirizine	>12 years	10 mg po bid
Zyrtec Syrup (Pfizer, New York, NY)	Cetirizine	6–11 years 2–5 years	10 mg po bid 5 mg po bid
Intranasal			
Astelin (Wallace Laboratories, Cranbury, NJ)	Azelastine HCL	5–11 years ≥12 years	1 spray/nostril bid 2 sprays/nostril bid

bid—twice daily
qd—daily

use in children 5 years of age and older with seasonal allergic rhinitis.

Topical corticosteroids, the most potent drugs for seasonal and perennial allergic rhinitis and first-line therapy for severe cases, effectively relieve all the symptoms of allergic inflammation [4••]. They prevent nasal inflammation during early- and late-phase reactions by inhibiting the release of mediators from basophils and the influx of eosinophils and other inflammatory cells, as well as regulating gene expression [43,44]. Due to their high topical/systemic ratios and rapid catabolism, the most recent additions to this class of compounds have limited systemic effects, although their onset of action is slow.

Six different topical corticosteroids are currently approved for use in children 6 years of age and older, and mometasone furoate was recently approved for children as young as 3 years (Table 9-5) [45,46•]. Studies in adults have shown them to have comparable efficacy; however, differences in dosing frequency, types of formulations, cost, and local side effects may deter-

mine preferences in children. Unfortunately, concern has been raised regarding their potential growth suppression in children, and results vary with the particular agent. One study of beclomethasone showed growth suppression of 1 cm in children treated for 1 year, but no such effects were found with mometasone furoate [47–49]. Intranasal beclomethasone has been shown to prevent bronchial hyperresponsiveness in patients with comorbid seasonal allergic rhinitis and asthma [31].

Two other classes of agents worthy of mention are decongestants and mast cell stabilizers. Nasal decongestants are α-adrenergic agents that cause vasoconstriction that impedes the blood supply to the turbinates; consequently, they are only effective for the congestion that results from turbinate swelling [44,46•]. While topical application is more effective and rapid in onset than oral administration, prolonged topical use can lead to rebound congestion [4••,5••]. Oral formulations are often used in combination with antihistamines. Another commonly used agent, cromolyn sodium, is a topically

TABLE 9-5. TOPICAL CORTICOSTEROIDS USED TO TREAT ALLERGIC RHINITIS

Drug	Delivery	Age	Dose
Beclomethasone			
Beconase (Glaxo Wellcome, Research Triangle Park, NC)	42 μg fluorocarbon aerosol	6–12 years 12 years	1 spray/nostril tid 1 spray/nostril bid–qd
Beconase AQ (Glaxo Wellcome, Research Triangle Park, NC)	42 μg liquid spray	6 years	1 or 2 sprays/nostril bid
Vancenase (Schering, Kenilworth, NJ)	42 μg fluorocarbon aerosol	6–12 years	1 spray/nostril tid
	Pockethaler	12 years	1 spray/nostril bid–qd or 2 sprays/nostril bid
Vancenase AQ (Schering, Kenilworth, NJ)	84 μg liquid spray	6 years	2 sprays/nostril qd
Budesonide			
Rhinocort (Astra, Westborough, MA)	32 μg fluorocarbon aerosol	6 years	2 sprays/nostril bid or 4 sprays/nostril qd
Flunisolide			
Nasarel (Dura Pharmaceuticals, San Diego, CA)	25 μg aqueous aerosol	6 years	1 spray/nostril tid or 2 sprays/nostril bid
Fluticasone propionate			
Flonase (Glaxo Wellcome, Research Triangle Park, NC)	50 μg aqueous spray	12 years	2 sprays/nostril qd or 1 spray/nostril bid; maintenance: 1 spray/nostril qd
Triamcinolone acetonide			
Nasacort (Aventis Pharmaceuticals, Parsippany, NJ)	55 μg fluorocarbon aerosol	>6 years	2 sprays/nostril qd–bid or 1 spray/nostril qid; maintenance: 1 spray/nostril qd
Nasacort AQ (Aventis Pharmaceuticals, Parsippany, NJ)	55 μg aqueous spray	>12 years	2 sprays/nostril qd; 1 spray/nostril qd
Mometasone furoate monohydrate			
Nasonex (Schering, Kenilworth, NJ)	50 μg aqueous spray	12 years 3–11 years	2 sprays/nostril qd; 1 spray/nostril qd

bid—twice daily
qd—daily
tid—three times daily

applied mast cell stabilizer that is particularly useful for the rhinorrhea, pruritus, and sneezing that occurs in seasonal allergic rhinitis or upon isolated exposure to a specific allergen [46•]. While it is one of the safest agents available, permitting its use in very young children, compliance issues may arise because of the need for prophylactic application and frequent administration because of its brief duration of action.

CONCLUSIONS

Because childhood allergic rhinitis continues to increase in prevalence, there is a compelling need to recognize and treat this most common chronic condition in the pediatric population. Appropriate management may curtail the development of asthma, which often coexists with allergic rhinitis, as well as other serious complications. A tripartite approach to management that includes allergen avoidance, immunotherapy, and pharmacologic treatment can reduce the progression of the inflammatory process and improve the child's quality of life.

REFERENCES AND RECOMMENDED READING

Papers of particular interest, published recently, have been highlighted as:
•   Of importance
••   Of major importance

1.   Newacheck PW, Stoddard JJ: Prevalence and impact of multiple childhood chronic illnesses. *J Pediatr* 1994, 124:40–48.

2.   Meltzer EO, Zeiger RS, Schatz M, Jalowayski AA: Chronic rhinitis in infants and children: etiologic, diagnostic, and therapeutic considerations. *Pediatr Clin North Am* 1983, 30:847–871.

3.   Settipane GA: Rhinitis: introduction. In *Rhinitis*. Edited by Settipane GA. Providence, RI: Oceanside Press Publications; 1991:1–11.

4.•• Dykewicz MS, Fineman S, Skoner DP, *et al.*: Diagnosis and management of rhinitis: complete guidelines of the Joint Task Force on practice parameters in Allergy, Asthma and Immunology. *Ann Allergy Asthma Immunol* 1998, 81:478–518.
This article provides a comprehensive set of practice parameters outlining the diagnosis and management of rhinitis.

5.•• Fireman P: Therapeutic approaches to allergic rhinitis: treating the child. *J Allergy Clin Immunol* 2000, 105:S616–S621.
This is an engaging review of allergic rhinitis tailored to the pediatric population.

6.• Lieberman P. Rhinitis. In *Expert Guide to Allergy and Immunology*. Edited by Slavin RG, Reisman RE. Philadelphia: American College of Physicians; 1999: 23–40.
This chapter gives an excellent overview of rhinitis.

7.•• Evans R III: Epidemiology and natural history of asthma, allergic rhinitis, and atopic dermatitis. In *Allergy: Principles and Practice* edn 4. Edited by Middleton E Jr, Reed CE, Ellis EF, *et al.* St. Louis: Mosby–Year Book; 1993:1109–1136.
This is a comprehensive review of the epidemiology of different atopic conditions throughout the world, as well as the natural history of atopy.

8.   Naclerio RM, Baroody F: Understanding the inflammatory processes in upper allergic airway disease and asthma. *J Allergy Clin Immunol* 1998, 101:S345–S351.

9.   Wang D, Smitz J, Waterschoot S, Clement P: An approach to the understanding of the nasal early-phase reaction induced by nasal allergen challenge. *Allergy* 1997, 52:162–167.

10. Wang D, Clement P, Smitz J, *et al.*: Correlations between complaints, inflammatory cells and mediator concentrations in nasal secretions after nasal allergen challenge and during natural allergen exposure. *Int Arch Allergy Immunol* 1995, 106:278–285.

11. Cook PR, Nishioka GJ: Allergic rhinosinusitis in the pediatric population. *Otolaryngol Clin North Am* 1996, 29:39–56.

12. Togias A: Unique mechanistic features of allergic rhinitis. *J Allergy Clin Immunol* 2000, 105:S599–S604.

13. Naclerio RM, Proud D, Togias AG, *et al.*: Inflammatory mediators in late antigen-induced rhinitis. *N Engl J Med* 1985, 313:65–70.

14.• Vinuya RZ: Specific allergen immunotherapy for allergic rhinitis and asthma. *Pediatr Ann* 2000, 29:425–432.
This is an up-to-date review of immunotherapy and its role in managing airway disease.

15. International Rhinitis Management Working Group. International consensus report on the diagnosis and management of rhinitis. *Allergy* 1994, 19:S5–S34.

16. Hagy GW, Settipane GA: Bronchial asthma, allergic rhinitis and allergy skin tests among college students. *J Allergy Clin Immunol* 1969, 44:323.

17. Malmberg H: Symptoms of chronic and allergic rhinitis and occurrence of nasal secretion granulocytes in university students, school children, and infants. *Allergy* 1981, 36:209.

18. Aberg N: Asthma and allergic rhinitis in Swedish conscripts. *Clin Exp Allergy* 1989, 19:59–63.

19. Rimpela AH, Savonius B, Rimpela MK, Haahtela T: Asthma and allergic rhinitis among Finnish adolescents in 1977–1991. *Scand J Soc Med* 1995, 23:60–65.

20. Gergen PJ, Mullally DI, Evans R III: National survey of prevalence of asthma among children in the United States, 1976–1980. *Pediatrics* 1988, 81:1.

21. Bjorksten B: Risk factors in early childhood for the development of atopic disease. *Allergy* 1994, 49:400–407.

22. Grossman J: One airway, one disease. *Chest* 1997, 111:11S–16S.

23. Corren J: Allergic rhinitis and asthma: how important is the link? *J Allergy Clin Immunol* 1997, 99:S781–S786.

24. Smith JM: Epidemiology and natural history of asthma, allergic rhinitis and atopic dermatitis (eczema). In *Allergy: Principles and Practice*. Edited by Middleton E. St. Louis: Mosby; 1988, 891–929.

25. Kapsali T, Horowitz E, Diemer F, Togias A: Rhinitis is ubiquitous in allergic asthmatics. *J Clin Allergy Immunol* 1997, 99:S138.

26. Settipane RJ, Hagy GW, Settipane GA: Long-term risk factors for developing asthma and allergic rhinitis: a 23-year follow-up study of college students. *Allergy Proc* 1994, 15:21–25.

27. Corren J: The association between allergic rhinitis and asthma in children and adolescents: epidemiologic considerations. *Pediatr Ann* 2000, 29:400–402.

28. Braman SS, Barrows AS, DeCotiis BA, *et al.*: Airway hyperresponsiveness in allergic rhinitis. *Chest* 1987, 91:671–674.

29. Corren J, Adinoff AD, Irvin CG: Changes in bronchial responsiveness following nasal provocation with allergen. *J Allergy Clin Immunol* 1992, 89:611–618.

30. Welsh PW, Stricker WE, Chu CP, *et al.*: Efficacy of beclomethasone nasal solution, flunisolide, and cromolyn in relieving symptoms of ragweed allergy. *Mayo Clin Proc* 1987, 62:125–134.

31. Corren J, Adinoff AD, Buchmeier AD, Irvin CG: Nasal beclomethasone prevents the seasonal increase in bronchial responsiveness in patients with allergic rhinitis and asthma. *J Allergy Clin Immunol* 1992, 90:250–256.

32. Aubier M, Levy J, Clerici C, *et al.*: Different effects of nasal and bronchial glucocorticoid administration on bronchial hyperresponsiveness in patients with allergic rhinitis. *Am Rev Respir Dis* 1992, 146:122–126.

33. Corren J, Rachelefsky GS: Interrelationship between sinusitis and asthma. *Immunol Allergy Clin North Am* 1994, 14:171–184.

34. Lieberman P: A pathophysiologic link between allergic rhinitis and asthma. *Pediatr Ann* 2000, 29:405–410.

35.• Meltzer EO: Treatment options for the child with allergic rhinitis. *Clin Pediatr* 1998, 37:1–10.
Treatment options are clearly outlined in this article.

36. Smith L: Special considerations for the child with airway disease. *J Allergy Clin Immunol* 1998, 101:S370–S372.

37. Bousquet J, Lockey RF, Malling HJ, *et al.*: World Health Organization Position Paper. Allergen immunotherapy: therapeutic vaccines for allergic diseases. *Eur J Allergy Clin Immunol* 1998, 44:23–27.

38.• Malling HJ, Weeke B: Immunotherapy: Position Paper of the European Academy of Allergology and Clinical Immunology. *Allergy* 1993, 48 (Suppl):9–35.
This paper presents guidelines from the European community regarding their use of immunotherapy.

39. Des Roches A, Paradis L, Menardo JL, *et al.*: Immunotherapy with a standardized *Dermatophagoides pteronyssinus* extract. VI. Specific immunotherapy prevents the onset of new sensitizations in children. *J Allergy Clin Immunol* 1997, 99:450–453.

40.• Davies RJ, Bagnall AD, McCabe RN, *et al.*: Antihistamines: topical vs. oral administration. *Clin Exp Allergy* 1996, 26:11–17.
This article provides a good assessment of antihistamine dosing and the implications for both topical and oral antihistamines.

41. Hurwitz ME: Treatment of allergic rhinitis with antihistamines and decongestants and their effects on the lower airway. *Pediatr Ann* 2000, 29:411–420.

42. Vuurman EFPM, van Veggel LMA, Uiterwijk MMC, *et al.*: Seasonal allergic rhinitis and antihistamine effects on children's learning. *Ann Allergy* 1993, 71:121–126.

43. Meltzer EO, Schatz M: Pharmacotherapy of rhinitis: 1987 and beyond. *Immunol Allergy Clin North Am* 1987, 7:57–91.

44. Naclerio RM: Allergic rhinitis. *N Engl J Med* 1991, 325:860–869.

45. Schenkel EJ, Berger WE: Treatment of allergic rhinitis with intranasal steroids and their effects on the lower airway. *Pediatr Ann* 2000, 29:422–424.

46.• Meltzer EO: Treatment options for the child with allergic rhinitis. *Clin Pediatrics* 1998, 37:1–10.
This paper clearly outlines treatment options.

47. Skoner DP, Rachelefsky GS, Meltzer EO, *et al.*: Detection of growth suppression in children during treatment with intranasal beclomethasone dipropionate. *Pediatrics* 2000, 205:2.

48. Schenkel EJ, Skoner DP, Bronsky EA, *et al.*: Absence of growth retardation in children with perennial allergic rhinitis after one year of treatment with mometasone furoate aqueous nasal spray. *Pediatrics* 2000, 105:2.

49. Allen DB: Influence of inhaled corticosteroids on growth: a pediatric endocrinologist's perspective. *Acta Paediatr* 1998, 87:123–129.

CHAPTER 10

Headache and Headaches of Nasal Origin

Mark Scarupa
Michael A. Kaliner

Headache is one of the most common complaints of patients seeking medical attention. While many headaches are due to phenomena in or around the skull, it is understood that head pain can also arise from infratentorial structures. These include but are not limited to the musculature of the neck and head, paranasal sinuses, or the nasal passages [1]. Rhinologic headaches, also called septal contact headaches, middle turbinate headache syndrome, or rhinopathic headaches, are headaches that arise from the nasal mucosa as a result of chronic septal-mucosal contact [2]. These contact points may be caused by changes in the nasal anatomy secondary to trauma, congenital septal deviation, or by mucosal inflammation as seen in allergic and vasomotor rhinitis.

Nasal mucosal edema seen in rhinitis can occlude the sinus ostea, interfering with drainage and predisposing to sinusitis. In fact, sinusitis without preceding or concomitant rhinitis is rare [3]. Both acute and chronic sinusitis cause headaches, and treating the underlying nasal mucosal inflammation is essential to effective management of sinusitis and the accompanying headaches. This chapter deals with rhinologic headache and discusses the role nasal inflammation plays in sinus headaches. The differential diagnosis of headache is reviewed, to place rhinologic headaches in the proper perspective.

HEADACHE

Headache is a universal human experience; seventy-six percent of women and 57% of men report at least one significant headache per month and 67% of patients with headache use over-the-counter analgesics to treat their symptoms [4]. The National Headache Foundation estimates the loss of productivity, absenteeism, and medical expenses due to headaches to be $50 billion annually in the United States. Although most headaches are usually not due to significant disease states, they can be severely debilitating. However, headaches may be the manifestation of serious illness, such as intracerebral tumor or aneurysm that requires immediate and aggressive diagnosis and treatment.

The differential for headache is extremely broad. In 1988, the International Headache Society (IHS) created a taxonomy of headache disorders. The taxonomy divided headache into thirteen categories with 129 subtypes (Table 10-1) [5]. Though their list is broad, the majority of primary headaches can be classified as tension, migraine, or cluster. Secondary headaches caused by underlying organic pathology include both sinus and rhinologic headaches.

The diagnosis of specific headaches relies greatly on taking a comprehensive history. The time profile of headache is perhaps the most important single piece of information and should include frequency, date of onset, periodicity, duration of each episode, and change of the pain quality over time [6••]. Additionally, a detailed understanding of the time leading up to a patient's headache (auras, mood, exertion), the exact location of the pain, and an assessment of pain quality is important. Any associated symptoms should be noted, such as focal neurologic deficits, nausea, photophobia, etc. The physical examination should include complete neurologic, ophthalmic, rhinoscopic, and temporomandibular joint examination.

TENSION-TYPE HEADACHE

Tension-type headaches comprise 90% of all adult headaches [7]. They are more prevalent in women with a lifetime prevalence of 90% versus 67% in men and a one-year prevalence rate of 86% versus 63% [8]. Prior to the IHS classification, tension-type headaches were called psychogenic headaches, ordinary headaches, stress headaches, muscle contraction headaches, and psychomyogenic headaches [9]. The IHS Classification Committee distinguishes between episodic tension-type headache (<180 episodes per year) and chronic tension-

TABLE 10-1. CLASSIFICATION AND DIAGNOSTIC CRITERIA FOR HEADACHE DISORDERS, CRANIAL NEURALGIAS, AND FACIAL PAIN

1 Migraine
2 Tension-type headache
3 Cluster headache and chronic paroxysmal hemicrania
4 Miscellaneous headaches unassociated with structural lesion
5 Headache associated with head trauma
6 Headache associated with vascular disorder
7 Headache associated with nonvascular intracranial disorder
8 Headache associated with substances or their withdrawal
9 Headache associated with noncephalic infection
10 Headache associated with metabolic disorder
11 Headache or facial pain associated with disorder of cranium, neck, eyes, ears, nose, sinuses, teeth, mouth, or other facial or cranial structures
12 Cranial neuralgias, nerve trunk pain, and deafferentiation pain
13 Headache not classifiable

Adapted from Headache Classification Committee of the International Headache Society [5].

type headache (>180 episodes per year). The criteria set by the IHS for the diagnosis of episodic tension headache include headaches occurring less than 15 days a month and lasting 30 minutes to 7 days; at least two of the following pain characteristics: a pressing or tightening (nonpulsating) quality, mild to moderate intensity, bilateral location, and not aggravated by routine nonstrenuous physical activity; no nausea, vomiting, or anorexia can be present; and either photophobia or phonophobia may be present, but not both. The criteria for chronic tension headache include headache occurring more 15 days a month and pain characteristics identical to episodic tension headache except that nausea may be present.

The classic tension-type headache is a continuous, dull, nonthrobbing bilateral or unilateral pain in the frontal, occipital, fronto-occipital, or hemicranial area [10]. The pain is usually a mild to moderate feeling of pressure, heaviness, or a sensation of band-like constriction. The mechanism of tension-type headaches has become increasingly complex as more is learned about the syndrome. Tension-type headaches were thought to be caused by extracranial muscle ischemia due to involuntary overactivity of pericranial muscles compressing small blood vessels [6••]. It is now thought that a combination of psychological, social, and physical factors play a role in aggravating tension-type headaches in patients susceptible to developing these headaches. Susceptible patients are prone to poor muscle control, which leads to prolonged pericranial muscle contraction, fatigue, and muscle tender spots [6••]. A possible continuum has been suggested between tension-type headache and migraine [11]. Unlike migraine headaches, there is no prophylactic treatment for tension-type headaches. Symptomatic administration of nonsteroidal anti-inflammatory drugs (NSAIDs) is generally the treatment of choice. Because patients are only mildly impaired, they rarely seek medical attention.

CLUSTER HEADACHE

Cluster headaches are far less common than migraine or tension-type headaches. They occur primarily in middle-aged or older men with a 6:1 male predominance [12]. Additionally, there is a correlation between cluster headaches and the use of cigarettes and alcohol. Prior to the IHS classification, cluster headaches were termed Horton's headaches, migrainous cranial neuralgias, and histamine headaches [13]. The criteria set by the IHS for the diagnosis of cluster headache include at least 5 attacks that are severe and unilateral, supraorbital, or temporal, lasting 15 to 180 minutes untreated; attacks occurring from 1 every other day to 8 daily; at least one of the following symptoms accompanying the headache pain: conjunctival injection, lacrimation, nasal congestion, rhinorrhea, forehead and facial sweating, miosis, ptosis, or eyelid edema.

Cluster headache pain is described as sudden, non-pulsatile, unexpected (without prodrome or aura), unilateral and burning affecting temporal, ocular, and frontal regions of the head [10]. They have been called the most painful of recurrent headaches, with pain often centered in the eye [14]. The attacks occur in clusters, frequently lasting for months, with daily or near-daily symptoms. Symptoms may wake patients from their sleep. According to IHS classification, there are also cluster variants including chronic paroxysmal hemicrania, chronic cluster headache, and cluster variant (cluster-tic syndrome).

The etiology of cluster headaches is unknown. There is evidence that alcohol, histamine, nitroglycerine, and other vasoactive substances play a role in cluster headache induction [6••]. Neuronal abnormalities involving the hypothalamus and circadian pacemaker functions of the suprachiasmic nuclei have been implicated by some researchers [14]. Like migraine headaches, cluster headaches have a wide variety of prophylactic and symptom-relieving therapies beyond the scope of this book.

MIGRAINE HEADACHE

Migraine headaches are reported by 15% to 20% of women and 7% to 10% of men [15]. In the United States there is approximately a 3:1 female predominance [16]. Historically, migraines were classified as classic (with an aura) or common (without an aura). Once again, the terminology changed after the IHS taxonomy divided the syndrome into migraine with and migraine without aura, then further broke the syndrome down into subtypes including ophthalmoplegic, retinal, and migraine associated with intracranial disorder. The IHS diagnostic criteria for migraine without aura include attacks lasting 4 to 72 hours; pain having two of the following characteristics: pulsating quality, unilateral location, moderate to severe intensity, or aggravation by movement or physical activity; the presence of at least one of the following associated symptoms: phonophobia, photophobia, or nausea or vomiting; or no evidence of organic disease. The IHS diagnostic criteria for migraine without aura include one or more transient neurological symptom (aura); gradual development of aura over more than 4 minutes, or multiple symptoms in succession; aura lasting 4 to 60 minutes; or headache following or accompanying aura within 60 minutes.

Migraine pain is best described as moderate to severe, pulsating and throbbing, and often accompanied by a sensation of pressure. Sixty per cent of migraine headaches are unilateral, most involving the whole hemicranium but may involve solely frontal, temporal, occipital, or more than one isolated locale [10]. Premonitory symptoms may occur hours or days before attacks and are separate from the migraine aura. These symptoms include changes in mood (euphoria, depression, nervousness, calm, irritability), changes in energy (drowsiness, hyperactivity, sluggishness), or autonomic phenomena (hunger cravings, anorexia, thirst, yawning) [17]. Similar symptoms following migraine attacks are termed postdromata.

Numerous triggers have been implicated in the provocation of migraine attacks. Stress or release from stress, too much or lack of sleep, bright lights, loud noises, smoke, strong smells, foods (chocolate, cheeses, cured meats containing nitrates, dairy, monosodium glutamate, aspartame, citrus), estrogen changes (oral contraceptives, menstruation, hormone replacement therapy), and head trauma have all been reported as triggers [18]. Unfortunately, many of these triggers are difficult or impossible to avoid. To determine if there is a specific migraine trigger, patients are advised to keep a headache diary. Even if a trigger is found, avoidance often does not put an end to migraine symptoms.

Migraine aura, neurologic symptoms preceding some migraine headaches, are localized to the cerebral cortex or brainstem. Almost all patients with migraine headaches with aura report visual disturbances (99%). Others additionally report sensory symptoms (31%), aphasia (18%), or motor disturbances (6%) [19]. The aura usually occur before the headache symptoms but may begin in the midst of head pain. Visual symptoms have been described as a flickering or shimmering light, a spot in front of the eyes, or a hole in the visual field [6••]. Visual disturbances are sometimes followed by sensory disturbances such as paresthesias, hyperesthesias, or dysesthesias often involving the upper extremities and face.

Like cluster and tension-type headaches, the exact mechanisms of migraine headache are poorly understood. Historically, it was thought that cerebral vasoconstriction was responsible for the migraine aura and that cerebral vasodilation resulted in throbbing headache pain [13]. While this may be in part true, more recent evidence further complicates the migraine pathophysiology, and there is now evidence for a number of migraine headache mechanisms. A more recent theory for the generation of migraine aura is that of cortical spreading depression, a depolarization wave that propagates across the brain cortex depressing spontaneous and evoked neuronal activity [20]. The depression is followed by a brief period of excitation with an efflux of amino acids from nerve cells and changes in vascular tone, all of which can produce symptoms of migraine aura.

Serotonin dysregulation, nitric oxide sensitivity, changes in brain stem blood flow (migraine generator), and cortical hyperexcitability all are theorized to be involved in migraine pathophysiology. Studies of serotonin (5-HT) regulation in migraine patients found that they have low plasma 5-HT levels between attacks compared to controls and that platelet 5-HT is released during attacks [21]. Nitric oxide infusion causes greater vasodilation in the middle cerebral arteries of migraine patients than in controls [22]. The migraine generator theory involves increased cerebral blood flow to the upper brain stem opposite the side of headache pain as seen in positron-emission tomography scans of migraine patients [23]. This area of increased flow remains after headache resolution and may be important in initiating migraines. Finally, multiple studies have documented a state of cortical hyperexcitability corresponding to the frequency of migraine attacks [24•].

The treatment of migraine headaches is complex, involving lifestyle modification, prophylactic pharmacotherapy, and pain management.

RHINOLOGIC HEADACHE

Headache of nasal origin, or rhinologic headache, has been discussed with some frequency in the otolaryngology literature since the early 1900s. In 1927, Sluder described a pain affecting the lower half of the head and face in a maxillary distribution (V2) of the trigeminal nerve. He termed this headache sphenopalatine neuralgia, Sluder's syndrome [1]. The best early direct evidence that nasal stimulation can be perceived as pain in the head was provided by Wolff, who applied noxious stimuli to both the structures of the ear and nasal passages. He then recorded the location where the pain was perceived by his patients. Wolff found that noxious stimuli (metal probe, faradic current, or adrenalin solution) applied to the mucosa of the middle turbinate is perceived under the eyes and along the

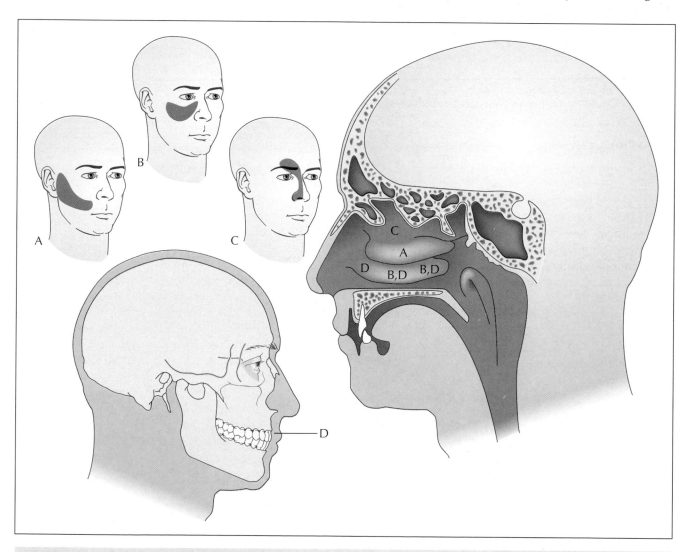

FIGURE 10-1.
Referred pain due to noxious stimuli applied to the middle turbinates. Wolff's 1948 experiments found that application of noxious stimuli to the middle turbinates caused referred pain both under the eyes and along the zygoma to the temple. *Adapted from* Wolff [25•].

zygoma (Fig. 10-1) [25•]. Thus, nasal irritation can be felt in the face or head.

The role of allergic rhinitis as a cause or contributor to mucosal-septal contact has been mentioned by many but rarely fully investigated [26–30]. An exception is Hoover, who attributed headache symptoms in her population of 80 patients suffering from rhinologic headache to inhalant and food allergies [31]. Though it has not been fully explored, it is easy to imagine that as the edema associated with rhinitis causes intranasal swelling, there is a greater likelihood that a point of contact with the nasal septum will be created.

A contact point created between the sensitive nasal mucosa and the relatively less innervated nasal septum is the universal anatomical feature found in rhinologic headache (Fig. 10-2). To understand the pathophysiology requires an understanding of the gross and neuroanatomy of the nasal passages. The inferior nasal turbinate is the largest of usually three but sometimes four (supreme turbinate anatomical variation) outpocketings in each nostril separated by the nasal septum. These turbinates are covered with a continuous mucous membrane. Above the superior turbinate the membrane is cuboid, squamous epithelium (olfactory epithelium) and below respiratory epithelium consisting of tall, columnar, psuedostratified, ciliated cells with mucus-secreting goblet cells and microvilli [27]. The superior nasal turbinate also creates the inferior distribution for the olfactory nerve (CN I). It is below the superior turbinate where the sensory innervation is exclusively provided by the trigeminal nerve (CN V) and where the contact points responsible for rhinologic headaches are created.

The sensory ganglionic cell bodies of the trigeminal nerve originate in the semilunar ganglion within the middle cranial fossa. The nerve then trifurcates where the maxillary (V2) division eventually innervates the nasal mucosa. The mucosa covering the turbinates has a rich sensory innervation, including C-fiber polymodal nociceptors of CN V2. The scalp, dura, and cranial vessels also have sensory innervation with sensory afferents converging on the projection neurons in the trigeminal nucleus. With sensory information from both the irritated nasal mucosa and supratentorial structures projecting on the same neuron, it is easy to understand how referred pain can occur. Additionally, the chronic irritation caused by the contact point can induce a state of hyperalgesia in which a stimulus of lower than normal intensity causes a sensation of pain [32••].

Rhinologic headache pain is frequently felt in a periocular location as demonstrated by Wolff's experiments [25•]. When the contact is created by mucosal edema, stimuli that worsen the inflammation may worsen both headache frequency and intensity. Patients with vasomotor rhinitis (VMR) often report that the noxious environmental stimuli worsen both VMR and headache symptoms. Patients with seasonal allergic rhinitis also may complain of seasonal headaches.

It was originally thought that most rhinologic headaches occurred in males, many of who had sustained significant nasal trauma. Schonsted-Madsen and Koch-Henriksen studied large populations both with a 2:1 male predominance [33,34]. Over time, nasal deformities in males may worsen due to more pronounced secondary growth, which in turn can create or worsen headache pain. Recently, a series of 73 patients found a significant female predominance (86.3%) [35]. The mucosal-septal contact points in these patients were predominantly caused by mucosal swelling associated with vasomotor rhinitis, a condition that is more common in women.

Diagnosis of rhinologic headache requires that there be a mucosal-septal contact point and a history suggestive of the disease. To confirm the diagnosis, nasal application of 4% lidocaine to the contact point should result in the rapid resolution of the headache. Oxymetazoline (Afrin; Schering-Plough, Kenilworth, NJ) sprayed into the nose during headache symptoms often has a similar effect.

Treatment of rhinologic headache focuses on reducing the mucosal-septal contact point. If that contact is caused by rhinitis-induced mucosal edema, then the

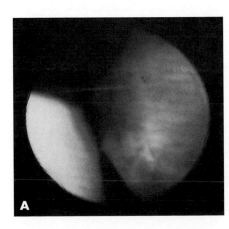 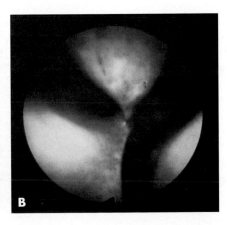

FIGURE 10-2.
Fiberoptic rhinoscopic views of mucosal-septal contact points. **A,** Septal-mucosal contact. **B,** Mucosal contact point created by a septal spur.

treatment focuses on reducing mucosal swelling and removing adherent mucus. For patients with allergic rhinitis as their primary diagnosis, a combination of nasal corticosteroids, saline nasal washings, and antihistamines (with or without decongestant) is employed. For acute headache, a topical decongestant (oxymetazoline, Afrin) can be used. In patients whose headaches persist after decongestant sprays, a solution of 4% lidocaine can be sprayed in the nose (2 sprays every 2 to 4 hours, as needed).

Patients with allergic rhinitis should receive instructions in allergy control measures and may benefit from immunotherapy. In patients with vasomotor rhinitis, a combination of nasal corticosteroids, saline nasal washings, and anticholinergic agents is employed, with decongestants, topical antihistamines, and lidocaine spray used when necessary. Refractory headaches, or rhinologic headaches in patients whose contact points are purely structural, may benefit from surgery.

SINUS HEADACHE

Headache is a frequent complaint of patients suffering from both chronic and acute sinusitis. As inflammation and swelling of the nasal mucosa usually precede sinusitis (see Chapter 11), it is worth briefly mentioning the prototypic head and facial pain associated with sinus headache. Sinusitis can occur in any of the four paranasal sinus cavities but most frequently occurs in the ethmoid. The location of headache pain is directly related to which sinus is involved, although more than one sinus is often affected. Maxillary sinus pain is often perceived over the involved sinus and in the teeth. Frontal sinus pain is usually localized above the eyes, over the frontal sinus, or in the temples or occiput. Ethmoidal sinusitis affects the eyes and medial orbit region. Finally, sphenoid sinus pain is referred to the teeth, vertex, occiput, or temples [36]. Regardless of the sinus or sinuses involved, sinusitis headaches have some unifying features including worsening with bending over, coughing or straining; a constant (nonthrobbing) pain lasting for hours; and no associated light or sound sensitivity [32••].

Once a sinus is infected, the mucosa swells, blood flow increases, neutrophils are attracted, and acute inflammation occurs. In the sinus environment, there is disrupted gas exchange leading to a stagnant environment favoring bacterial growth [37]. Additionally, the cilia become less active, making bacterial clearance more difficult. As the pressure within the sinus builds it can either cause pain directly or indirectly. Treatment of sinus headache involves treating the underlying sinusitis, often by treating the underlying rhinitis. The treatment of sinusitis itself is covered in Chapter 11.

CONCLUSIONS

Headaches are a universal human experience. For some patients they are truly debilitating. The majority of headaches are primary headaches including tension-type, migraine, or cluster headaches. Secondary headaches should be suspected during the work up of patients with headache pain. In patients with rhinitis symptoms and headaches, both rhinologic and sinus headaches should be considered. Treating the underlying nasal inflammation and swelling often provides great relief and can be quite rewarding.

REFERENCES AND RECOMMENDED READING

Papers of particular interest, published recently, have been highlighted as:
- • Of importance
- •• Of major importance

1. Sluder G: Vacuum frontal headaches with eye symptoms only. In *Nasal Neurology, Headaches and Eye Disorders.* Edited by Kimpton H. St. Louis: Mosby; 1927:31–67.

2. Saunte C, Soyka D: Headaches related to ear, nose and sinus disorders. In *The Headaches.* Edited by Olesen J. New York: Raven Press Ltd; 1993:753–757.

3. Lund VJ, Kennedy DW: Quantification for staging sinusitis: the Staging Therapy Group. *Ann Otol Rhinol Laryngol* 1995, 167:17–21.

4. Saper JR: Headache disorders. *Med Clin North Am* 1999, 83(3):663–690.

5. Headache Classification Committee of the International Headache Society: Classification and diagnostic criteria for headache disorders, cranial neuralgias, and facial pain. *Cephalalgia* 1988, 8(suppl 7):1–96.

6.•• Olesen J, Bonica JJ: Headache. In *The Management of Pain* edn 2. Edited by Bonica JJ. Philadelphia: Lea & Febiger; 1990:687–726.
   This chapter gives an excellent summary of the IHS classification. Both authors are leaders in their field and have a fantastic grasp of even the most obscure of the 129 subtypes of headache classified by the IHS.

7. Diamond S: The management of migraine and cluster headaches. *Compr Ther* 1995, 21(9):492–498.

8. Rassmussen BK, Jensen R, Schroll M, Olesen J: Epidemiology of headache in a general population—a prevalence study. *J Clin Epidemiol* 1991, 44:1147–1157.

9. Silberstein SD: Tension-type headaches. *Headache* 1994, 34:S2–S7.

10. Bonica JJ: General considerations of pain in the head. In *The Management of Pain* edn 2. Edited by Bonica JJ. Philadelphia: Lea & Febiger; 1990:651–675.

11. Silberstein SD: Tension-type and chronic daily headache. *Neurology* 1993, 43:1644–1649.

12. Mathew NT: Advances in cluster headache. *Neurol Clin* 1990, 8:867–890.

13. Johnson CJ: Headaches and facial pain. In *Principles of Ambulatory Medicine* edn 5. Edited by Barker LR, Burton JR, Zieve PD. Baltimore: Williams & Wilkins; 1999:1214–1229.

14. Walling AD: Cluster headache. *Am Fam Physician* 1993, 47(6):1457–1463.

15. Olesen J, Tfelt-Hansen P, Welch KMA: *The Headaches*. New York: Raven Press, 1993.

16. Stewart WF, Lipton RB, Celentano DD, Reed ML: Prevalence of migraine headache in the United States. Relation to age, income, race and other sociodemographic factors. *JAMA* 1992, 267:64–69.

17. Solomon S: Migraine diagnosis and clinical symptomatology. *Headache* 1994, 34:S8–S12.

18. Bartleson JD: Treatment of migraine headaches. *Mayo Clinic Proc* 1999, 74:702–708.

19. Russell MD, Oleson J: A nosographic analysis of the migraine aura in a general population. *Brain* 1996, 119:355–361.

20. Lauritzen M: Pathophysiology of the migraine aura. The spreading depression theory. *Brain* 1994, 117:199–210.

21. Ferrari MD, Saxena PF: On serotonin and migraine: a clinical and pharmacological review. *Cephalalgia* 1993, 13:151–156.

22. Olesen J, Thomsen LL, Lassen LH, Olesen IJ: The nitric oxide hypothesis of migraine and other vascular headaches. *Cephalalgia* 1995, 15:94–100.

23. Weiller C, May A, Limmroth V, *et al.*: Brain stem activation in spontaneous human migraine attacks. *Nat Med* 1995, 1:658–660.

24.• Ferrari MD: Migraine. *Lancet* 1998, 351:1043–1051.
This excellent review article on migraine headaches contains both an up-to-date discussion of migraine treatment as well as details on the future direction of migraine therapy.

25.• Wolff HG: *Headache and other head pain*. Edited by Wolff HG. New York: Oxford University Press; 1948:446–471.
Dr. Wolff's 1948 experiments, summarized in great detail in this book chapter, create the foundation for understanding rhinologic headache pathophysiology.

26. Baker DC: Intranasal procedures of value in the management of patients with headache. *Headache* 1966, 5:116–119.

27. Goldsmith AJ, Zahtz GD, Stegnjajic A, Shikowitz N: Middle turbinate headache syndrome. *Am J Rhinol* 1993, 7(1):17–23.

28. Moore GF, Massey JD, Emanuel JM, *et al.*: Head pain secondary to nasal allergies. *Ear Nose Throat J* 1987, 66:41–53.

29. Graham JK: Headache of nasal origin. *J La State Med Soc* 1970, 122:375–379.

30. Ryan RE, Kern EB: Rhinologic causes of facial pain and headache. *Headache* 1978, 18(1):44–50.

31. Hoover S: Nasal pathophysiology of headaches and migraines. *Rhinology* 1987, 26(suppl 2):3–23.

32.•• Clerico DM: Rhinopathic headaches: referred pain of nasal and sinus origin. In *Diseases of the Sinuses*. Edited by Gershwin ME, Incaudo GA. Totowa, NY: Humana Press; 1996:403–423.
This chapter explores rhinologic headaches in great detail. The author gives pages of anatomy review as well as a fascinating historical prospective of the disease.

33. Schonsted-Madsen U, Stoksted P, Christensen PH, Koch-Henriksen N: Chronic headache related to nasal obstruction. *J Laryngol Otol* 1986, 100:165–170.

34. Koch-Henriksen N, Gammelgaard N, Hvidegaard T, Stoksted P: Chronic headache: the role of deformity of the nasal septum. *Br Med J* 1984, 288:434–435.

35. Scarupa MD, Economides A, Kaliner MA: Rhinologic headache and rhinitis. *J Allergy Clinical Immunol* 2001, 107(2):S262.

36. Lucente FE: Headache and facial pain. In *Otolaryngology–Head and Neck Surgery*. Edited by Meyerhoff WL, Rice DH. Philadelphia: W.B. Saunders; 1992:119–127.

37. Slavin RG: Complications of allergic rhinitis: implications for sinusitis and asthma. *J Allergy Clin Immunol* 1998, 101:S357–S360.

CHAPTER 11

Medical Management of Rhinosinusitis

Michael A. Kaliner

Sinusitis is an inflammatory process involving one or more of the paranasal sinuses. The inflammation may be infectious in nature, from viral, bacterial, or fungal growth, or due to a self-perpetuating inflammatory process. Because of the contiguous anatomical relationships, it is hard to conceive of inflammation of the sinuses that does not involve the adjoining nasal mucosa. Therefore, it is probably more appropriate to refer to this condition as rhinosinusitis [1••].

Sinusitis affects 31 to 35 million Americans, accounting for 25 million office visits in 1991 [2]. In a recent symposium on sinusitis, it was estimated that the direct annual cost of sinusitis was more than $2.4 billion, excluding the cost of surgery [1••]. Surgical intervention probably adds another $1 billion to this estimate [3••]. More recent evidence, which takes into account some of the indirect costs of sinusitis, suggests a cost exceeding $6 billion [4]. It is currently estimated that sinusitis is the third most frequent diagnosis for which antibiotics are prescribed [5]. Thus, sinusitis is both extremely common and extremely expensive (Table 11-1). Along with allergic rhinitis, asthma, and other allergic diseases, sinusitis is increasing in prevalence, and the importance of these common diseases to the health of America is being recognized.

THE NORMAL FUNCTIONS OF THE NOSE

The nose functions as the preferred airway, provides the sense of smell, contributes to the sense of taste, purifies air so that only particle-free air reaches the lungs, and eliminates all trapped particles by mucociliary action (Table 11-2). The mucus secreted by the nose is a very complex mixture of proteins and carbohydrates that lubricates the surface of the nose, humidifies air before it reaches the lungs, and provides critical host-defense functions [6]. Thus, mucus contains proteins, such as lysozyme, which kill potentially harmful bacteria, and also contains antibodies secreted by the mucus-producing glands that kill both viruses and bacteria [7]. Ordinary mucus is clear to light yellow in color. Infections cause the mucus to thicken and darken in color. During a cold, the mucus might become a deep yellow color; however, with bacterial infections, such as occur in sinusitis, the mucus frequently becomes a green or dark grey color. The color reflects the presence of many neutrophils as well as the bacteria growing in the mucus. Mucus is odorless, but bacteria growing in mucus may provide a rank smell. In fact, foul-smelling mucus may indicate the presence of gram-negative bacteria, such as *Escherichia coli* or pseudomonas, and should be treated with appropriate antibiotics.

Rhinitis is a universally experienced condition that ranges from a cold to chronic rhinosinusitis with complications. Disorders of the nose and nasal function are among the most common causes of medical disability, with an estimated 17% of the population suffering with allergic rhinitis, 10% with vasomotor (nonallergic) rhinitis, and 100% experiencing upper respiratory tract infections during the course of each year. For allergic rhinitis alone, the estimated costs range from $1.8 to $5.9 billion per year in 1996 dollars [8,9]. One of the more common dilemmas facing physicians is differentiating between rhinitis and sinusitis (discussed later).

The paranasal sinuses are four paired cavities in the skull that surround the eye sockets. The maxillary and ethmoid sinuses develop in utero and are present at birth, the frontal sinuses develop during the first year of life, and the sphenoid sinus develops during the first several years of life [10]. The maxillary and ethmoid sinuses drain into the middle meatus area under the middle turbinate. The ostia of the maxillary sinus is above the floor of the sinus, and mucociliary clearance sweeps the mucus in the sinus along the walls of the sinus through the opening. The frontal sinus drains through a recess into the most anterior and superior aspect of the middle meatus. The sphenoid sinus drains along the posterior wall of the nasal cavity into the pharynx.

The physiologic reasons for the presence of paranasal sinuses are not clear. The sinuses act to lighten the weight of the skull and provide resonance to the voice, as well as participate in the production of the mucous

blanket, which constantly clears the nose of trapped particulate materials. The sinuses are lined with the same type of mucous membrane that lines the whole respiratory tract, a pseudostratified columnar epithelium with submucous glands and goblet cells. One of the major functions of this type of mucous membrane is the production of mucus. A total of two quarts of mucus are made every day by the nose and sinuses. Although we are not aware of it, we constantly swallow mucus from our nose and sinuses as part of the mechanisms that keep particles in the air from being inspired into the lungs. A particle of material trapped on the anterior tip of the inferior turbinate takes 10 to 15 minutes to travel to the pharynx (approximately 1 cm per minute) [6].

PATHOPHYSIOLOGY OF ACUTE SINUSITIS

The classification of sinusitis is arbitrarily separated into acute sinusitis (symptoms present for 4 weeks or so) and chronic sinusitis (symptoms present for 8 to 12 weeks or longer). Subacute sinusitis is the stage from 4 to 12 weeks. Recurrent acute sinusitis indicates four or more episodes per year for two or more years, with resolution of symptoms between episodes.

The current dogma on the pathophysiologic mechanisms causing sinusitis suggests that obstruction of the ostiomeatal complex combined with the presence of pathogenic bacteria in the obstructed cavity are the critical events [11••]. Ordinarily, bacteria are swept from the sinuses through mucociliary clearance; however, when the ostia are obstructed, ordinarily innocuous bacteria remain in the sinus cavity and multiply. The mucous membrane inside the cavity becomes swollen, inflamed, and infiltrated with inflammatory cells, leading to filling of the cavity with inflammatory secretions. The resultant symptoms include pain and pressure over the infected sinus, nasal congestion, purulent drainage, and fever (Table 11-3). Infections in the frontal sinuses cause pain to be felt above the eyes. If the ethmoid sinuses are involved, the discom-

TABLE 11-1. RHINOSINUSITIS

Facts:

14.7% incidence in United States population
Incidence increased by 18% over past 11 years
26 million office visits for sinusitis in 1997
>21 million antibiotic prescriptions in 1997
Third most common diagnosis for antibiotics
>70 million restricted activity days in 1992
250,000 surgeries per year

Costs:

Hospital days	= 143,000	($220 million)
Antibiotics	= 21,000,000	($600 million)
Physician visits	= 11,500,000	($1.7 billion)
Hospital admissions	= 84,000	($500 million)
Surgery	= 250,000	($1.2 billion)
Direct costs	= >$4 billion	
Total costs	= >$6 billion	

TABLE 11-2. FUNCTIONS OF THE NOSE

Nasal airway
Olfaction
Taste
Humidification of inspired air
Filtration of inspired air
Warming of inspired air
Mucociliary clearance of trapped particulates
Local host defenses
    Antibody secretion (IgA)
    Mucous secretion with anti-infective activities (lysozyme)
Resonance

fort is felt between the eyes. Maxillary sinusitis is associated with pain in the face and teeth, and sphenoid sinusitis causes pain at the top, back, or sides of the head.

The ostiomeatal complex is that area under the middle meatus into which the anterior ethmoid, frontal, and maxillary sinuses drain (Fig. 11-1). The middle turbinate protrudes into the nasal passage, acting as an air baffle, causing inspired air to become turbulent during respiration. The turbulence helps the nose cleanse, warm, and humidify air before it travels to the lungs. The location of the frontal, ethmoid, and maxillary ostia under the middle turbinate suggests that this structure protects the sinuses from inspired particles, such as infectious or allergic agents. The space lateral to the middle turbinate (into which the sinuses drain) is known as the middle meatus, and the functional anatomy of this space is critical to normal sinus drainage. Thus, the term *ostiomeatal complex* has been termed to signify the functional relationships between the space and the ostia that drain into it.

The most common sequence begins with a cold that acutely obstructs the sinus outflow track because of mucosal swelling, followed by a sinus infection. It is estimated that up to 10% of colds in children are followed by bacterial sinusitis and that each child experiences 6 to 8 colds per year [12•]. It has been estimated that up to

17% of children presenting to physicians for treatment of severe cold symptoms have sinusitis [13•]. Computed tomography (CT) scans of patients with viral upper respiratory infections reveal a striking incidence of abnormalities [14••], and 90% of volunteers with experimentally-induced viral upper respiratory infections demonstrate abnormal CT scans. Thus, the sinuses are infected during a cold nearly half the time; however, these abnormal CT scans do not indicate that a bacterial infection is present, and the abnormalities generally resolve spontaneously within 2 weeks [14••].

Smears of nasal secretions during a sinus infection usually show sheets of neutrophils, but on occasion, eosinophils are found. In such patients, biopsy of the sinus mucosa may reveal an eosinophil-rich infiltrate and the presence of eosinophil-derived products, such as major basic protein. Several studies have shown the sinus mucosa to contain IL-5, a cytokine that promotes eosinophil migration, activation, and survival. In these patients, the mucosa can be abnormally predisposed to developing sinusitis because of the presence of the ongoing eosinophil-rich inflammation [1••]. The inciting event for developing acute sinusitis still involves obstruction of the outflow tract, but the presence of an eosinophil-rich inflammation in the mucosa is a predisposing factor. The eosinophil-rich inflammation responds to a cold, an allergic event, or for no recognized reason with a prolonged, self-perpetuating, inflammatory response that causes the same symptoms as an infectious sinusitis, but cultures may be negative [15–17].

Certain groups of patients appear to be particularly predisposed to this type of reaction, particularly those

TABLE 11-3. SIGNS AND SYMPTOMS OF SINUSITIS
Acute sinusitis (symptoms present 2 to 8 weeks)
Primary symptoms
Persistent upper respiratory infection (> 7 to 10 days)
Congestion
Mucopurulent nasal or posterior pharyngeal discharge
Cough
Secondary symptoms
Fever
Headache
Facial pain
Chronic sinusitis (symptoms persisting 8 to 12 weeks or more)
Primary symptoms
Persistent nasal obstruction
Purulent nasal and posterior pharyngeal discharge
Postnasal drip
Cough
Secondary symptoms
Fetor oris
Hyposmia, anosmia
Sore throat
Malaise
Fever
Headache
Facial fullness

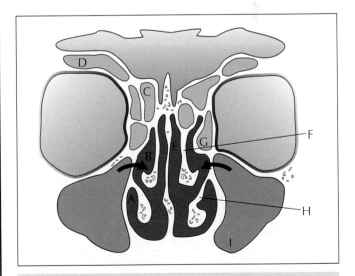

FIGURE 11-1.
The structures of the sinuses. **A**, Inferior meatus, **B**, middle meatus; **C**, ethmoidal air cells; **D**, frontal sinus; **E**, olfactory cleft; **F**, middle turbinate; **G**, ethmoidal bulla; **H**, inferior turbinate; **I**, maxillary sinus.

subjects with sensitivity to aspirin and other non-steroidal anti-inflammatory drugs (NSAIDs); however, many other patients with recurrent acute or chronic sinusitis, especially when it is associated with nasal polyps, have this eosinophil-rich inflammatory infiltrate in their mucosa.

The bacteria found in sinusitis are exactly the same as are found in ear infections. Most commonly they include *Streptococcus pneumonia*, *Haemophilus influenza*, and *Moraxella catarrhalis*. Both adults and children have *Pneumococcus* and *Haemophilus* infections, whereas children are much more likely to have *Moraxella* infections [18•,19••]. Other bacteria sometimes found include *Staphylococcus*, Streptococcus spp, *Pseudomonas*, and *E. coli*, among other gram-negative infections. About 7% of isolates are anaerobic.

There are many different fungi that may be found in fungal sinusitis, although this is believed to be a less common problem. A recent study from the Mayo Clinic demonstrated that fungi can regularly be cultured from the nose and sinuses of both normal volunteers and patients with chronic rhinosinusitis. In this study, 96% of 210 patients with chronic sinusitis and 14 out of 14 normal volunteers were found to have fungi that could be obtained by washing the nose and sinuses [20••]. Allergic fungal sinusitis generally is diagnosed by the following criteria: (1) nasal polyposis, (2) allergic mucin, (3) chronic sinusitis by CT scan, (4) positive fungal culture or histology, and (5) allergy to fungi by history, skin test, or serology [21•]. About 7% of surgical cases of sinusitis are

eventually diagnosed as fungal sinusitis. The Mayo Clinic article suggests that a strikingly higher number might have fungi obtainable from the nose, but the presence of the same fungi in normal volunteers makes this observation's meaning much less certain.

DIAGNOSIS OF ACUTE SINUSITIS

The decision that the patient actually has sinusitis is based upon the symptom complex and confirmatory physical findings, taking into account the differential diagnosis of rhinitis (Table 11-4). Assuming that the cardinal signs and symptoms, including congestion and purulent drainage, direct the physician toward the diagnosis of sinusitis (see Table 11-3 for the symptoms of acute and chronic sinusitis), a careful examination of the anterior aspect of the nose with an otoscope should reveal the presence of purulent secretions.

Some physicians employ nasal smears in assessing sinusitis. Most sinus infections cause a neutrophil-rich secretion whereas colds produce a relatively acellular secretion. Nasal cultures have often been disappointing because they have not provided information that was useful in directing therapy against specific bacteria. The nasal cavity is coated with a number of bacteria, the "normal" nasal flora, which are harmless. Moreover, swabbing the inside of the nose usually leads to contamination with these bacteria and useless culture results. The best source of culture would be to aspirate the sinus itself by puncturing the cavity and washing out the secretions within. Unfortunately, this is not an easy procedure and is not done frequently in the United States. Alternatively, we have had very good success by using pediatric urethral culture swabs (calcium alginate on a thin wire that can be bent to assist in accessing mucus under the turbinate or posteriorly in the nose) and trying to place the culture swab directly into secretions guided by direct endoscopic visualization. Done well, the results of this type of culture have been quite useful in many patients and show a reasonable correlation with intra-sinus cultures.

If possible, examination of the posterior two thirds of the nose by flexible rhinoscopy can be performed in order to observe purulent drainage from the middle meatus or from the sphenoid ostia. Sometimes, the presence of purulent secretions posteriorly in the nose or in the piriform sinuses are the only visible evidence of sinusitis. Rhinoscopy allows the examiner to directly determine if an anatomical defect which predisposes to sinusitis is present.

In most instances of acute sinusitis, the diagnosis is made by a suggestive clinical history and supportive physical findings, and treatment is initiated empirically, with disease resolution within a few days.

TABLE 11-4. DIFFERENTIAL DIAGNOSIS OF RHINITIS

Infections	Rhinitis secondary to
Upper respiratory tract	Pregnancy
Sinusitis	Hypothyroidism
Allergic	Horner's syndrome
Seasonal	Wegener's granulomatosis
Perennial	Anatomical abnormalities causing rhinitis
Nonallergic rhinitis	Foreign body
Vasomotor rhinitis	Nasal polyps
Aspirin intolerance	Nasal septal deviation
Eosinophilic nonallergic rhinitis	Enlarged tonsils and adenoids
Rhinitis medicamentosa	Concha bullosum and other abnormalities of the middle turbinates
Decongestants	Tumors
β-blockers	Cerebral spinal fluid rhinorrhea
Birth control pills	
Antihypertensives	

CHRONIC SINUSITIS

Chronic sinusitis is the symptom complex caused by a persistent sinus infection or inflammation, lasting 8 to 12 weeks or more. Often, chronic or persistent sinusitis overlaps with recurrent sinusitis (four episodes of sinusitis per year for two or more years). In fact, when questioned, many patients with recurrent sinusitis claim that they never actually feel that their sinus symptoms completely resolve or that the symptoms recur shortly after each course of antibiotics. The classic symptoms of chronic sinusitis are nasal congestion, purulent drainage, and headache, along with the other symptoms listed in Table 11-3. Patients with chronic sinusitis may have a chronic bacterial or fungal infection of the sinuses, often superimposed upon a self-perpetuating inflammatory process in the sinuses that combine to produce the symptoms of sinusitis [1••]. The bacteria that cause chronic sinusitis include the same spectrum found in acute sinusitis, plus Staphylococcal spp, gram-negative bacteria, anaerobic bacteria, and fungi.

DIAGNOSIS OF CHRONIC SINUSITIS

In most instances, the diagnosis of chronic sinusitis is suggested by the symptom complex and confirmed by examination of the anterior and posterior aspect of the nose with otoscopy or flexible rhinoscopy. The presence of purulent drainage in the nose and throat supports the diagnosis, and when combined with the appropriate symptom complex, leads to treatment. In addition to rhinoscopy, transillumination of the frontal and maxillary sinuses may be helpful in both the diagnosis and follow-up of patients with sinusitis. Whereas the absolute confirmation of the diagnosis requires a radiologic examination, many physicians only use CT scans of the sinuses to examine patients who have failed initial treatment in order to confirm the diagnoses before intensifying the treatment plan. In the clinical population seen in our office, less than 20% of the sinusitis patients eventually undergo CT examination [22••]. Thus, the diagnosis is made on a presumptive basis, supported by history, physical findings, and rhinoscopy, and therapy is initiated. If the patient's clinical problems resolve, then the diagnosis is presumed to be correct and no radiologic examination is done. If the symptoms persist or worsen, then the CT is warranted, as are other facets of the work-up.

For the purposes of confirming the presence of sinusitis, only a limited CT of the sinuses in the coronal plane is necessary. Full sinus scans are required only at the time of surgery, when careful analysis of anatomic variations that might affect surgery must be reviewed. At our center, the limited coronal plane CT of the sinuses costs about the same as the "sinus series," four views of the sinuses done by standard radiologic techniques; however, the information yielded by the CT is infinitely more useful.

NASAL POLYPS

Nasal polyps are benign inflammatory growths that arise from the nose and sinuses and indicate the presence of rhinosinusitis. In a large series of patients with chronic sinusitis, nasal polyps were found in 10% [22••]. Moreover, most aspirin-sensitive patients have nasal polyps, as do those patients with cystic fibrosis, IgG or IgA deficiency, allergic fungal sinusitis, or abnormalities of ciliary function. Polyps most frequently arise in the region of the maxillary and ethmoid sinuses, although they can come from the turbinates as well. Sometimes polyps are found on CT scan deep within the sinus cavity. Polyps form from the swollen inflamed tissue inside the sinuses near the ostia or from the inflamed turbinates. Microscopically, polypoid tissue looks like normal sinus tissue except for the presence of eosinophils and the absence of normal submucosal glands. Polyps are richly endowed with blood vessels (and often bleed heavily when removed) but no pain fibers. They range in size from pea-sized to thumb-sized or larger. Some polyps grow posteriorly and extend into the posterior choana, blocking breathing.

The presence of polyps is suggested by persistent congestion and loss of the sense of smell. Polyps have a characteristic dusky grey color that distinguishes them from the pink nasal mucous membrane. It has been our experience that the underlying sinus infection will not resolve until the polyps have been reduced in size, either medically or surgically. Unfortunately, polyps recur. In fact, those patients who develop nasal polyps seem to perpetually carry the tendency for new polyp growth and recurrent sinus disease after any insult, from a cold to nasal congestion after exposure to strong smells. In one study of 200 patients with polyps, 115 had evidence of recurrence within a few years [23]. Thus, patients with polyps need to be warned that although polyps may be effectively treated medically or surgically, they have to be followed periodically for regrowth of polyps.

Often, the first sign of polyp recurrence is loss of the sense of smell. The sense of smell is mediated by the olfactory epithelium located high in the nose above the superior turbinate (Fig. 11-1). While extreme nasal congestion in rhinitis may reduce the sense of smell, sinusitis almost always reduces the sense of smell. Often the hyposmia or anosmia persists until the inflammatory condition is totally clear. In fact, many patients note that a change in their sense of smell is the earliest sign of an impending sinus infection. Nasal polyps almost always cause hyposmia, and a patient who describes persistent and profound anosmia should be carefully examined for the presence of polyps. Endoscopic examination of the nose can reveal the presence of asymptomatic polyps, which can be effectively treated before any symptoms develop.

The presence of unilateral polyposis or CT evidence of unilateral sinusitis should alert the physician to the possibility of additional diagnoses. In this situation the physician should consider the possibility of allergic fungal sinusitis or an intranasal or sinus tumor. The most frequent intra-nasal tumor is a benign but destructive inverted papilloma that resembles a polyp but can (rarely) undergo malignant transformation. Allergic fungal sinusitis can be suspected by the presence of a thick, brown mucus (described as resembling peanut butter) and thick dense secretions on CT scan.

DIFFERENTIATING SINUSITIS FROM RHINITIS

The differential diagnosis of rhinitis detailed on Table 11-4 is employed in determining if a patient has sinusitis and not rhinitis. The most common signs and symptoms differentiating noninfectious rhinitis from sinusitis are summarized in Table 11-5. Sinusitis involves inflammation of the sinuses, including those which drain primarily down the throat (the sphenoids and posterior ethmoids), causing postnasal drip, whereas rhinitis generally involves the anterior structures in the nose, leading to rhinorrhea. Thus, postnasal drip, the need to clear the throat, and a throat cough are usually found in sinusitis, and less so in rhinitis. The sense of smell is located high in the nose, near the superior turbinate (Fig. 11-1, olfactory cleft). While extreme nasal congestion in rhinitis may reduce the sense of smell, usually for relatively brief periods, sinusitis nearly always reduces the sense of smell, and often the hyposmia persists until the inflammatory condition is totally clear. Headaches can be caused by the pressure and fullness within an impacted or inflamed sinus cavity much more readily than in rhinitis.

It is important to differentiate the pain syndromes that might be confused with sinusitis. Migraine headaches usually are felt on one side of the head, are associated with nausea and light and sound sensitivity, last for hours to days, are throbbing in nature, and are often preceded by an aura. Pain from an inflamed temporomandibular joint (TMJ) is felt in the temples and worsened by jaw movement or chewing. Tension headaches usually are felt in the back of the neck or the sides of the head. Cluster headaches are rare, felt in one eye or the other, and associated with a runny nose and eye symptoms. The characteristic headache associated with sinusitis is steady (as opposed to throbbing), lasts for a few hours, is felt over the affected sinus, and is worsened by head movement. Most often there is no nausea or aura preceding the headache. Additionally, although pain is common in acute sinusitis, it is uncommon in chronic disease. The chronically thickened inflamed mucosa is less sensitive to pain. In fact, the most common symptoms of chronic sinusitis are not pain (Table 11-3) but a feeling of fullness in the face over the affected sinus.

One confounding syndrome should be noted. Some patients may present with "recurrent sinusitis" manifested as purulent postnasal drip accompanied by headaches. These patients are often thin, young women who have a very crowded nasal cavity. The syndrome they experience is due to nasal congestion leading to direct opposition of nasal mucosal surfaces upon each other. A layer of mucus may form between the opposing mucous membranes, which may even take on a purulent color and fool the physician into repeated courses of antibiotics. These patients generally retain their sense of smell, have limited postnasal drip and coughing, and have normal transillumination examinations of their sinuses. Absolute confirmation of this "rhinologic headache," as we call it (also known as a rhinopathic headache, Sluder's headache, and sphenopalatine headache [24••]), requires a CT examination, which is normal in the face of severe "sinus" symptoms. The application of topical anesthetics into the nose may reduce the "sinus headaches" experienced by these patients, and this procedure can be employed as a diagnostic test.

DISEASES WHICH PREDISPOSE TO DEVELOPING SINUSITIS

While an upper respiratory tract infection is the most common precipitating event in acute sinusitis, allergic and nonallergic rhinitis are the most common underlying causes of chronic or recurrent sinusitis (Table 11-6).

TABLE 11-5. SIGNS AND SYMPTOMS OF RHINITIS VERSUS SINUSITIS

Symptom	Rhinitis	Sinusitis
Congestion	++++	++++
Sneezing	+++	+
Itching	+++	-
Rhinorrhea		
Clear	++++	+
Purulent	+	++++
Postnasal drip	+ or ++	++++
Headache	+	+++
Facial pressure	+	++ to ++++
Anosmia, hyposmia	+ or ++	+++ or ++++
Cough	+	+++
Throat clearing	+	+++
Fever	- or +	++

In a series of 200 consecutive cases with chronic sinusitis, allergic rhinitis was found in 56% of the patients, whereas vasomotor rhinitis was believed to be the underlying cause in another 26% [22••]. The term *vasomotor rhinitis* (VMR) is used to describe a frequent and underappreciated diffuse nasal hyperreactivity syndrome of nasal congestion and rhinorrhea that is precipitated in response to environmental irritants, such as cold air, strong smells (perfume, cleaning solutions, paint), tobacco smoke, changes in the weather (particularly increases in humidity and barometric pressure as occur when storms move into the area), or from drinking beer or wine. This syndrome occurs primarily in women, most commonly of middle age, and may occur more often during the luteal phase of the menstrual cycle. About 10% of the time, VMR is found in men. VMR can overlap with allergic rhinitis and is invariably found in aspirin-sensitive patients.

Allergic disease is certainly the most common underlying cause of sinusitis because of the edema associated with allergies (with closure of the ostia) as well as the eosinophilic inflammatory infiltrate in the nasal and sinus mucosa [22••,25]. Moreover, allergic rhinitis leads to nasal mucosa hyperresponsiveness to nonspecific irritants and accentuates the tendency to VMR. An appropriate evaluation for underlying allergies is indicated in any patient with chronic or recurrent sinusitis, particularly if any of the signs suggesting allergies are present: seasonal disease, concomitant eczema or asthma, positive family history, pale nasal mucosa, associated conjunctivitis, disease exacerbated by exposure to allergens, such as dust or pets, or moderate eosinophilia.

Aspirin sensitivity is most commonly found in patients with asthma, moderate eosinophilia, nonallergic or allergic rhinitis, chronic or recurrent sinusitis, and nasal polyps. In 200 consecutive atients with chronic sinusitis, 10% were aspirin sensitive [22••]. It has always been believed that aspirin-sensitive patients are the most difficult patients with sinusitis to treat, in part because they do not always respond to antibiotics. If sinusitis is conceptualized as an inflammatory condition caused either by infection or alternatively as a self-perpetuating condition independent of infection, then the approach to aspirin sensitivity is somewhat clarified. In our experience, if it can be convincingly demonstrated that no infection is present, the use of oral corticosteroids, usually on an every-other-day basis, is employed and the disease tends to become somewhat less difficult to manage (discussed later).

Data exist suggesting that the long-term use of aspirin desensitization might be useful in managing these patients [26]. Aspirin desensitization is the progressive exposure of patients to increasing doses of aspirin until they are able to take two aspirin tablets twice a day [27]. The usual progression is 1, 5, 25, 81, 325, and 650 mg given orally at 90- to 120-minute intervals in a setting where vital signs can be monitored closely and emergency medical response is available. The other circumstance where a limited desensitization is required is when an aspirin-sensitive patient needs cardiac doses of aspirin for coronary disease.

Medications, either local or systemic, can cause nasal congestion and predispose to sinusitis. A careful history should alert the physician to this possibility. Examination of the nasal mucosa may occasionally raise the same possibility: the mucosa is often beefy red and irritated in response to repeated abuse of nasal decongestants, leading to rhinitis medicamentosa. Treatment of topical decongestant abuse involves local corticosteroids (although systemic corticosteroids may also be required).

The most frequent anatomical abnormalities predisposing to sinusitis are nasal septal defects and variations in the size and location of the middle turbinate. Nearly everyone has some nasal septal deviation; these variations become significant when they push the middle turbinate into the middle meatus, causing obstruction of the sinus outflow track. In determining whether a septal deviation might be severe enough to warrant resection, a simple test is suggested. Topical application of a decongestant is applied, and if the septum and turbinate separate sufficiently for air and secretions to flow, then medical management might suffice. Thereafter, a trial of

TABLE 11-6. CONDITIONS THAT PREDISPOSE TO CHRONIC SINUSITIS

Common conditions which cause sinusitis

Allergic and nonallergic rhinitis
Anatomic abnormality of the sinus outflow track
  Septal deviation
  Concha bullosum
  Paradoxical curvature of the middle turbinate
  Haller cells
Aspirin sensitivity
Common variable immunoglobulin deficiency
  IgG deficiency
  Specific antibody deficiency
  IgG subclass deficiency
  IgA deficiency
AIDS

Less common conditions which cause sinusitis:

Cystic fibrosis
Ciliary dyskinesia, Kartagener's syndrome, Young's syndrome
Bronchiectasis
Rhinitis medicamentosa
Cocaine abuse
Wegener's granulomatosis

topical nasal corticosteroids, plus consideration for an oral decongestant or prudent use of topical decongestants (no more than 3 days per week), is in order.

A concha bullosum is the presence of an extra sinus-like air cell within the middle turbinate which results in the turbinate becoming enlarged and often encroaching on the middle meatus. About 20% of normal subjects have this anatomic variation; thus, the presence of a concha bullosum, like the presence of nasal septal deviation, is not an indication for surgery. In patients with sinusitis, however, there is an increased frequency of concha bullosa, septal deviation, paradoxical curvature of the middle turbinate, Haller cells, and other anatomic variations [28].

Whenever a patient has recurrent or persistent sinusitis, especially when combined with bronchitis or otitis, an immunologic evaluation is in order. Patients who fail to make an adequate antibody response to bacterial infections usually develop sinusitis as the presenting disease. The major circulating antibody we produce is IgG, and clinically significant deficiencies in IgG levels nearly always lead to sinusitis. The major antibody designed to protect mucous membranes is IgA. IgA is produced by lymphocytes congregated around the submucosal glands in the lamina propria. IgA secreted by the lymphocytes is taken up by serous cells in the seromucous glands, an additional piece of protein (the secretory piece) is added conjoining two IgA molecules, and the secretory IgA is then secreted as a component of mucus. The secreted IgA functions to kill viruses and bacteria. Absence of IgA may lead to sinusitis in some patients, but not everyone deficient in IgA develops clinical problems. It is not uncommon to find abnormally low levels of both IgG and IgA in patients with recurrent or chronic sinusitis, especially if bronchitis is present as well.

The screening tests suggested include determining the serum concentrations of IgG, IgA, and IgM, the three major circulating antibodies [7]. Some sinusitis patients have the pattern of somewhat reduced IgG and IgA along with increased amounts of IgM. Unless the levels of IgG or IgA are grossly reduced (more than 20% below normal), the critical question is whether the patient can make an antibody response to appropriate bacteria. Thus, the evaluation of such patients includes immunization with Pneumovax (Merck & Co., West Point, PA) (the vaccine developed to reduce the incidence of pneumonia) and measurement of antibodies directed at the various serotypes of Pneumococci 2 months later. The post-immunization titers should either fall within the therapeutic range or increase from baseline by four-fold to sixfold. Thus, using Pneumovax immunizations determines if the patient can make an adequate antibody response, and at the same time may help protect the patient from infections caused by the Pneumococcal bacteria. In our office, we routinely immunize with Pneumovax for chronic or persistent sinus disease.

Sometimes patients are also immunized with *H. influenzae* B conjugated to protein (ProHIBiT; Aventis Pasteur, Swiftwater, PA) or tetanus toxoid in order to determine if the patient can make antibodies to these proteins as well. Both Haemophilus and tetanus raise a specific type of IgG antibody called IgG1, whereas Pneumovax raises an IgG2 response. Thus, using these different immunizations allows an allergist-immunologist to assess the adequacy of immune responses in these patients. It is not recommended that physicians go to the bother and expense of these measurements unless the patient has recurrent or persistent disease, and there is a consideration for the use of IgG replacement therapy.

The sinus disease in some patients with IgG deficiency cannot be managed without correcting the antibody deficiency. In our experience, those patients whose total IgG is more than 20% below the lowest limit of normal IgG values, or who cannot make adequate antibody responses to immunizations, may require IgG replacement therapy. This population represents about 25% to 50% of those patients with IgG deficiency; the remainder of the patients do quite well with good medical management (see below) and do not need IgG replacement therapy to stay well.

IgG is prepared from a large pool of healthy normal subjects (up to 10,000 donors are pooled). The IgG is isolated by a number of steps designed to remove and inactivate any possible infectious agents (such as HIV); however, there are some data suggesting that a few patients in the United States might have contracted hepatitis C from IgG during the early 1990s. IgG is infused intravenously in order to raise the IgG to levels consistently above normal in the patient's blood. In most subjects, infusing IgG at 400 mg/kg results in normal IgG levels for 4 weeks or longer. Generally, IgG is infused monthly, and the trough level is maintained at the lowest limit of normal levels.

Because such a large pool of IgG donors is used, essentially every IgG antibody directed against all bacteria and viruses should be present in the IgG preparation. Unfortunately, not everyone who gets IgG replacement has an adequate outcome, and if patients are still having infections after 6 months of replacement therapy, the cost and inconvenience of IgG replacement have to be weighed against the therapeutic response. IgG is quite expensive, and even with good insurance, it costs some patients $4000 to $8000 per year.

TREATMENT
Pharmacologic treatment of acute sinusitis

The decisions of when and how to treat patients with sinusitis are determined by the patient's age, the acuteness of the infection, the underlying disease which predisposed toward sinusitis, and the history of previous treatments. Acute and chronic or recurrent sinusitis are treated differently, and the presence of nasal polyposis, IgG or IgA deficiency, or aspirin sensitivity definitely influences the treatment plan.

The treatment of acute sinusitis includes an antibiotic given in sufficient dosage for an adequate period of time. Our "rule of thumb" is to treat the patient until he or she is well, plus an additional 7 days. For acute sinusitis, that usually means 10 to 14 days. The antibiotics suggested reflect our experience with antibiotic resistance and the prevalence of uncomfortable side effects. In a community-based practice, a short course of amoxicillin (500 mg three times daily for 3 days, or 40 mg/kg/d in three divided doses for children) as a first order of therapy is appropriate. If the patient has an initial response (feels much better and secretions are diminishing and clearing in color), continue the treatment until he or she is well, plus 7 additional days. If the patient fails to respond after 3 days, switch to these more broadly active (and more expensive) products; they have proven effective and are listed here roughly in the order of preference in our experience: cefuroxime axitil (250 mg twice daily) and amoxicillin-clavulanate (875 mg twice daily) have been the most reliable choices; clarithromycin (1000 mg/d) is a good next choice in selected individuals, and gatifloxicin (400 mg/d) or levofloxacin (500 mg/d) is an excellent choice if the other antibiotics fail. Additional antibiotics that can be employed include trimethoprim/sulfamethoxazole (one double-strength twice daily), clindamycin (Cleocin [Pharmacia & Upjohn, Kalamazoo, MI], 300 mg three times daily), and other second- or third-generation cephalosporins. Azithromycin is an excellent antibiotic for certain infections but a single course has not proven adequate in sinusitis. Ceclor (Eli Lilly and Company, Indianapolis, IN) was an excellent choice for the treatment of sinusitis in the past, but the incidence of resistant bacteria has made this antibiotic a less attractive choice.

The choices of antibiotics suggested are based both upon their proven efficacy and the increasing pattern of penicillin-resistance exhibited by the bacteria most commonly aspirated from the sinuses of acutely infected subjects. Although the incidence of antibiotic resistance was below 20% a decade ago, current data suggest that 50% of *S. pneumoniae*, 42% of *H. influenzae*, and more than 90% of *M. catarrhalis* are either moderately or highly resistant to penicillin [29•]. Why then might one select amoxicillin as the starting antibiotic? Approximately 50% of acute sinusitis infections tend to resolve in a few days without the need for antibiotics (probably indicating a self-limited viral infection), and about 50% of those infected with either pneumococcus or *Haemophilus* will respond to amoxicillin. Thus, about 75% of patients should respond to this relatively safe and inexpensive antibiotic; however, failure to have an initial response (after 3 days) should lead to

the use of the potent beta-lactamase–resistant antibiotics listed previously.

A sinus infection usually indicates both bacterial overgrowth and obstruction to drainage from the sinus outflow track. Thus, the treatment plan should have two components: an antibiotic and a strategy to open and drain the sinuses. A decongestant, either applied topically (such as Afrin [Schering-Plough, Kenilworth, NJ], 1–2 sprays twice daily for 3–7 days) or orally (such as pseudoephedrine 30–60 mg, two to four times daily), is recommended in order to facilitate drainage from the sinuses. First-generation antihistamines usually are not used in this circumstance because of their drying actions. The exception to this rule is sinusitis in an allergic subject experiencing allergic symptoms, including swelling of the nasal mucosa, which might contribute to obstruction of the sinus outflow track. In this circumstance, a nonsedating antihistamine, such as fexofenadine (Allegra [Aventis Pharmaceuticals, Kansas City, MO], 180 mg/d) or loratidine (Claritin [Schering, Kenilworth, NJ], 10 mg/d), is selected because these agents do not cause mucus inspissation.

To help clear secretions, patients are advised to drink six to eight full glasses of liquid per day and to lavage their nasal cavities with saline (Table 11-7). To open the ostia and reduce swelling in the nose, one of the topical corticosteroid preparations available may also be employed.

Thus, the treatment for acute sinusitis may include oral hydration, an antibiotic, a topical (or less often,

---

TABLE 11-7. NASAL LAVAGE

To wash the nose (and sinuses), patients lavage their noses in the morning and at night, sometimes after one to two sprays of a long-acting nasal decongestant. As a rule of thumb, use topical decongestants for up to 3 consecutive days or as often as every other day. The easiest method involves:

1) Prepare saline solution using a half-teaspoon salt (non-iodized salt may be used to avoid stinging), 8 oz warm tap water, and a pinch of baking soda. For some patients, one to two teaspoons of providone-iodine (Betadine*) are added to the saline washes.

2) Lean over the sink and, using an ear bulb syringe, expel the solution into each nostril, repeatedly aspirating and washing the nose until all secretions are washed out.

Alternatives include using a cold-steam vaporizer to create a "steam tent" for 15 minutes; a facial sauna; or long, hot showers. For recurrent disease, especially after surgical enlargement of the ostia, the purchase of a Waterpik† with a Grossan‡ nasal adapter may be warranted.

Purdue Frederich Company, Norwalk, CT
† Water Pik Technologies, Inc., Fort Collins, CO
‡ HydroMed Inc., Sherman Oaks, CA

systemic) decongestant, nasal lavage, and a topical corticosteroid. There are no adequate trials of "muco-evacuants," and our experience has not supported their usefulness.

CHRONIC SINUSITIS

Chronic sinusitis is treated in a similar way as acute sinusitis except that the antibiotics may be given for a longer period of time (up to 3–6 weeks), and the nasal treatment includes the chronic use of a topical nasal corticosteroid preparation (Table 11-8). The choice of antibiotics for chronic sinusitis usually does not include amoxicillin; instead, the broad-spectrum antibiotics listed above are begun with the intent of treating for 3 to 4 weeks or more, until the patient is completely well.

The use of topical corticosteroids prevents rhinitis medicamentosa from developing from the topical decongestant, and therefore the decongestants may be used for a longer period of time. There are at least five topical nasal corticosteroid preparations on the market in the United States today and all are effective for treating the

---

TABLE 11-8. APPROACH TO THE TREATMENT OF CHRONIC SINUSITIS

1) Hydration (six to eight glasses of water per day)
2) Antibiotics (21 days or longer; until patient is well plus 7 days)

    Cefuroxime axetil (Ceftin; Glaxo Wellcome, Research Triangle Park, NC)

    Amoxicillin and clavulanate (Augmentin; SmithKline Beecham Pharmaceuticals, Philadelphia, PA)

    Clarithromycin (Biaxin; Abbott Laboratories, North Chicago, IL)

    Levofloxacin (Levaquin; Ortho-McNeil Pharmaceutical, Raritan, NJ)
3) Topical long-acting decongestants, twice daily for 7 to 14 days

    Oxymetazoline (Afrin; Schering-Plough, Kenilworth, NJ)
4) Nasal lavage using saline applied via ear bulb syringe or Waterpik (Water Pik Technologies, Inc., Fort Collins, CO) plus Grossan adapter (HydroMed Inc., Sherman Oaks, CA) twice daily
5) Topical corticosteroids* (aim toward the eye and away from the nasal septum)

    Three sprays twice daily for 2 weeks

    Two sprays twice daily for 2 to 8 weeks until symptomatically well

    One to two sprays, one to two times daily until sinusitis is resolved

Choice of nasal corticosteroid may be determined by patient preference. Dry sprays are administered by metered-dose canister, whereas wet sprays are hand-activated pumps. All of the current nasal corticosteroid preparations are effective.

---

underlying rhinitis. The data supporting topical corticosteroids in the management of chronic sinusitis are limited, but appear to be rational based upon our understanding of the disease. The choice of topical corticosteroid is predicated on patient preference for a dry or wet spray, or one that does not smell. There are suggestions that some corticosteroids might have less systemic absorption than others (mometesone [Nasonex; Schering, Kenilworth, NJ] and fluticasone [Flonase; GlaxoWellcome Inc., Research Triangle Park, NC]). Some patients prefer odorless products (triamcinolone [Nasacort AQ; Aventis Pharmaceuticals, Parsippany, NJ] or budesonide [Rhinocort Aqua; AstraZeneca, Wilmington, DE]). Another consideration is the wide range in pricing that might affect compliance.

There has been a very disturbing observation of a reduction in linear growth in children treated with nasal beclomethasone sprays for a year [30••]. Thus, prescribing topical corticosteroids should be done with an eye for the safety of the product and its cost and presumed usefulness. A reasonable plan is to use the topical corticosteroids at high dose until the symptoms are resolved and then to use the lowest dose possible thereafter. Generally, we maintain sinusitis patients with 1 to 2 sprays of nasal corticosteroids per day for extended periods and increase the dosing whenever an episode occurs.

Our experience indicates that topical corticosteroids act to keep the sinus outflow track open and prevent recurrence of disease. There is evidence suggesting that the distribution and retention of the steroid sprays is increased if the patient administers the medications in a "head down" position. This position can be accomplished by having the patient assume a kneeling position with the neck flexed forward, or by lying prone on a bed with the neck flexed next to a pillow or hyperextended back over a pillow. When administering topical corticosteroids, the patient is instructed to direct the corticosteroid spray away from the nasal septum and toward the eye in order to reduce the risk of a septal perforation. Septal perforations usually are heralded by nose bleeds and some irritation. Steroid irritation of the septum can be treated by placing a small amount of petroleum jelly on the septum prior to nasal washing and corticosteroid usage, and by reminding the patient to aim the steroid out toward the eye. If a septal perforation does occur, it is often only of cosmetic importance, and we do not recommend surgical repair. When considerable symptomatology does occur, repair may be affected by surgical closure or a prosthetic button.

If the patient does not improve or experiences a recurrence after a relatively brief asymptomatic phase, the most prudent option is to consider a second course of antibiotics (either the same antibiotic or one chosen with a different spectrum of activity) while continuing the other components of treatment (Table 11-8). In this circumstance, a CT scan is indicated. It is possible that the patient might have a tumor or other process mimicking sinusitis, or a fungal sinusitis. Fungal sinusitis requires surgical intervention plus aggressive medical antifungal treatment. Alternatively, some patients experience sinusitis-like symptoms, but their sinuses are normal or minimally involved. Such patients may have the "rhinologic syndrome" described earlier. About 75% of patients with recurrent sinusitis treated medically will respond to initial treatment with improvement, some permanently [22••].

Some patients fail to respond to initial therapy because they have an anaerobic infection of their sinuses. The suspicion for an anaerobic infection may be raised by the results of culture of sinus secretions, the presence of foul breath or a fetid odor from the nasal cavity, or by the prior use of repeated courses of broad-spectrum antibiotics. In this circumstance, it might be appropriate to try a combination of broad-spectrum antibiotics plus metronidizole (500 mg four times daily for 14 days) or, alternatively, clindamycin (500 mg three times daily).

Some patients have recurrent symptoms despite apparent resolution initially. These patients may respond only if maintained on long-term antibiotics. Good success has been seen with doxycycline (50 mg daily or twice daily) for prolonged periods. In such patients, if an episode of acute sinusitis should occur despite the prophylactic doxycycline, a second antibiotic is administered for the usual course and the doxycycline is temporarily suspended. In such patients, a CT scan and a consultation with an experienced otolaryngologist is appropriate. Patients who have negative cultures may have a sterile inflammatory process that requires systemic corticosteroids along with topical corticosteroids. In these patients, an initial course of oral corticosteroids given on a daily basis is followed by treatment every other day, employing the lowest dose which maintains remission. Often, 5 to 15 mg of prednisone every other day, given along with nasal lavage and topical nasal corticosteroids, can maintain a relatively asymptomatic state.

Aspirin sensitivity is caused by an abnormal production of leukotrienes, associated with an exaggerated response to leukotrienes [31]. Three medications are available in the United States which interfere with leukotrienes, either by inhibiting leukotriene synthesis (zileuton [Zyflo; Abbott Laboratories, North Chicago, IL]) or by receptor blockade (zifirlukast [Accolate; AstraZeneca, Wilmington, DE] and montelukast [Singulair; Merck & Co., West Point, PA]). In patients with aspirin sensitivity, a trial of either Accolate (20 mg twice daily on an empty stomach), Singulair (10 mg at night), or Zyflo (600 mg four times daily) may be attempted. Some of the patients in whom these medicines have been tried appear to have less nasal symptoms and require fewer courses of antibiotics for acute

infections. Zyflo is associated with increased liver enzymes in about 4% of patients, and liver function tests need to be monitored if there is an initial response. Neither product is licensed for use in sinusitis, but both are worth trying in difficult-to-manage patients, especially if they have polyposis or aspirin sensitivity.

COMPLICATIONS OF SINUSITIS

With proper management, complications of sinusitis today are rare and more common with acute bacterial sinusitis than with chronic sinusitis. The adolescent male without a prior history of sinusitis is more at risk for intracranial complications, whereas young children are more at risk for orbital complications. In untreated patients with chronic sinusitis, the disease process may destroy adjacent bony walls. Indeed, some recent studies suggest that the bone does become actively involved during sinus infections. Some of the complications of sinusitis are summarized on Table 11-9. Microbial infections of the sinuses may destroy adjacent bony walls and dissect into the orbit, brain, or one of the major nerves or arteries which pass through the sinuses (the carotid artery and optic nerve both pass through the sphenoid sinus).

Sinusitis and nasal polyposis are associated with loss of the sense of smell and partial to significant loss of the sense of taste. Mouth breathing introduces unfiltered air into the lungs and may play a role in the frequent association between sinusitis and asthma. Asthma occurs in about 5% of the population, but is found in 20% to 35% of patients with chronic sinusitis. Conversely, sinusitis is found in up to 75% of moderate to severe asthmatics. There are several hypotheses as to frequent coexistence of asthma and sinusitis. As mentioned, mouth breathing may introduce allergen-laden air to the lungs and predispose toward the development of allergic asthma; however, many asthmatics who have sinusitis do not have apparent allergies, and in fact may only experience asthma when their sinuses are infected. It is possible that concordant nasal, sinus, and bronchial disease could reflect contiguous diseases affecting the upper and lower respiratory track. There is also evidence for a sino-nasal-bronchial reflex that would account for lower respiratory airflow obstruction when

TABLE 11-9. COMPLICATIONS OF SINUSITIS	
CNS infections	Cavernous sinus thrombosis
Orbital cellulitis	Optic neuritis
Reactive meningitis	Carotid aneurysm
Osteomyelitis	Anosmia

the sinuses are inflamed. Other possible reasons for this association include drainage of purulent secretions into the bronchi with resultant bronchitis. In offices where moderate to severe asthma is treated, identification and treatment of concomitant sinusitis markedly enhances the treatment of asthma.

SURGERY IN THE MANAGEMENT OF RHINOSINUSITIS

Surgery is indicated in severe acute rhinosinusitis that has not responded to appropriate medical therapy or when the development of complications is suspected. In general, the risk of complications from sinusitis is greater in acute frontal or acute sphenoid sinusitis, and therefore these patients require more intense monitoring, and earlier consideration should be given to otolaryngologic consultation should these patients fail to respond appropriately to medical therapy. In chronic and recurrent acute sinusitis, surgery usually is reserved for those patients who have failed adequate medical therapy and have persistent disease or recurrent symptoms after several courses of antibiotics and other appropriate medical intervention; however, earlier surgical consultation should be sought in patients with suspected fungal sinusitis or in patients with unilateral disease that may be suspicious for a neoplasm.

In general, sinus surgery is now performed endoscopically, working through the nose. The goals of surgery are to remove both obstructive mucosal disease and osteitic bone in areas of disease, remove inspissated mucus and pus, and restore normal mucociliary clearance. With our improved knowledge of the pathogenesis of sinusitis, significant care and attention is now directed during surgery to avoiding stripping mucosa and exposing bone.

The extent of surgery is dependent upon the extent of disease present and may vary between a very limited opening of a maxillary sinus ostium to an extensive resection of the ethmoid air cells and opening and removal of disease from the frontal and sphenoid sinuses. In general, however, care should be taken to preserve the normal anatomic structures inasmuch as this is possible with any given extent of disease. We generally prefer to preserve the normal turbinate structures when these are not involved in the disease process to maintain normal nasal function. The inferior turbinates, in particular, are dynamic structures, responding with congestion to both environmental stimuli and to the presence of sinus inflammation, as well as controlling the normal nasal airflow cycle. Additionally, there is some evidence to suggest that inappropriate inferior turbinectomy may increase the risk of maxillary sinus disease [32]. When a septal deformity either appears to be contributing to the disease process or limits access to areas of disease, a septoplasty is performed. Unfortunately, patients who have formed polyps tend to have polyp regrowth after

surgery, and it is appropriate to warn them that they may require prolonged use of nasal washings and topical nasal corticosteroids despite surgical resection.

With current endoscopic techniques, postsurgical pain, discomfort, and swelling are generally minimal, and the surgery itself can frequently be performed under local anesthesia. Because of the location of the sinuses and their immediate anatomical relationships, there are serious potential risks from sinus surgery. These potentially devastating complications include diplopia or even loss of vision, or cerebrospinal fluid leak with attendant risk of meningitis or intracranial injury; however, in the hands of a skilled endoscopic sinus surgeon, the incidence of such major complications is very low [33,34]. The primary issues in the surgical decision-making process are therefore the expected degree of improvement in the disease process and the effort and discomfort involved in performing endoscopic follow-up and necessary office débridement. The latter is required to ensure that persistent inflammation does not lead to restenosis and recurrent disease. Particularly in more extensive disease, surgery should be considered as an adjunct rather than an alternative to appropriate medical therapy.

Several days prior to surgery, patients with extensive polyposis, very reactive nasal mucosa, or concomitant asthma should be started on oral steroid therapy to reduce mucosal hyperreactivity and bleeding and to minimize any risk of bronchospasm. Postoperatively, the steroids in these patients should be tapered based upon the endoscopic appearance of sinus mucosa, but they should be tapered sufficiently slowly to ensure that early obstruction and adhesions do not reform. Broad-spectrum antibiotics usually are provided in the postoperative period during the time that mucociliary clearance remains compromised and small areas of bone may be exposed. Because there is evidence to suggest that the bone becomes significantly involved in chronic sinusitis and in the presence of severe disease, oral antibiotic courses may be prolonged, and in some cases, parenteral antibiotics may be advocated [35••]. Typically, it is recommended that all patients continue their topical nasal steroid sprays until such time as it is clear from nasal endoscopy that the mucosa within the sinuses is both stable and normal in appearance. In a number of cases, topical steroid therapy will be continued long term. In the early postoperative period, topical nasal saline sprays or saline or antibiotic irrigations may be recommended to reduce postoperative crusting. Finally, patients usually are required to return for frequent follow-up for nasal endoscopy and office cleaning of the cavity under topical anesthesia, until such time that the cavity has healed.

Overall, the results from such surgical intervention, combined with appropriate medical therapy, are excellent. In a prospective study performed at the University of Pennsylvania, 98.4% of patients reported subjective improvement on long-term follow-up (mean 7.8 years postsurgery), and 90% of patients with asthma reported significant improvement [35••,36••]. Oral steroid and antibiotic use was also decreased despite the fact that the cohort largely consisted of a group of tertiary referral patients with disease that had been previously recalcitrant to both prior medical and surgical therapy. Other studies have similarly demonstrated both significant improvement in disease-specific symptom scores and in overall quality of life following sinus surgery [37,38]. On the other hand, it is important not to confuse symptomatic improvement in this disease with cure.

Surgery, therefore, should be considered as an approach with a high success rate for patients with recalcitrant disease; however, it should be recognized that surgical intervention, per se, does not result in disease resolution, especially in advanced disease. Surgery should be considered as adjunctive to the patient's overall medical management, and postoperative endoscopic observation is required for persistent asymptomatic disease that may result in recurrent symptoms over time. Even after surgery, and in the face of continued medical management, some patients will continue to experience episodes of sinusitis. Continued research into the pathophysiology of sinusitis will be required before we understand how best to manage these patients. Additionally, we need to develop a better understanding of the most appropriate timing and patient selection for surgical intervention and improved understanding of the natural course of this all-too-common disorder [1••]. None of these studies will be carried out until the medical and lay communities recognize the importance of sinusitis in terms of economic cost and quality of life and urge funding of additional research and prospective clinical trials.

REFERENCES AND RECOMMENDED READING

Recently published papers of particular interest have been highlighted as:
• Of interest
•• Of outstanding interest

1.•• Kaliner MA, Osguthorpe JD, Fireman P, et al.: Sinusitis: bench to bedside. J Allergy Clin Immunol 1997, 99:S829–S848.
A concise, provocative summary of what is known and what is not understood about acute and chronic sinusitis. This paper represents our current state of knowledge and is heavily cited.

2. Collins JG: Prevalence of selected chronic conditions: United States, 1986–1988. National Center for Health Statistics. Vital Health Stat 1993, 10:1–87.

3.•• Kaliner MA: Allergy care in the next millennium: Guidelines for the specialty. J Allergy Clin Immunol 1997, 99:729–734.
My Presidential address to the American Academy of Allergy, Asthma, and Immunology. This paper lays out the reasons for referring sinusitis patients to specialists and what a referring physicians should learn from the referral.

4. Ray NF, Baraniuk J, Thamer M, et al.: Healthcare expenditures for the treatment of sinusitis in 1996: contributions of asthma, rhinitis and other airway disorders. J Allergy Clin Immunol 1999, 103:408–414.

5. McCraig LF, Hughes JM: Trends in antimicrobial drug prescribing among office-based physicians in the United States. JAMA 1995, 273:214–219.

6. Raphael GD, Baraniuk JN, Kaliner MA: How the nose runs and why. J Allergy Clin Immunol 1991, 87:457–467.

7. Kaliner MA: Human nasal host defense and sinusitis. In Diseases of the Sinuses. Edited by Gershwin ME, Incaudo GA. Humana Press: Totowa NJ; 1996:53–6.

8. McMenamin P: Costs of hay fever in the United States in 1990. Ann Allergy 1994, 73:35–39.

9. Ray NF, Thamer M, Rinehart CS, et al.: Medical expenditures for the treatment of allergic rhinoconjunctivitis in the United States in 1996. J Allergy Clin Immunol 1999: 103:401-407.

10. Peynegre R, Rouvier P: Anatomy and anatomical variations of the paranasal sinuses: influence on sinus dysfunction. In Diseases of the Sinuses. Edited by Gershwin ME, Incaudo GA. Totowa, NJ: Humana Press; 1996:3–33.

11.•• Messerklinger W: Endoscopy of the Nose. Baltimore: Urban and Schwarzenberg; 1978.
A classic book describing the functional anatomy of the nose and sinuses. This book introduced the concepts of functional endoscopic surgery to the United States.

12.• Berg O, Carenfelt C, Rystedt G, Anggard A: Occurrence of asymptomatic sinusitis in common cold and other acute ENT-infections. Rhinology 1986, 24:223–225.

13.• Aitken M, Taylor JA: Prevalence of clinical sinusitis in young children followed up by primary care pediatricians. Arch Pediatr Adolesc Med 1998, 152:244–248.

14.•• Gwaltney JM Jr, Phillips CD, Miller RD, Riker DK: Computed tomographic study of the common cold. N Engl J Med 1994, 330:25–30.

15. Hamilos DL, Leung DYM, Woods R, et al.: Chronic hyperplastic sinusitis: association of tissue eosinophilia with mRNA expression of granulocyte-macrophage colony stimulating-factor and interleukin-3. J Allergy Clin Immunol 1993, 92:39–48.

16. Hamilos DL, Leung DYM, Wood R, et al.: Evidence for distinct cytokine expression in allergic versus nonallergic chronic sinusitis. J Allergy Clin Immunol 1995, 96:537–544.
This paper shows how frequently colds lead to radiologic evidence of sinusitis.

17. Denburg JA, Gauldie J, Dolovich J, et al.: Structural cell-derived cytokines in allergic inflammation. Int Arch Allergy Appl Immunol 1991, 94:127–132.

18.• Gwaltney JM, Scheld WM, Sande MA, Sydnor A: The microbial etiology and antimicrobial therapy of adults with acute community-acquired sinusitis: a fifteen year experience at the University of Virginia. J Allergy Clin Immunol 1992, 90:457–462.

19.•• Wald ER: Microbiology of acute and chronic sinusitis in children and adults. Am J Med Sci 1998, 316:13–20.
Antral puncture cultures in children reveal the incidence of specific bacterial infections.

20.•• Ponokau JU, Sherris DA, Kern EB, et al.: The diagnosis and incidence of allergic fungal sinusitis. Mayo Clin Proc 1999, 74:877–884.
Cultures of the nose and sinuses of patients with sinusitis reveal a wide range of fungi. This article is certain to lead to diagnostic and therapeutic trials.

21.• Bent JP III, Kuhn FA: Diagnosis of allergic fungal sinusitis. Otolaryngol Head Neck Surg 1994, 111:580–588.

22.•• McNally PA, White MV, Kaliner MA: Sinusitis in an allergist's office: analysis of 200 consecutive cases. Allergy Asthma Proceedings 1997, 18:169–176.
The largest study of the medical evaluation and treatment of patients with chronic sinusitis. A must read for anyone managing sinusitis.

23. Drake-Lee AB, Lowe D, Swanston A, et al.: Clinical profile and recurrence of nasal polyps. J Laryngol Otol 1984, 98:783–793.

24.•• Clerico DM: Rhinopathic headaches: referred pain of nasal and sinus origin. In *Diseases of the Sinuses*. Edited by Gershwin ME, Incaudo GA. Humana Press: Totowa, NJ; 1996:403–424.
A fascinating review of headaches and sinusitis.

25. Pelikan Z: The role of allergy in sinus disease. In *Diseases of the Sinuses*. edited by Gershwin ME, Incaudo GA. Humana Press: Totowa, NJ; 1996: 97–166.

26. Stevenson DD: Commentary: the American experience with aspirin desensitization for aspirin-sensitive rhinosinusitis and asthma. *Allerg Proc* 1992, 13:185–192.

27. Mathison DA, Simon RA, Stevenson DD: Aspirin, sulfur dioxide/sulfite, and other chemical sensitivities and challenges in asthmatic patients. In *Provocation Testing in Clinical Practice*. Edited by Spector SL. New York: Marcel Dekker; 1995:599–622.

28. Zinreich SJ: Radiologic diagnosis of the nasal cavity and paranasal sinuses. In *Sinusitis: Pathophysiology and Treatment*. Edited by Druce HD. New York: Marcel Dekker; 1994:57–72.

29.• Gruneberg RN, Felmingham D, the Alexander Project Group: Results of the Alexander Project: a continuing, multicenter study of the antimicrobial susceptibility of community-acquired lower respiratory tract bacterial pathogens. *Diagn Microbiol Infect Dis* 1996, 25:169–181.

30.•• Rachelefsky GS, Chervinsky P, Meltzer EO, *et al.*: An evaluation of the effects of beclomethasone diproprionate aqueous nasal spray (Vancenase AQ) on long-term growth in children. *J Allergy Clin Immunol* 1998, 109:S236.

31. Kowalski ML: Pathophysiology of rhinosinusitis in aspirin-sensitive patients. In *Progress in Allergy and Clinical Immunology*, vol 4. Edited by Oehling AK, Huerta Lopez JG. Seattle: Hogrefe and Huber; 1997:174–178.
An extremely important study that demonstrates growth suppression in children taking normal doses of nasal beclomethasone.

32. Berenholz L, Kessler A, Sarfati S, *et al.*: Chronic sinusitis: a sequela of inferior turbinectomy. *Am J Rhinol* 1998, 12:257–261.

33. Kennedy DW: Prognostic factors, outcomes and staging in ethmoid sinus surgery. *Laryngoscope* 1992, 102:1–18.

34. Stankiewicz JA: Complications in endoscopic intranasal ethmoidectomy: an update. *Laryngoscope* 1989, 99:686–690.

35.•• Senior BA, Kennedy DW, Tanabodee J, *et al.*: Long-term results of functional endoscopic sinus surgery. *Laryngoscope* 1998, 108:151–157.
The largest long-term analysis of functional endoscopic sinus surgery. These are the undisputed leaders in sinus surgery in the United States.

36.•• Senior BA, Kennedy DW, Tanabodee J, *et al.*: Long-term impact of functional endoscopic sinus surgery on asthma. *Otolaryngol Head Neck Surg* 1999, 121:66–68.
This study confirms and extends earlier work by Ray Slavin on the usefulness of sinus treatment in the management of asthma.

37. Gliklich RE, Metson R: The health impact of chronic sinusitis in patients seeking otolaryngologic care. *Otolaryngol Head Neck Surg* 1995, 113:104–109.

38. Hoffman SJ, Dersarkissian RM, Buck SH, *et al.*: Sinus disease and surgical treatment: a results oriented quality assurance study. *Otolaryngol Head Neck Surg* 1989, 100:573–577.

CHAPTER 12

Conjunctivitis and Allergic Eye Diseases

Leonard Bielory
Patrick Ambrosio

The eye can often be viewed as a common target of allergic and immunologic disorders. Primary care physicians are usually the first to correlate ocular diagnosis with systemic findings in a patient and formulate a treatment plan.

Ocular inflammation often presents itself in the form of a "red eye." The most common etiologies include allergic or infectious agents. In the majority of cases, a thorough history and physical examination focusing on signs and symptoms will yield a presumptive diagnosis. Other etiologies will need to be considered in patients with atypical clinical signs and symptoms and in patients who do not respond to standard therapy. This chapter reviews conjunctivitis in its many different forms as well as other allergic ocular disorders.

CATEGORIES OF OCULAR INFLAMMATION AND OCULAR MAST CELLS

The eye is a complex organ usually involved in allergic and immunologic disorders. The conjunctiva is often described as the most immunologically active tissue of the external eye [1••]. Histologically, it is divided into two layers—the epithelial and substantia propria. Mast cells, Langerhans' cells, CD3+ lymphocytes, cytotoxic antibodies, and immune complexes are all involved in the ocular immunological hypersensitivity reactions (Table 12-1) [2•].

Mast cells are the principal cell type that initiates inflammatory responses, which are associated with immediate hypersensitivity reactions. Histamine, leukotrienes, prostaglandins, proteoglycans, and neutral proteases (tryptase, chymase) are all mediators that are released by mast cells upon activation. Two different types of mast cells exist, based on their tryptase-chymase content. Ocular mast cells are normally of the tryptase-positive, chymase-positive type, which is commonly designated as the connective tissue type mast cell. We currently have strong evidence for the role of the mast cell in chronic inflammatory diseases of the eye because examination of conjunctival tissue reveals invasion by mast cells with release of mast cell mediators in tear fluid [3••]. Vernal conjunctivitis, giant papillary conjunctivitis (GPC), and atopic keratoconjunctivitis are disorders in which increased concentrations of mast cells have been reported [3••,4••].

HISTORY AND PHYSICAL EXAMINATION

Obtaining an accurate and detailed history is by far the key element in making a differential diagnosis between allergic and nonallergic diseases of the eye. Patients may reveal recent exposure to individuals with upper respiratory tract illnesses or conjunctivitis, either at home or at the workplace. Obtaining a sexual history may further reveal clues to suggest chlamydial or neisserial infection. A complete past medical history may give the clinician clues to associated ocular conditions, such as in rheumatoid arthritis or other collagen vascular disorders. Patients will often present to a physician with ocular symptoms consisting of low-grade ocular and periocular itching, tearing, burning, stinging, photophobia, and watery discharge. Patients most commonly complain of a red and itchy eye. Symptoms tend to be better during cool and rainy weather and are generally worse when the weather is warm and dry. Symptoms, such as tearing, irritation, stinging, burning, and photophobia, tend to be nonspecific. Pruritus is an essential element of allergic conjunctivitis. It is, by far, the most important feature distinguishing allergic from nonallergic eye disorders. Patients should point out the location of itching in order to distinguish conjunctival versus itching of the eyelid skin. Itching related to eyelid skin may be related to a contact allergy affecting both the skin and conjunctiva. Discharge may also be present in patients complaining of a red and itchy eye. The discharge can be variably described from watery (serous) to purulent. A purulent discharge with morning crusting indicates an infectious etiology. A stringy, ropy discharge is usually present in allergic disorders.

Environmental allergens commonly affect both eyes simultaneously. Ocular pain is not usually associated with allergic disorders and should be referred to an ophthalmologist to rule out other causes.

A thorough examination of the eye is necessary to confirm a diagnosis. One need not be an experienced ophthalmologist in order to perform a routine ocular examination. Evidence of eyelid involvement including blepharitis, dermatitis, swelling, discoloration, and ptosis should be noted. Conjunctival involvement may take the form of chemosis, hyperemia, palpebral and bulbar papillae, cicatrization, and presence or absence of secretions (Fig. 12-1) [5••]. A glossary of ophthalmologic terms used in this chapter is given in Table 12-2. A funduscopic evaluation will reveal evidence of uveitis, an inflammation commonly seen in collagen vascular and autoimmune disorders or cataracts, that may be associated with atopic dermatitis or chronic steroid use [3••].

The conjunctiva should be thoroughly examined. To examine the bulbar conjunctiva, ask the patient to look up and down while gently retracting the opposite lid. Examine the palpebral (tarsal) conjunctiva by grasping the upper lid at its base with a cotton swab on the upper portion of the lid while the patient looks down, and the lower tarsal conjunctiva by everting the lower eyelid while placing a finger near the lid margins and drawing downward. If a beefy, red conjunctiva as well as purulent discharge is present, a bacterial etiology is indicated. If edema is present and severe, patients will usually exhibit periorbital edema, which is more prominent around the lower lids secondary to gravity. Allergic shiners, which are ecchymotic areas thought to result from impaired venous return from the skin and subcutaneous tissues, have also been described in allergic patients.

The superior limbus and superior tarsal conjunctiva should also be examined, because these are the areas

TABLE 12-1. CATEGORIES OF OCULAR INFLAMMATION

Category	Recognition component	Cellular response	Associated disease
IgE/mast cell	IgE	Eosinophils	Allergic conjunctivitis
		Neutrophils	Anaphylaxis
		Basophils	Atopic keratoconjunctivitis
Cytotoxic antibody	IgG	Neutrophil	Vernal keratoconjunctivitis
	IgM	Macrophage	Mooren's ulcer
			Pemphigus
			Pemphigoid
Immune complex	IgG	Neutrophils	Corneal immune rings
	IgM	Eosinophils, lymphocytes	Serum sickness
			Lens-induced uveitis
			Behçet's syndromep
Delayed hypersensitivity	T lymphocytes	Lymphocytes	Vaculitis
	Monocytes	Monocytes	Corneal allograft rejection
		Eosinophils	Sympathetic ophthalmia
		Basophils	Sarcoid-induced uveitis

where Trantas' dots and giant papillae form in more severe ocular allergies.

OPHTHALMIC EXAMINATION

In addition to a thorough history and physical examination, an ophthalmic examination should be performed to help determine the presence of ocular allergic disease. The examination will help to differentiate between viral and bacterial conjunctivitis as well as allergic ocular disorders versus a more serious ocular disease (Table 12-3).

Thorough observation of a patient should be done prior to any hands-on assessment. This approach can often help the physician or health-care provider determine the appropriate examination and testing techniques needed for diagnosis [6]. Facial features may reveal forehead and eyelid vesicular eruptions often seen in ophthalmic zoster. A

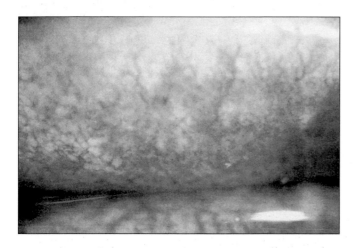

FIGURE 12-1.
Chemosis, injection, and papillae of the lower conjunctiva. (*Courtesy of* Marc Dinowitz, Newark, NJ.)

TABLE 12-2. GLOSSARY OF OPHTHALMIC TERMS

Term	Definition
Blepharitis	Inflammation of eyelid margins, which may have an infectious or inflammatory etiology. Clinical features include telangiectasia, lash collars and rosettes, thickening, crusting, and ulceration of eyelid margin.
Chemosis	Edema of the conjunctiva due to transudate leaking though fenestrated conjunctival capillaries.
Keratitis	Inflammation and infection of the corneal surface, stroma, and endothelium, with numerous causes.
Papillae	Large, hard, polygonal, flat-topped excrescences of the conjunctiva seen in many inflammatory and allergic ocular conditions.
Photophobia	Extreme sensitivity of the eye to light.
Proptosis	Forward protrusion of the eye or eyes.
Ptosis	Drooping of the eyelid, which may have neurogenic, muscular, or congenital causes. Conditions specific to the eyelid that may cause a ptotic lid include chalazia, tumors, and preseptal cellulitis.
Trantas' dots	Pale, grayish-red, uneven nodules with a gelatinous composition seen at the limbal conjunctiva in vernal conjunctivitis.

TABLE 12-3. DIFFERENTIAL DIAGNOSIS OF CONJUNCTIVAL INFLAMMATORY DISORDERS

Disorder	Seasonal	Itching	Tearing	Discharge	Bilateral	Cell type	Cobblestoning
Allergic conjunctivitis	+	+++	++	Mucoid	Yes	Mast cell; eosinophil	-
Bacterial conjunctivitis	No	No	±	Mucopurulent	Variable	PMN	-
Viral conjunctivitis	Variable	No	+/++	Watery; clear mucoid	Yes	PMN, lymphocyte, monocyte	±
Vernal conjunctivitis	Yes	+++	++	Stringy mucoid	Yes	Lymphocyte, eosinophil	++
Giant papillary conjunctivitis	Variable	++	++	Clear white	Variable	Lymphocyte, eosinophil	++

clue to a diagnosis of systemic lupus erythematosus may be a malar rash. Proptosis and lid lag is often seen in Graves' ophthalmopathy. Sjögren's syndrome is associated with enlarged parotid glands and extreme dryness of the mouth and lips. A patient's extremities should also be examined for signs of flexor contracture deformities, which may be seen in rheumatoid arthritis, or of Raynaud's phenomenon, which is seen in scleroderma.

The next step in the examination is the formal ocular examination. A patient's visual acuity should be assessed using a Snellen chart. The chart is usually placed 20 feet from the patient under appropriate lighting. Normal visual acuity is expressed as 20/20.

In examining patients for ocular allergy, the eyelids and lashes are assessed first, followed by the sclera and conjunctiva. The cornea and precorneal tear film are assessed last. Illumination and magnification are essential for appropriate examination; use a penlight, pocket flashlight, or a hand-held magnifying lens. A direct ophthalmoscope (Welch-Allyn; Tycos, Arden, NC) combines the essentials of both illumination and magnification [7]. This instrument is a light source connected to a magnified viewing system. Magnification is produced by a series of built-in "plus" and "minus" lenses, which are selected by moving the dial of the Kekoss disk found on the sides of the ophthalmoscope head piece. "Plus" lenses are color-coded with green numbers, whereas "minus" lenses are coded with red numbers. Larger images can be produced with the more powerful "plus" lens or higher green number used. A "plus 10" lens or greater is used frequently to examine external ocular disease or ocular allergy.

Proper positioning is very important in an ophthalmologic examination. Typically, direct ophthalmoscopy is performed with the eye that corresponds to the patient eye being examined. The eyelids and eyelashes are examined under the maximal intensity of light that can be tolerated by the patient. The superficial lid structures are examined by moving the ophthalmoscope light beam from the lateral to the medial canthus.

The examination of the conjunctiva includes examination of the palpebral, limbal, and bulbar conjunctiva. The palpebral conjunctiva is examined after lid eversion [8]. This procedure is performed by asking the patient to look up while gently pressing the skin below the lower lid with a cotton-tipped applicator and pulling downward. The upper conjunctiva is assessed by gently pulling the upper lid margin away from the globe by grasping the eyelashes while the patient looks down. A cotton-tipped applicator is placed at the upper lid crease. The upper eyelid is gently pulled down and out while the applicator stick is lightly dragged downward against the upper eyelid. This will give a good view of the upper conjunctiva. After completion of this examination, release the upper eyelid and ask the patient to look up.

The limbal and bulbar conjunctiva are examined under diffuse illumination. Fluorescein and rose bengal can be used to evaluate denuded and damaged epithelial cells of the conjunctiva. Fluorescein pools in surface irregularities of the cornea and conjunctiva. Rose bengal stains dead and degenerating epithelium and evaluates the ocular surface. Direct ophthalmoscopy can be used to evaluate abnormalities of the cornea. For optimal viewing, the ophthalmoscope light beam should be held near the temporal limbus and shined across the front of the eye toward the nose.

The precorneal tear film is evaluated after instillation of fluorescein. After the patient blinks several times (this allows a uniform spread of fluorescein over the corneal surface), the cobalt blue filter is used to measure the tear film breakup time (TBUT). The TBUT is a measure of tear film stability and is determined as the period between the opening of the eyes and the first appearance of a defect (black spot) in the green fluorescein layer. The average normal TBUT is 20 seconds, with a normal range between 15 to 35 seconds. An abnormal TBUT is less than 10 seconds [9].

CONJUNCTIVITIS

Conjunctivitis can be defined as a broad group of ocular clinical disorders involving inflammation of the conjunctiva. It can often result from viral or bacterial infections that involve the eyelids, cornea, or conjunctivae, or from ocular allergy.

Bacterial conjunctivitis

Patients with bacterial conjunctivitis usually do not follow a seasonal pattern. Ocular itching is usually not present in this disorder. Ocular inflammation and its degree

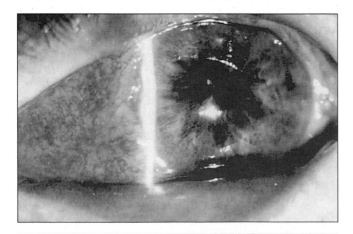

FIGURE 12-2.
Patient with conjunctivitis. A mucopurulent discharge, irritation, and redness of the conjunctiva are present. (*Courtesy of* Marc Dinowitz, MD, Newark, NJ.)

often correlate with the causative pathogen. Certain systemic diseases often manifest as conjunctivitis. Examples include Kawasaki disease and infectious mononucleosis.

Common signs and symptoms that tend to lead to a diagnosis of bacterial conjunctivitis include morning crusting with difficulty opening the eyelid, as well as ocular stinging or burning and purulent secretions. *Streptococcus* or *Haemophilus* species commonly produce acute catarrhal conjunctivitis in children. A mucopurulent discharge, as well as irritation and redness of the conjunctiva, is often present (Fig. 12-2). In the newborn period, conjunctivitis caused by *Neisseria gonorrhoeae* should always be included in the differential diagnosis. It often produces a profuse and purulent discharge. Chronic bacterial conjunctivitis can usually be attributed to *Staphylococcus* or *Moraxella* species.

Ocular conjunctivitis caused by a bacterial organism is seen in both adults and children, although the etiologies between the two groups differ. *Streptococcus pneumoniae* and *Haemophilus influenzae* are common pathogens seen in the pediatric population. Adults frequently encounter *Staphylococcus* species as the main etiologic organism.

The treatment of bacterial conjunctivitis is aimed at preventing patient discomfort, reducing infection, and preventing the spread to others. Several antimicrobial ophthalmic preparations are available. Treatment is typically empiric because cultures are often not obtained in acute cases of conjunctivitis. Broad spectrum antimicrobial preparations are often used in the treatment of bacterial conjunctivitis. These agents include trimethoprim-polymyxin B, bacitracin-neomycin, sulfacetamide, tobramycin, fluoroquinolones, and erythromycin. Topical corticosteroid and antibiotic-corticosteroid combinations should be avoided. Trimethoprim sulfate and

polymyxin B combination is often well tolerated and provides excellent coverage for both gram-positive and gram-negative organisms. Agents such as tobramycin should be limited to use in more serious infections. Topical fluoroquinolones have also become available for use in severe cases of bacterial conjunctivitis.

Viral conjunctivitis

Viral conjunctivitis often presents itself with redness, itching, and, occasionally, a nonpurulent, serous discharge in one or both eyes. In examining the eye, one may note follicular hypertrophy and preauricular lymphadenopathy (Fig. 12-3). Adenovirus types 8, 19, and 37 are the likely etiologies of viral conjunctivitis in school-age children. Adenovirus types 3, 4, and 7 often produce a triad of symptoms including pharyngitis, conjunctivitis, and fever, which is often referred to as the PCF triad. Infection is usually self-limited and dissipates in 7 to 10 days. Subconjunctival hemorrhages, which are commonly benign (*ie*, they look worse than they are), can also be seen with viral conjunctivitis. Enterovirus species commonly cause acute hemorrhagic conjunctivitis. Treatment for viral conjunctivitis is primarily symptomatic.

Allergic conjunctivitis

Allergic conjunctivitis is a common clinical problem, affecting approximately 25% of the general population [3••]. The mast cell plays an important role in allergic conjunctivitis because millions of mast cells are contained in the conjunctiva. Seasonal and perennial allergic conjunctivitis are commonly seen, and cases of seasonal allergic conjunctivitis outweigh perennial allergic conjunctivitis. Grass pollen has been found to produce ocular symptoms, especially during the spring season. Common signs and symptoms include itchy or burning eyes with a watery discharge that may become stringy in the chronic form. Papillary hypertrophy of the tarsal conjunctiva can be seen in severe cases (Fig. 12-4). Signs and symptoms are commonly bilateral and recurrent in nature. Photophobia or visual disturbances are not often seen in allergic conjunctivitis. On physical examination, injection of the conjunctival surface with chemosis may be noted (Fig. 12-5). Lid edema may occur as well. Tear-fluid IgE is present in almost all (96%) of the tear fluid samples [3••,10]. Conjunctival cytology has revealed eosinophilic infiltrates in 25% of seasonal allergic conjunctivitis [11]. Interestingly, recent studies have shown that the nervous system may have a role in the inflammatory process in allergic conjunctivitis because elevated levels of substance P have been found in tears of patients with allergic conjunctivitis [12].

As the name implies, perennial allergic conjunctivitis persists throughout the year. Dust mites and animal dander are often the etiologic allergens. Like seasonal allergic conjunctivitis, mast cell–mediated hypersensitivity occurs.

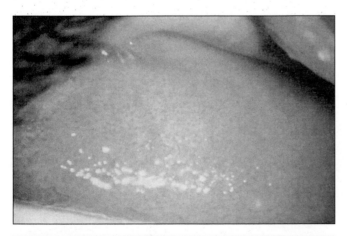

FIGURE 12-3.
Follicular reaction of the lower conjuctiva. Follicular hypertrophy and preauricular lymphadenopathy are apparent.
(*Courtesy of* Marc Dinowitz, MD, Newark, NJ.)

Both seasonal and perennial allergic conjunctivitis are similar with reference to age range and length of history.

Primary treatment of allergic conjunctivitis includes avoidance, cold compresses, and lubrication. Cold compresses provide considerable symptomatic relief, especially from pruritus. Secondary treatment of ocular allergies is based largely on the interference in the patient's quality of life. Topical agents available for treatment include antihistamine drops, vasoconstricting drops, and mast cell stabilizers. The medications are often used in combinations and their effectiveness varies from patient to patient. The choice of agent depends on the health of the eye, drug cost, use of contact lenses, as well as the potential for compliance. The vasoconstrictors and antihistamine formulations together provide relief of the erythema and itching associated with ocular allergy. Newly available medications have dual actions in one drug that provides effective relief of symptoms. H_1 stimulation principally mediates the symptom of pruritus in the conjunctiva.

A review of the drugs to be used in the treatment of ocular allergies reveals many options for the patient. Olopatadine hydrochloride (Patanol; Alcon, Fort Worth, TX), an ocular allergy medication, possesses properties of a mast-cell stabilizing drug and antihistaminic activity. The dual mechanism of activity may be the reason it has an efficacy advantage in the control of the symptoms of ocular allergy [13]. It has proven to be one of the most widely prescribed ocular allergy medications and has been shown to be significantly more effective than placebo in relieving itching and redness for up to 8 hours. Another medication with a dual mechanism of action is Ketotifen (Zaditor; Novartis Pharmaceuticals, East Hanover, NJ), a new topical antihistamine and mast cell stabilizer. It has been used in Europe for the treatment of asthma. It is being dosed in ophthalmic solution as a single drop every 8 to 12 hours. A relatively new drug with a single mechanism of action is levocabastine (Livostin; Novartis Pharmaceuticals, East Hanover, NJ), whose antihistamine properties are to block the H_1 receptor. It is potent in its action and relieves ocular itching with only a minor irritant side effect. Ketorolac (Acular; Allergan, Irvine, CA) is in the family of the nonsteroidal anti-inflammatory drugs (NSAIDs) and has been used in the treatment of ocular allergies. The mechanism of action is to inhibit prostaglandin E synthesis, thus allowing analgesic, anti-inflammatory, and antipruritic effects. It has also been proven to reduce the ocular itching of seasonal allergic conjunctivitis [14]. A common side effect of this drug has been the transient burning and stinging upon administration of the drug into the eye. Ketorolac is currently the only NSAID approved by the Food and Drug Administration for use in acute seasonal allergic conjunctivitis. Pemirolast (Alamast; Santen, Napa, CA) is a mast cell stabilizer that was recently approved for use in the United States for the treatment of ocular allergies. It has been used in Japan on patients as young as 2 years of age with no serious side effects. The Japanese have used pemirolast in the treatment of allergic rhinitis, bronchial asthma, and allergic and vernal conjunctivitis for many years with success. Its potency is 100 times that of disodium cromoglycate. Lodoxamide (Alomide; Alcon, Fort Worth, TX) is a mast cell stabilizer that is 2500 times more potent than cromolyn in preventing histamine release. It has been shown to deliver greater and earlier relief in patients with more chronic forms of conjunctivitis. Nedocromil (Alocril; Allergan, Irvine, CA) is a mast cell stabilizer with inhibitory effects on both mast cells and eosinophils. It improves ocular pruritus and irritation with a safety profile comparable to sodium cromoglycate but it is more potent and can be given just twice daily. Azelastine has been available as a nasal spray for

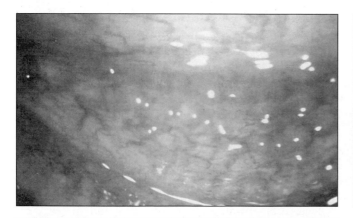

FIGURE 12-4.
Papillary hypertrophy. Everted lid revealing papillary hypertrophy of the tarsal conjunctiva. (*Courtesy of* Marc Dinowitz, MD, Newark, NJ.)

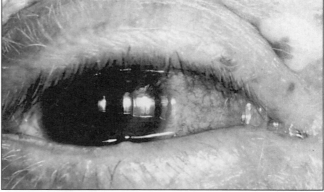

FIGURE 12-5.
Patient with allergic conjunctivitis. Injection of the conjunctival surface with chemosis is noticeable. (*Courtesy of* Marc Dinowitz, MD, Newark, NJ.)

the treatment of seasonal allergic rhinitis and vasomotor rhinitis (Astelin; Wallace Laboratories, Cranbury, NJ), and has recently been approved for use in allergic conjunctivitis (Optivar; Muro Pharmaceutical, Tewksbury, MA) [15••]. It functions as a selective H_1-receptor antagonist, which has been proven to reduce the symptoms of allergic conjunctivitis at the higher concentration (0.05%).

Tertiary treatment of ocular allergy includes the use of topical steroids and immunotherapy. Topical steroid use should be reserved for use by an eye care specialist such as ophthalmologist or allergist experienced in these conditions because the associated complications of these agents far outweigh their benefits for use in allergic conjunctivitis. Allergen immunotherapy is well established for allergic conjunctivitis and rhinitis. Immunotherapy for ragweed, molds, animal dander, and Japanese cedar has been shown to decrease ocular symptoms and sensitivity to specific pollen exposure as well as the need for oral medications to control allergy symptoms.

Vernal conjunctivitis

Vernal conjunctivitis is a perennial disorder that has a noticeable increase in spring. Symptoms include bilateral itching, tearing, photophobia, and mucus discharge. The disorder is a childhood disease that affects prepubertal males more than females. The disease has been linked to gender-related influences, and studies have shown that tarsal and bulbar conjunctival biopsy specimens stain positive for estrogen and progesterone receptors. Therefore, hormones may possibly influence eosinophilic activity in patients with vernal conjunctivitis [13]. The pruritus seen in vernal conjunctivitis seems to be exacerbated by time, wind, bright light, hot weather, or physical exertion. Photophobia and lacrimation are also seen. On physical examination, conjunctival hyperemia with papillary hypertrophy ("cobblestoning") on the superior tarsal conjunctiva is seen. A thin, copious, milk-white, fibrinous secretion is usually composed of eosinophils, epithelial cells, and Charcot-Leyden granules. Conjunctival or limbal "yellow-white points," also known as Horner's points and Trantas' dots, can be present. In severe cases, the epithelium can break down and form corneal ulcerations, which are more common in children and can cause severe visual disturbances if scarring should result. Follicles are usually not present in this disorder. The disease is self-limited for the great majority of patients. Medical therapy includes antihistamines, vasoconstrictors, mast cell stabilizers, and NSAIDs. Corticosteroids can be considered for short-term management in resistant cases but only under the supervision of an ophthalmologist. Surgical measures should also be considered in resistant cases [16••]. Therapy using laser phototherapeutic keratectomy is beneficial in removing superficial corneal scars. Vernal plaques may be removed using superficial keratectomy in the hope that reepithelialization of the cornea occurs.

Giant papillary conjunctivitis

Giant papillary conjunctivitis (GPC) is a syndrome that has been directly linked to contact lens use or use of other foreign materials, such as sutures or ocular prosthetics. A mast cell-mediated as well as a lymphocyte-mediated process has been implicated [17]. Symptoms usually include decreased lens tolerance, mucus production upon awakening that chronically becomes thick and stringy, redness, burning, and itching. On physical examination, inflammation and papules can be seen, mainly on the upper tarsal conjunctiva. Patients may also develop Trantas' dots, limbal infiltration, and bulbar conjunctival hyperemia and edema.

Giant papillary conjunctivitis may develop from wearing any type of contact lens; after insertion in the eye, contact lenses develop a coating often seen in GPC. The cause of GPC and whether it is purely an immunologic disorder or result of mechanical trauma are unknown. It has been hypothesized that the coating on the contact lens stimulates an inflammatory reaction that results in GPC [17].

The treatment of GPC consists of contact lens discontinuation in severe cases. Other modalities are aimed at contact lens care, including daily cleaning, weekly enzymatic treatment, and daily-wear lenses. Cromolyn sodium has been used with great success in treating GPC, and NSAIDs have also been reported to be effective. In a recent study done on patients with contact lens–associated GPC, the use of loteprednol etabonate was found to have a rapid therapeutic response [16••]. Again, the chronic use of topical steroids should be reserved for use by experienced ophthalmologists.

FUTURE DEVELOPMENTS

Drugs still under development for use in the treatment of ocular allergies include medications that are widely used in organ transplantation. Cyclosporine is a fungal antimetabolite that has been used as an anti-inflammatory drug. Its action is on IL-2, which has an immunomodulatory effect on the activation of T-lymphocytes. Recent studies and reports of the use of topical cyclosporine in cases of vernal keratoconjunctivitis have demonstrated marked and lasting improvement in symptoms [18]. Tacrolimus/FK506 (Prograf; Fujisawa Healthcare, Deerfield, IL) is a hydrophobic macrolide lactone that that has been effective in the treatment of immune-mediated ocular diseases such as corneal graft rejection, keratitis, scleritis, ocular pemphigoid, and uveitis. The drug is approximately 100 times as potent as cyclosporine. Tacrolimus and cyclosporine have both been shown, in vitro, to inhibit histamine release [19].

An alternative delivery system for the topical agents, a liposomal drug delivery system, is currently under development. Liposomal-encased compounds have been shown to have a greater penetrating effect into the cornea, aqueous humor, vitreous humor, and conjunctiva. Other areas of future research include cytokine antagonists and anti-IgE therapy [20••].

REFERENCES AND RECOMMENDED READING

Recently published papers of particular interest have been highlighted as:
• Of interest
•• Of outstanding interest

1.•• Bielory L, Wagner RS: Allergic and immunologic pediatric disorders of the eye. *J Invest Allergol Clin Immunol* 1995, 5:309–317.
This is an excellent article giving a general review of the anatomy of the eye, related allergic disorders of the eye, and a few pediatric immunologic ocular disorders.

2.• Irani AA: Ocular mast cells and mediators. *Immunol Allergy Clin North Am* 1997, 17:1–13.
This article focuses on mast cells and their mediators as they relate to ocular disorders. The different types of mast cells and their significance to ocular disorders are reviewed.

3.•• Bielory L, Friedlaender MH: Allergic conjunctivitis. *Immunol Allergy Clin North Am* 1997, 17:19–31.
This is a comprehensive review of allergic conjunctivitis. It includes an excellent discussion on treatment options in allergic conjunctivitis and a detailed discussion on history and physical examination as they pertain to allergic conjunctivitis.

4.•• Friedlaender MH: A review of the causes and treatment of bacterial and allergic conjunctivitis. *Clin Ther* 1995, 17:800–809.
This article summarizes important differences between allergic and bacterial conjunctivitis, and gives important clinical clues in distinguishing between the two disorders.

5.•• Bielory L: Allergic and immunologic disorders of the eye. Part I: Immunology of the eye. *J Allergy Clin Immunol* 2000, 106:805–816.
This article focuses on mechanisms by which mast cells, T cells, eosinophils, cytokines, and other inflammatory constituents contribute to the unique features of eye disease.

6. Wilson FM: *Practical Ophthalmology: A Manual for Beginning Residents.* San Francisco: American Academy of Ophthalmology; 1996.

7. Luff A, Elkington A: Better use of the ophthalmoscope. *Practitioner* 1992, 236:161–165.

8. Knoop K, Trott A: Ophthalmologic procedures in the emergency department part 3: slit lamp use and foreign bodies. *Acad Emerg Med* 1995, 2:224–230.

9. Toda I, Shimazaki J, Tsubota K: Dry eye with only decreased tear, but is sometimes associated with allergic conjunctivitis. *Ophthalmology* 1995, 102:302–309.

10. Hoffmann-Sommergruber K, Ferreira ED, Ebner C, *et al.*: Detection of allergen-specific IgE in tears of grass pollen–allergic patients with allergic rhinoconjunctivitis. *Clin Exp Allergy* 1996, 26:79–87.

11. Middleton E Jr, Reed CE, Ellis EF, *et al.*: *Allergy Principles and Practice*, edn 5. New York: Mosby; 1998:1151–1152.

12. Fujishima H, Takeyama M, Takeuchi T, *et al.*: Elevated levels of substance P in tears of patients with allergic conjunctivitis and vernal keratoconjunctivitis. *Clin Exp Allergy* 1997, 27:372–378.

13. Yanni JM, Miller ST, Gamache DA, *et al.*: Comparative effects of topical ocular anti-allergy drugs on human conjunctival mast cells. *Ann Allergy Asthma Immunol* 1997, 79:541–545.

14. Friedlander MH: The current and future therapy of allergic conjunctivitis. *Curr Opin Ophthalmol* 1998, 9:54–58.

15.•• Bielory L: Allergic and immunologic disorders of the eye. Part I: Immunology of the eye. *J Allergy Clin Immunol* 2000, 106:805–816.
This article focuses on mechanisms by which mast cells, T cells, eosinophils, cytokines, and other inflammatory constituents to the unique features of eye disease.

16.•• Lee Y, Raizman M: Vernal conjunctivitis. *Immunol Allergy Clin North Am* 1997, 17:33–51.
This article gives a comprehensive review of vernal conjunctivitis, including clinical signs and symptoms, pathogenesis, differential diagnosis, laboratory evaluation, and treatment options. The article ends with an excellent discussion on individual therapeutic treatment options used in treating ocular allergies.

17. Bonini S, Lambiase A, Schiavone M, *et al.*: Estrogen and progesterone receptors in vernal keratoconjunctivitis. *Ophthalmology* 1995, 102:1374–1379.

18. Mendicute J, Aranzasti C, Eder F, *et al.*: Topical cyclosporine A 2% in the treatment of vernal keratoconjunctivitis. *Eye* 1997, 11:75–78.

19. Sperr WR, Agis H, Semper H, *et al.*: Inhibition of allergen induced histamine release from human basophils by cyclosporine A and FK-506. *Int Arch Allergy Immunol* 1997, 114:68–73.

20.•• Bielory L: Allergic and immunologic disorders of the eye. Part II: Ocular allergy. *J Allergy Clin Immunol* 2000, 106:1019–1032.
This article provides an overview of the spectrum of ocular allergy ranging from acute seasonal allergic conjunctivitis to variants of chronic keratoconjunctivitis.

CHAPTER 13

Role of Pollution in Rhinitis

David B. Peden

Allergic rhinitis is a very common disease worldwide and is influenced by both genetic and environmental factors. Exposure to environmental allergens is the most significant environmental factor in development and exacerbation of allergic rhinitis. However, air pollutants that are not allergens may affect allergic inflammation in the nasal airway. The nasal airway also possesses a number of defense mechanisms to deal with environmental irritants. This chapter examines the effect of ozone and particulate air pollution on T_H2-type inflammation in the airway and how nasal defenses protect the upper and lower airway from adverse effects of pollutants.

INTRODUCTION

The nasal airway has a number of important functions, including warming and humidifying inhaled ambient air, olfaction, participating in airway host defense, and filtering inhaled air of particulate agents [1]. The nasal airway may also be important as an initial site for sensitization to airborne antigens. As the initial region that encounters ambient air, the nasal airway is also the first region that encounters ambient air pollutants. A number of occupational and human exposure studies have shown that exposure to noxious agents, such as airborne endotoxin or ozone, is associated with increased neutrophilic airway inflammation [2]. Thus, ambient air pollutants can be expected to have an impact on nasal function and physiology.

Perhaps the most common chronic inflammatory disorder of the nasal airway is allergic rhinitis [3]. In the United States, allergic rhinitis has a substantial impact on healthcare costs, quality of life, workplace and school performance, and other airway diseases such as asthma and sinusitis [4]. A number of factors are known to influence the severity of allergic rhinitis, including environmental exposure to allergens and genetic risk factors for the development of atopy [5,6]. Less well appreciated is the impact of nonspecific inflammatory agents, such as air pollutants, on allergic rhinitis.

Epidemiologic studies of the impact of air pollutants tend to focus on lower airway outcomes, such as asthma, rather than morbidity in the upper airway attributable to allergic rhinitis. Nonetheless, such studies demonstrate that air pollution certainly has an impact on allergic airway disease. Increases in ambient air levels of ozone or particulate matter has been linked with increased asthma morbidity, as indicated by need for rescue medication, visits to the emergency room, or hospital admissions. Additionally, these changes are often observed 1 or more days after the increased level of air pollutants is encountered. This time lag between exposure and health effect suggests that inflammatory changes, rather than immediate reflex responses, account for correlation between pollutant exposure and asthma morbidity [7••].

Allergic disorders of the airway are characterized by eosinophilic inflammation and increased reactivity to nonspecific irritants. Underlying this inflammation is development of primary immune responses to antigens that exhibit a T_H2 phenotype [8]. Although environmental pollutants induce neutrophilic inflammation in nonallergic persons, they may impact atopic inflammation either by promoting primary T_H2 responses to antigens or exacerbating such inflammation in those already sensitized.

Challenge studies of human volunteers with allergic rhinitis have provided the clearest demonstration of the impact of air pollutants on T_H2 inflammation in the nasal airway. As outlined below, it can be argued that pollutants impact nasal allergy, and that atopic persons may be more sensitive to the effects of air contaminants. A number of studies demonstrating the interaction between pollutant effects and allergic processes in the human nasal airways are reviewed in this chapter. Pollutants that are emphasized include ozone and selected components of particulate air pollution—diesel exhaust particles (DEP) and endotoxin—because these pollutants represent a significant percentage of pollutants encountered in the United States.

COMMONLY ENCOUNTERED AIR POLLUTANTS

The United States Environmental Protection Agency (EPA) oversees monitoring of specified air pollutants as outlined in the Clean Air Act of 1970, which was most recently amended in 1990. The EPA proposed updated standards in 1997 although at the time of this writing legal action has delayed their implementation. Including the proposed 1997 modifications, the monitored (or criteria) pollutants include carbon monoxide, lead, sulfur dioxide (SO_2), nitrogen dioxide (NO_2), ozone (O_3), particulate matter less than 10 μm (PM10) and 2.5 microns (PM2.5) in diameter [9,10].

Except for carbon monoxide and lead, each of these pollutants (or classes of pollutants) can impact asthma or allergic disease. It is important to recognize that particulate air pollution (PM10 and PM2.5) is composed of a variety of different entities which are less than 10 μm in diameter and derive from a number of different sources. Thus, any number of chemical or biological entities could account for the effect of particulate matter on nasal airway inflammation.

Ozone and Rhinitis

As with many irritants, exposure to ozone has been shown to induce inflammation in the nasal airway. Investigators

at the EPA [11,12] reported that 0.4-ppm ozone exposure induces a neutrophilic inflammation in nonallergic volunteers. Ozone was found to induce increased levels of tryptase, suggesting that mast cell degranulation might occur with ozone exposure. This finding also suggested that the effect of ozone in allergic subjects might be more significant than in nonallergic subjects.

Bascom *et al.* [13] demonstrated that subjects with allergic rhinitis exposed to 0.5-ppm ozone for 4 hours have an inflammatory response to ozone, characterized not only by neutrophils but by eosinophils as well. When allergen challenge was performed after exposure to ozone, there was no reported effect on allergen-induced eosinophilia. Nonetheless, this study demonstrated that allergic subjects had a unique response (eosinophilia) in the nasal airway following ozone exposure.

In allergic asthmatic patients, ozone (0.4 ppm for 2 hours without exercise) was again shown to directly induce both neutrophil and eosinophil influx to the nasal airway [14•]. Unlike those with allergic rhinitis, asthmatics also had increased numbers of eosinophils and eosinophil cationic protein following allergen challenge when allergen challenge was preceded by ozone exposure. Additionally, there was a suggestion that allergic subjects had an increased immediate response to allergen following ozone exposure. However, in a study designed to focus on the impact of ozone on the immediate response to allergen, no impact on mast cell response to allergen was observed [15].

Another study examined the relative sensitivity of atopic and nonatopic subjects to ozone exposure. In this study, subjects were exposed to 0.12- and 0.24-ppm ozone, and nasal lavage fluid (NLF) was recovered. In the atopic subjects, there were increased numbers of granulocytes present in NLF following ozone exposure, which were not observed in nonatopic subjects. Further, there was a correlation between interleukin (IL)-8 and polymorphonuclear neutrophil concentrations in NLF after exposure to 0.24-ppm ozone. This study suggests that atopic subjects have increased responses to ozone than nonatopic subjects [16].

Field studies have also examined the effect of ambient air exposure on nasal inflammation, primarily in children. Although there is variation between these studies, ambient ozone exposure in atopic subjects has been associated with increases in nasal neutrophils, eosinophils, epithelial cells, and IL-8 levels [17•]. In a series of studies examining nasal airway inflammation in Mexico City, children (not defined as allergic or nonallergic) exposed to ozone were reported to have increased nasal polymorphonuclear concentrations and increased expression of β-2 intergins. Additionally, DNA damage was reported in chronically exposed children, suggesting that ozone may have effects on airway mucosal repair as well. This suggestion has been strengthened by a study of nasal neoplasms in Mexico City [18–20].

Taken together, these studies indicate that ozone induces nasal inflammation in atopic subjects that is greater than that observed in nonatopic subjects. Furthermore, ozone can enhance IgE-mediated responses to allergens, and chronic exposure to ozone has been linked to DNA changes in the nasal airway. Clearly, ozone clearly impacts allergic rhinitis.

Endotoxin and nasal inflammation

Environmental lipopolysaccharide (LPS) derives from gram-negative bacteria, which are common contaminants in indoor and outdoor environments [1]. Occupational settings that include exposure to animal waste (*eg*, swine confinement and poultry facilities) or plant matter (*eg*, cotton dust and corn dust) have increased levels of ambient air endotoxin [21]. In office buildings, ambient LPS levels of 254 ng/m^3 (range, 100 to 408 ng/m^3) are associated with sick building syndrome [22]. Ambient air pollution particles also are rich in LPS activity [23•]. Thus, exposure to ambient LPS might be expected to enhance nasal inflammation.

Lipopolysaccharide has also been measured in house dust, and levels of LPS in house dust are have been reported to correlate with asthma severity in mite-sensitive asthmatics independently of the concentration of mite allergen [24]. This observation suggests that endotoxin responses in the nasal airway might be modified by allergic inflammation.

A number of occupational and inhalation studies have shown that endotoxin induces neutrophilic inflammation in nasal and lower airway inflammation in nonatopic subjects [1,21,22]. A number of molecules participate in response to endotoxin, including signaling molecules such as CD14 and TLR4 [25]. Recent studies of the lower airway suggest that inhaled allergen challenge can enhance the amount of CD14 present in the airway, possibly modifying the response to LPS [26,27••]. Indeed, in one study there was a strong correlation between eosinophil influx and soluble CD14 expression. Thus, there is a mechanistic rationale for an interaction between allergic and endotoxin-mediated inflammation in the nasal airway.

Studies from our group have shown that low-level (1 µg) LPS challenge induces eosinophil responses in some atopic subjects but no nonallergic subjects. Those atopic subjects with nasal responses to LPS had eosinophils and neutrophils and were in season for locally encountered tree pollens. Furthermore, the amount of granulocyte-macrophage colony-stimulating factor present at baseline correlated well with nasal eosinophils after LPS. Thus, ongoing nasal allergic inflammation may contribute to increased response to this pollutant [28].

In a subsequent study, atopic subjects underwent nasal allergen challenge before LPS challenge to examine the effect of allergen on LPS response. The dose of allergen employed was not enough to induced nasal symptoms. It was found that allergen followed by LPS yielded increased nasal neutrophils and eosinophils compared with the effect of allergen alone, LPS alone, or control [29•]. Taken together, these studies indicate that allergic inflammation enhances response to LPS.

Diesel exhaust particles and nasal allergy

Diesel exhaust particles (DEPs) are some of the most commonly encountered particulate air pollutants encountered in the United States, Europe, and Japan. As outlined below, nasal challenge studies of human volunteers have shown that DEPs can induce nasal airway inflammation, enhance immediate- and late-phase response to nasal allergen challenge, and, unlike any reported effect of ozone, can contribute to initial sensitization to a neoantigen.

Diesel exhaust particles have a clear impact on IgE homeostasis. In 1994, Diaz-Sanchez *et al.* [30••] reported that nasal IgE production was enhanced after exposure to 0.3 mg of DEP. The volunteers included four atopic and seven nonatopic subjects. There was no effect on IgG, IgA, or IgM production in the nasal airway. This effect was very dose specific; only a dose of 0.3 mg (but not 1.0 or 0.1 mg) of DEP caused this result. Additionally, this effect was only observed 4 days after initial challenge.

Cytokine production by cells recovered in lavage fluid is also modified by DEP challenge. Cells recovered under baseline conditions were found to have detectable mRNA levels for interferon-γ, IL-2, and IL-13. DEP challenge induced message for IL-2, IL-4, IL-5, IL-6, IL-10, IL-13, and interferon-γ in recovered cells. IL-4 protein was also measured in postchallenge lavage fluid [31]. Although it was unclear in this study what cell type accounted for increased cytokine message, it was not thought to be due to increased lymphocyte numbers. The general conclusion is that DEPs do appear to enhance T$_H$2-type inflammation.

When coupled with ragweed allergen challenge, DEP was found to enhance allergen-specific responses in ragweed-sensitive subjects. DEP plus allergen induced a marked increase in ragweed-specific IgE and IgG4 without an increase in either total IgE and IgG. Compared with DEP alone, this combination also induced increased expression of IL-4, IL-5, IL-6, IL-10, and IL-13 and decreased expression of interferon-γ and IL-2, generally favoring an atopic (T$_H$2) profile [32].

Recent studies demonstrate that the effect of DEP on IgE-mediated responses in the nasal airway result from modification of mast cell biology. In one study, atopic subjects underwent DEP plus allergen challenge, and flow cytometry was used to define the characteristics of IL-4–positive cells recovered in NLF. The cell marker profile of IL-4–positive cells 4 hours after dual challenge was most consistent with mast cells, whereas 18 hours after challenge, IL-4–positive cells were increasingly lymphocytes. This study indicates that initial responses to DEP and allergen are mediated by mast cells [33].

Diesel exhaust particles also modify allergen-induced mast cell degranulation. Subjects were found to have increased symptoms and increased histamine release following allergen challenge when DEP preceded such challenge. Without allergen, DEP did not induce histamine release. This observation was confirmed in vitro using a murine mast cell [34•]. In a separate study, nasal steroids were found to inhibit allergen-induced nasal inflammation, but did not have an effect on the adjuvant effect of DEP [35].

Perhaps the most provocative observation on the effect of DEP on allergen response in humans is the ability of DEP challenge to shift primary immune response to a neoantigen from a T_H1 towards a T_H2 response. In these studies, atopic human subjects underwent nasal immunization to keyhole limpet hemocyanin (KLH). Some subjects were pretreated with DEP and others were not. In the non–DEP-treated group, local anti-KLH IgG was produced. However, in the DEP-treated group, anti-KLG IgE was produced following immunization [36••].

Compared to other pollutants, such as ozone and endotoxin, DEP appears to be unique in its effect on IgE production and primary sensitization to neoantigens. The in vivo effect of DEP on IgE isotype switch can be replicated in vitro with extracts from DEP containing the polyaromatic hydrocarbon (PAH) fraction from these particles, and the specific PAH compounds phenanthrene and 2,3,7,8-tetracholorodibenzo-p-dioxin [37•]. Thus, PAHs appear to play a central role in the effect of DEPs on allergic inflammation. This may be relevant because a number of other combustion products, including tobacco smoke, are rich in such chemicals.

NASAL FUNCTION AND UPPER AND LOWER AIRWAY RESPONSE TO POLLUTANTS

A significant function of the nasal airway is to warm, humidify, and cleanse inhaled air so that the air is physiologically compatible with the lower airway. It has been argued that abnormalities in nasal physiology might impede this function. Such abnormalities could include inflammation due to allergic rhinitis, which might modify nasal function or impede nasal airflow such that mouth breathing occurs, thus allowing air to bypass the nasal airway.

Uric acid is a significant antioxidant that interacts with ozone. Urate is a major antioxidant in nasal air-

way secretions [38]. Secretion of nasal urate appears to be a function of nasal glands, which likely take up urate from plasma pools. Treatment of the volunteers with probenecid, which depletes plasma urate via excretion in the urine, decreases nasal glandular levels of urate [39]. Thus, nasal glands may provide a significant antioxidant function.

Other studies have shown that urate in epithelial lining fluid is an important ozone scavenger [40]. It has also been shown that nasal urate is depleted following ozone exposure, suggesting that urate scavenges ozone. It is not yet clear if ozone uptake in the nasal airway is an important antioxidant defense against ozone in the lower airway or if this function is modified in persons with nasal allergic disorders. However, the relatively high concentration of ozone in proximal airway regions suggests such a role [40].

Another commonly encountered pollutant is SO_2. SO_2 causes an immediate drop in lung function in asthmatics but not in nonasthmatic subjects. It has been observed that nasal breathing largely eliminates the bronchospastic effect of SO_2 inhalation in asthmatic patients. This is thought to be due to uptake of this water-soluble gas by the nasal mucosa. Without exercise, most airflow occurs through the nasal airway except in those with nasal obstruction such as occurs in allergic rhinitis. Exercise causes in a shift from nasal breathing to combined oral-nasal breathing, resulting in less inspired air interacting with the nasal mucosa. It has been argued that this results in more SO_2 reaching the lower airway. This may account for the observed effect of exercise on the response of asthmatics to SO_2 [41].

The nasal airway is also rich in cilia, which remove particles from the airway. This can be important in relation to the effect of pollutants on nasal allergy (with cilia clearing allergens from the nasal airway) and to cilia being unable to remove pollution particles from the nasal airway. Ciliary beat may be decreased in allergic rhinitis [42], suggesting that allergic inflammation of the nasal airway may decrease clearance of inhaled particulates. Ozone damages ciliary function in rodents, suggesting that pollutant exposure may allow particulates containing allergens to have prolonged contact with the nasal mucosa [43]. Mucous cell hyperplasia, mucin production, and epithelial cell hyperplasia may also be enhanced after ozone exposure, further affecting nasal function [44].

Nitrogen dioxide is another agent that may impact allergic inflammation in the nasal airway. Although it is usually considered as a precursor to ozone, this gas has been shown to be able to enhance allergen-induced eosinophil responses in atopic subjects [45]. Taken together, these examples show that persons with allergic rhinitis may be more prone to the effect of ambient air pollutants and, conversely, that pollutants may modify nasal mechanisms that allow clearance of allergens from the nasal airway.

CONCLUSIONS

This chapter gives examples of how responses to pollutants are modified by allergic inflammation in the nasal airway. Pollutants also modify responses to allergen in the nasal mucosa. Although treatment strategies have not been extensively studied, it seems that control of nasal allergy by conventional therapies such as topical corticosteroids may the most useful therapy for minimizing interactions between allergic inflammation and pollutants.

The full impact of allergic rhinitis on either upper or lower airway response is poorly appreciated. However, it seems likely that nasal physiology provides an important defense against the effect of ambient air pollutants. There is some appreciation that nasal allergic inflammation enhances lower airway hyerresponsiveness in asthmatics. Furthermore, some investigators have shown that treatment of nasal inflammation is an important adjunct to treatment of the lower airway in asthma [46]. Although several investigators have focused on nasal allergy as a model for events that likely occur in the lower airway, the potential impact of nasal allergy on lower airway inflammation and responses may be quite significant. Thus, the effect of air pollutants on nasal allergy may ultimately be important for exacerbation of asthma as well as rhinitis.

REFERENCES AND RECOMMENDED READING

Papers of particular interest, published recently, have been highlighted as:
- Of importance
- • Of major importance

1. Togias A: Unique mechanistic features of allergic rhinitis. *J Allergy Clin Immunol* 2000, 105:S599–S604.

2. Anonymous: Health effects of outdoor air pollution. Committee of the Environmental and Occupational Health Assembly of the American Thoracic Society. *Am J Resp Crit Care Med* 1996, 153:3–50.

3. Nathan RA, Meltzer EO, Seiner JC, Storms WC: Prevalence of allergic rhinitis in the United States. *J Allergy Clin Immunol* 1997, 99:S808–S814.

4. Weiss KB, Sullivan SD: The health economics of asthma and rhinitis. I. Assessing the economic impact. *J Allergy Clin Immunol* 2001, 107:3–8.

5. Weiss ST: Environmental risk factors in childhood asthma. *Clin Exp Allergy* 1998, 28:29–34.

6. Holgate ST: Genetic and environmental interaction in allergy and asthma. *J Allergy Clin Immunol* 1999, 104:1139–1146.

7.•• Peden DB: Controlled exposures of asthmatics to air pollutants. In *Air Pollution and Health*. Edited by Holgate S, Koren H, Samet J. London: Academic Press; 1999:865–880.
This is a review of the effect of air pollutants on airway inflammation as demonstrated by human challenge studies. Included is discussion of inflammatory effects of ozone, diesel exhaust, and other pollutants in the upper and lower airway.

8. Durham SR: Mechanisms of mucosal inflammation in the nose and lungs. *Clin Exp Allergy* 1998, 28:11–16.

9. Lippmann M, Maynard RL: Air Quality Guidelines and Standards. In *Air Pollution and Health*. Edited by Holgate ST, Samet JM, Koren HS, Maynard RL. San Diego: Academic Press; 1999:983–1017.

10. National ambient air quality standard for ozone final rule. Washington DC: US Congress; 1997 [*Fed Reg* 62:38856–38896].

11. Graham DE, Koren HS: Biomarkers of inflammation in ozone-exposed humans. Comparison of the nasal and bronchoalveolar lavage. *Am Rev Respir Dis* 1990, 142:152–156.

12. Koren HS, Hatch GE, Graham DE: Nasal lavage as a tool in assessing acute inflammation in response to inhaled pollutants. *Toxicology* 1990, 60:15–25.

13. Bascom R, Naclerio RM, Fitzgerald TK, *et al.*: Effect of ozone inhalation on the response to nasal challenge with antigen of allergic subjects. *Am Rev Respir Dis* 1990, 142:594–601.

14.• Peden DB, Setzer RW Jr, Devlin RB: Ozone exposure has both a priming effect on allergen-induced responses and an intrinsic inflammatory action in the airways of perennially allergic asthmatics. *Am J Respir Crit Care Med* 1995, 151:1336–1345.
This article describes the effect of ozone on allergen-induced eosinophilic inflammation in the nasal airway and the direct effect of ozone on nasal eosinophils, following up on the initial observation by Bascom [13].

15. Michelson PH, Dailey L, Devlin RB, Peden DB: Ozone effects on the immediate phase response to allergen in the nasal airways of allergic asthmatics. *Otolaryngol Head Neck Surg* 1999, 120:225–232.

16. McBride DE, Koenig JQ, Luchtel DL, *et al.*: Inflammatory effects of ozone in the upper airways of subjects with asthma. *Am J Respir Crit Care Med* 1994, 149:1192–1197.

17.• Kopp MV, Ulmer C, Ihorst G, *et al.*: Upper airway inflammation in children exposed to ambient ozone and potential signs of adaptation. *Eur Respir J* 1999, 14:854–861.
This paper demonstrates that ozone induces nasal inflammation in children in "real-life" settings associated with natural exposure to ozone, not in experimental challenge.

18. Calderon-Garciduenas L, Rodriguez-Alcaraz A, Garcia R, *et al.*: Nasal inflammatory responses in children exposed to a polluted urban atmosphere. *J Toxicol Environ Health* 1995, 45:427–437.

19. Calderon-Garciduenas L, Delgado R, Calderon-Garciduenas A, *et al.*: Malignant neoplasms of the nasal cavity and paranasal sinuses: a series of 256 patients in Mexico City and Monterrey. Is air pollution the missing link? *Otolaryngol Head Neck Surg* 2000, 122:499–508.

20. Calderon-Garciduenas L, Wen-Wang L, Zhang YJ, *et al.*: 8-hydroxy-2'-deoxyguanosine, a major mutagenic oxidative DNA lesion, and DNA strand breaks in nasal respiratory epithelium of children exposed to urban pollution. *Environ Health Perspect* 1999, 107:469–474.

21. Wang Z, Larsson K, Palmberg L, *et al.*: Inhalation of swine dust induces cytokine release in the upper and lower airways. *Eur Respir J* 1997, 10:381–387.

22. Teeuw KB, Vandenbroucke-Grauls CM, Verhoef J: Airborne gram-negative bacteria and endotoxin in sick building syndrome. A study in Dutch governmental office buildings. *Arch Intern Med* 1994, 154:2339–2345.

23.• Bonner JC, Rice AB, Lindroos PM, *et al.*: Induction of the lung myofibroblast PDGF receptor system by urban ambient particles from Mexico City. *Am J Respir Cell Mol Biol* 1998, 19:672–680.
This article identifies endotoxin as a competent of ambient air particles.

24. Michel O, Kips J, Duchateau J, *et al.*: Severity of asthma is related to endotoxin in house dust. *Am J Respir Crit Care Med* 1996, 154:1641–1646.

25. Martin TR: Recognition of bacterial endotoxin in the lungs. *Am J Respir Cell Mol Biol* 2000, 23:128–132.

26. Dubin W, Martin TR, Swoveland P, *et al.*: Asthma and endotoxin: lipopolysaccharide-binding protein and soluble CD14 in bronchoalveolar compartment. *Am J Physiol* 1996, 270:L736–L744.

27.•• Virchow JC, Julius P, Mattys H, *et al.*: CD14 expression and soluble CD14 after segmental allergen provocation in atopic asthma. *Eur Respir J* 1998, 11:317–323.
This is an important demonstration of the ability of allergen exposure to upregulate response to endotoxin, a stimulus which does not activate inflammation via IgE.

28. Peden DB, Tucker K, Murphy P, *et al.*: Eosinophil influx to the nasal airway after local, low-level LPS challenge in humans. *J Allergy Clin Immunol* 1999, 104:388–394.

29.• Eldridge MW, Peden DB: Allergen provocation augments endotoxin-induced nasal inflammation in subjects with atopic asthma. *J Allergy Clin Immunol* 2000, 105:475–481.
This report describes the ability of allergen-induced inflammation to enhance response to endotoxin, which is found in particles, suggesting that nasal atopy may be a risk factor in enhancing response to a pollutant.

30.•• Diaz-Sanchez D, Dotson AR, Takenaka H, Saxon A: Diesel exhaust particles induce local IgE production in vivo and alter the pattern of IgE messenger RNA isoforms. *J Clin Invest* 1994, 94:1417–1425.
This report demonstrates that diesel exhaust particles can induce IgE production. It suggests that DEPs, unlike many other pollutants, can contribute to development of allergy versus exacerbation of allergic inflammation.

31. Diaz-Sanchez D, Tsien A, Fleming J, Saxon A: Combined diesel exhaust particulate and ragweed allergen challenge markedly enhances human in vivo nasal ragweed-specific IgE and skews cytokine production to a T helper cell 2-type pattern. *J Immunol* 1997, 158:2406–2413.

32. Fujieda S, Diaz-Sanchez D, Saxon A: Combined nasal challenge with diesel exhaust particles and allergen induces in vivo IgE isotype switching. *Am J Respir Cell Mol Biol* 1998, 19:507–512.

33. Wang M, Saxon A, Diaz-Sanchez D: Early IL-4 production driving Th2 differentiation in a human in vivo allergic model is mast cell derived. *Clin Immunol* 1999, 90:47–54.

34.• Diaz-Sanchez D, Penichet-Garcia M, Saxon A: Diesel exhaust particles directly induce activated mast cells to degranulate and increase histamine levels and symptom severity. *J Allergy Clin Immunol* 2000, 106:1140–1146.
This report demonstrates that DEPs can directly augment mast cell degranulation in vivo. This has not been observed in humans with other agents.

35. Diaz-Sanchez D, Tsien A, Fleming J, Saxon A: Effect of topical fluticasone propionate on the mucosal allergic response induced by ragweed allergen and diesel exhaust particle challenge. *Clin Immunol* 1999, 90:313–322.

36.•• Diaz-Sanchez D, Garcia MP, Wang M, *et al.*: Nasal challenge with diesel exhaust particles can induce sensitization to a neoallergen in the human mucosa. *J Allergy Clin Immunol* 1999, 104:1183–1188.
This report demonstrates more directly that DEPs promote an IgE-type response to a neoantigen, suggesting that DEPs contribute to development of allergy, not only simply exacerbation of allergic inflammation.

37.• Diaz-Sanchez D: The role of diesel exhaust particles and their associated polyaromatic hydrocarbons in the induction of allergic airway disease. *Allergy* 1999, 52:52–56.
This review discusses the effect of specific compounds found in diesel exhaust that impact IgE switch mechanisms.

38. Peden D, Hohman R, Brown ME, *et al.*: Uric acid is a major antioxidant in human nasal airway secretions. *Proc Natl Acad Sci USA* 1990, 87:7638–7642.

39. Peden DB, Swiersz M, Ohkubo K, *et al.*: Nasal secretion of the ozone scavenger uric acid. *Am Rev Respir Dis* 1993, 148:455–461.

40. Linn WS, Shamoo DA, Spier CE, *et al.*: Respiratory effects of 0.75 ppm sulfur dioxide in exercising asthmatics: influence of upper-respiratory defenses. *Environ Res* 1983, 30:340–348.

41. Mudway IS, Blomberg A, Frew AJ, *et al.*: Antioxidant consumption and repletion kinetics in nasal lavage fluid following exposure of healthy human volunteers to ozone. *Eur Respir J* 1999, 13:1429–1438.

42. Ohashi Y, Nakai Y, Kihara S, *et al.*: Ciliary activity in patients with nasal allergies. *Arch Otorhinolaryngol* 1985, 242:141–147.

43. Harkema JR, Morgan KT, Gross EA, *et al.*: Consequences of prolonged inhalation of ozone on F344/N rats: collaborative studies. Part VII: Effects on the nasal mucociliary apparatus. *Res Rep Health Eff Inst* 1994, (65 Pt 7):3–26; discussion 27–34.

44. Cho HY, Hotchkiss JA, Bennett CB, Harkema JR: Neutrophil-dependent and neutrophil-independent alterations in the nasal epithelium of ozone-exposed rats. *Am J Respir Crit Care Med* 2000, 162:629–636.

45. Wang JH, Devalia JL, Duddle JM, *et al.*: Effect of six-hour exposure to nitrogen dioxide on early-phase nasal response to allergen challenge in patients with a history of seasonal allergic rhinitis. *J Allergy Clin Immunol* 1995, 96:669–676.

46. Corren J: The relationship between allergic rhinitis and bronchial asthma. *Curr Opin Pulm Med* 1999, 5:35–37.

CHAPTER 14

The New Antihistamines in Allergic Rhinitis

Robert A. Nathan

Antihistamines are an integral part of pharmacologic therapy for patients with allergic rhinitis, chronic urticaria, atopic dermatitis, and other allergic disorders. For years, the customary first-line pharmacotherapeutic approach for the treatment of patients with allergic rhinitis consisted of antihistamines despite their pronounced unwanted side effects. New or second-generation antihistamines are now the focus of therapy, largely because these agents are nonsedating or less sedating than their predecessors.

Although various inflammatory mediators play a role in producing clinical signs and symptoms of allergic rhinitis, histamine still is recognized as the primary mediator in this disorder. Histamine is released within minutes after contact between an allergen and specific IgE molecules on the surface of mast cells. Once released from mast cells and basophils, histamine produces vascular permeability and vasodilation in the skin (Table 14-1) [1••]. In the nose, histamine stimulates sensory nerves, causing itching and sneezing. Histamine also increases mucosal blood flow, resulting in nasal congestion, and increases goblet cell secretion and vascular permeability, evoking symptoms of rhinorrhea (Table 14-1) [1••].

Antihistamines act in the skin to suppress the wheal and flare response by inhibiting histamine binding at its receptors on nerves, vascular smooth muscle, endothelium, and mast cells. In the nose, antihistamines competitively inhibit histamine receptors on nasal mucosa cells, diminishing the early phase reaction.

PHARMACOKINETICS

Collectively, the second-generation oral and topical antihistamines are similar in their ability to competitively antagonize histamine at its receptors. Individually, these agents differ considerably in their pharmacokinetic and pharmacodynamic profiles (Table 14-2) [2••,3]. Second-generation antihistamines possess a similar core moiety, but the side chains adjoining the core determine their pharmacokinetic properties.

Pharmacokinetic profiles of second-generation antihistamines allow for once- or twice-daily treatment. All new agents are well absorbed after oral administration, with peak plasma concentrations generally occurring within 1 to 2 hours. Terfenadine, astemizole, and loratadine are metabolized extensively in the liver, each with active metabolites. Cetirizine (the carboxylated metabolite of hydroxyzine), fexofenadine (the active metabolite of terfenadine), and acrivastine are poorly metabolized and excreted largely unchanged. Desloratadine (the active metabolite of loratadine), a new selective H$_1$-receptor antagonist, is metabolized minimally in the liver to 3OH-desloratadine [4,5].

Most new antihistamines have a rapid onset of action—defined as a significant therapeutic effect within 1 to 2 hours—and duration of action 12 to 24 hours after a single dose. One exception is the second-generation antihistamine astemizole. This drug has an onset of action within 2 days and a prolonged duration of action. Steady-state plasma levels of astemizole are reached in as long as 4 weeks, with the wheal response taking as long as 8 weeks to recover to normal [6••].

Typically, the onset of action of antihistamines is determined by suppression of histamine-induced wheal and flare in the skin. However, Day *et al.* [7•] at Kingston General Hospital (Kingston, Ontario) recently used the environmental exposure unit (EEU) to investigate the onset of action of terfenadine, astemizole, cetirizine, and loratadine in patients with seasonal allergic rhinitis. The EEU is designed to eliminate confounding factors (*eg*, seasonal and geographic variations in pollen counts) encountered during evaluation of antihistamines by exposing individuals to a predetermined, controlled, constant level of airborne pollen. Essentially, the unit is a modified classroom with a feeder system that delivers controlled levels of commercially available ragweed pollen into a study area (Fig. 14-1). A modified laser counter measures the grains emitted and records concentrations using a com-

TABLE 14-1. PHYSIOLOGIC RESPONSES TO HISTAMINE CHALLENGE AND MECHANISMS UNDERLYING THESE RESPONSES IN THE SKIN AND NASAL MUCOSA

	Response	Mechanism
Skin		
Wheal	Increased vascular permeability	H$_1$-receptor–mediated endothelial cell contraction (via EDRF (NO)/PGI$_2$)
Flare	Vasodilation	H$_1$/H$_2$-receptor–mediated axonal reflex (substance P/CGRP/NKA-mediated)
Nasal mucosa		
Itch	Sensory nerve activation	H$_1$-receptor–mediated trigeminal nerve activation
Congestion	Increased mucosal blood flow (vasodilation)	H$_1$/H$_2$-receptor–mediated stimulation of sympathetic nerves; VIP release from parasympathetic (?) nerves
Rhinorrhea	Increased goblet cell secretion, increased vascular permeability	H$_1$-receptor interaction with parasympathetic nerves (goblet cells); H$_1$-receptor–mediated increase in engorgement (sympathetic) of highly fenestrated capacitance vessels.

EDRF—endothelium-derived relaxing factor; NO—nitric oxide; PGI$_2$—prostaglandin I$_2$; P/CGRP—substance P/calcitonin gene-related peptide; NKA—neurokinin A; VIP—vasoactive intestinal peptide.
Adapted from *Monroe et al. [1••].*

TABLE 14-2. PHARMACOKINETIC PROPERTIES OF SELECTED SECOND-GENERATION ANTIHISTAMINES

Antihistamine	Dosage*	Elimination half-life	Active metabolite	Onset of action	Duration of action, *h*	Metabolized in liver	Protein binding, %
Astemizole	10 mg qd	20 h 7 to 10 d †	Yes	2 to 4 d	>24	Yes	~97
Cetirizine	5 or 10 mg qd	7 to 10.6 h	No	<1 h	12 to 24	Minimally	93
Fexofenadine	60 mg bid	14.4 h	No	1 h	12	Minimally	60 to 70
Loratadine	10 mg qd	8 to 11 h	Yes	1 to 3 h	>24	Yes	~97
Terfenadine	60 mg bid	20 h	Yes	1 to 2 h	12	Yes	97
Desloratadine	5 mg qd	27 h	Yes	<1 h	>24	Minimally	~85
Azelastine	2 sprays per nostril bid (1.1 mg/day)	~54 h	Yes	2 to 3 h	12	Yes	97

*Adult
† Biphasic half-life: 20 h for distribution, 7 to 10 days for elimination.
bid—twice daily; qd—once daily

puter. Fans circulate room air continuously, while six impact-type particle samplers determine pollen levels in the patients' seating area. Patients are moved every 30 minutes, ensuring that they spend an equal amount of time in each section of the chamber. Day's group [7•] found no significant ($P = 0.119$) difference among antihistamines in the time to onset of clinically important relief (mean range, 1:45 to 2:28 h), with the quickest to slowest agents being cetirizine, terfenadine, astemizole, and loratadine, respectively. They also used the EEU to study fexofenadine. Using a "relaxed" criteria of clinically important relief (slight to complete relief rather than marked or complete relief), they showed that fexofenadine (60- and 120-mg doses) had a median time to onset of clinically important relief of 60 minutes [8•]. With desloratadine, Horak *et al.* observed an onset of action of less than one hour in responding subjects in a similar environmental unit, the Vienna Challenge Chamber [9].

EFFICACY

The clinical effects of antihistamines in allergic rhinitis result primarily from competitive inhibition of H_1 receptors in the nasal mucosa during an allergic response.

Antihistamines are most effective when occupying the H_1 receptor site before histamine is released. Hence, maximum therapeutic benefits are gained through prophylactic treatment before allergen exposure.

Several methods are used to assess the potency and activity of antihistamines. The most popular method is the suppression of epicutaneous histamine-induced wheal and flare. All H_1 antihistamines inhibit wheal and flare response but differ in the strength of their effect, time to peak effect, and duration of action. Investigators previously have suggested that the inhibition of wheal and flare by antihistamines correlates with relief of allergic rhinitis symptoms [10,11].

Recently, however, Monroe *et al.* [1••] challenged the reliability of antihistamine suppression of histamine-induced wheal and flare as a predictor of clinical effect. The authors concluded, based on a comprehensive literature review, that the method is useful in determining dose-response relationships for individual drugs, but correlates poorly with the ability of various antihistamines to modify clinical responses (Tables 14-3 and 14-4). Histamine, although an important mediator of allergic response in the skin, is just one of a number of significant mediators and cells involved in an allergic reaction.

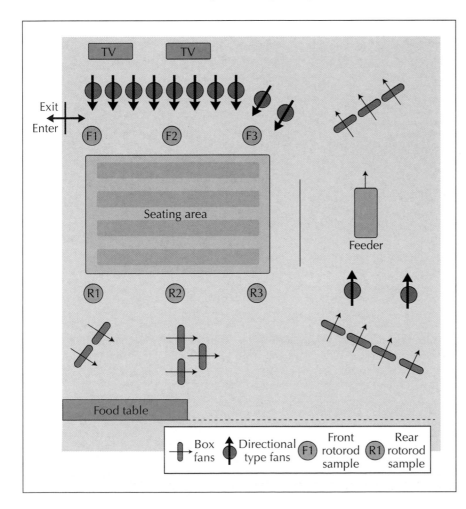

FIGURE 14-1.
Representation of the environmental exposure unit. *Adapted from* from Day JH, *et al.* [7•].

TABLE 14-3. ANTIHISTAMINE SUPPRESSION OF CUTANEOUS HISTAMINE-INDUCED WHEAL AND FLARE REACTIONS: DOUBLE-BLIND, PLACEBO-CONTROLLED, PHARMACODYNAMIC STUDIES

Investigator	Antihistamine and dose	Patients, n	Duration	Suppressive effects*
Roman et al., 1986	L 10, 20, 40 mg qd; Chl 12 mg qd	60	4 wk	Wheal: L 40 mg > L 20 mg > L 10 mg > P=Chl
Small, 1993	C 10 mg qd; L 10 mg qd	51	1 wk	C = L > P
Paul et al., 1994	C 10 mg qd; L 10 mg qd; T 60 mg bid; Cl 2 mg qd	24	3 d	C > T > L > Cl > P
Simons et al., 1990	C 10 mg qd; L 10 mg qd; T 60, 120 mg qd; Ast 10 mg qd; Chl 4 mg qd	20	1 d	C > T 120 mg > T 60 mg > L > Ast > Chl
Rosenzweig et al., 1994	C 10 mg qd; L 10 mg qd; T 120 mg qd; M 10 mg qd	15	1 d	Wheal: M > T > C > L Flare: C > T > M > L
Lever et al., 1994	C 10 mg qd; L 10 mg qd; T 120 mg qd	12	1 d	T = C > L > P
Kontou-Fili et al., 1989	C 10 mg qd; L 10 mg qd	10	1 d	C > L > P
Pechadre et al., 1988	C 10 mg qd; T 60 mg qd	9	1 d	C > T > P
Rihoux and Dupont, 1987	C 10 mg qd; T 180 mg qd	9	1 d	C > T > P
Fadel et al., 1990	L 10 mg qd; C 10 mg qd	7	1 d	C > P > L
Simons and Simons, 1997	F 60 mg bid; F 120 mg qd; L 10 mg qd	20	1 d	F 120 mg = F 60 mg bid > L 10 mg > P

*> sign means the first antihistamine suppresses wheal and flare more effectively than the second antihistamine; = sign means antihistamines are not significantly different from each other.
Ast—astemizole; bid—twice daily; C—cetirizine; Chl—chlorpheniramine; Cl—clemastine; F—fexofenadine; L—loratadine; M—mizolastine; qd—once daily; T—terfenadine.
Adapted from Monroe et al. [1••].

TABLE 14-4. COMPARATIVE DOUBLE-BLIND, PLACEBO-CONTROLLED TRIALS OF ANTIHISTAMINE EFFICACY IN THE TREATMENT OF PATIENTS WITH SEASONAL ALLERGIC RHINITIS

Investigator	Antihistamine and dose	Patients, n	Duration, wk	Symptom control*
Davies et al., 1989	C 10 mg AM; C 10 mg PM; T 60 mg bid	487	8	C > T (eye symptoms)
Bousquet, 1987	L 10 mg bid; Ast 10 qd	452	2	L > Ast > P
Kemp et al., 1985	T 60 mg bid; Chl 4 mg tid	397	1	T = Chl > P
Dockhorn et al., 1987	L 10 mg qd; Cl 1 mg qd	321	2	L = Cl > P
De Carpio et al., 1989	L 10 mg qd; T 60 mg bid	317	2	L = T > P
Kemp et al., 1987	L 10 mg qd; Chl 1 mg qd	313	2	L = Cl > P
Siegal et al., 1988	L 5 to 10 mg qd; Chl 2 to 4 mg qd	271	2	L = Chl > P
Reed et al., 1991	C 10 mg qd; Ast 10 mg qd	270	3	C = Ast > P
Horak et al., 1988	L 10 mg qd; T 60 mg bid	256	2	L = T > P
Alexander et al., 1994	C 10 mg qd; L 10 mg qd	241	2	C = L > P
Buckley et al., 1988	T 60 mg bid; Chl 4 mg tid	215	1	T = Chl > P
Backhouse and Rosenberg, 1987	T 60 mg bid; Chl 4 mg tid	138	6	T = Chl > P
Backhouse et al., 1982	T 60 mg bid; Chl 8 mg bid	136	1	T = Chl > P
Oei, 1988	L 10 mg qd; Ast 10 mg qd	65	2	L > Ast > P
Skassa-Brociek et al., 1988	L 10 mg qd; Meq 5 mg bid	64	2	L = Meq > P
Brandon and Weiner, 1980	T 20 mg tid; Chl 4 mg tid	60	1†	T > Chl > P
Brostoff and Lockhart, 1982	T 60 mg bid; Chl 8 mg bid	60	2	T = Chl > P
Grossman, 1988	C 10 mg qd; T 60 mg bid	53	4	C = T > P
Howarth et al., 1999	F 120 mg qd; F 180 mg qd; C 10 mg qd	842	2	F = C > P

* > sign means the first antihistamine suppresses symptoms of seasonal allergic rhinitis more effectively than the second antihistamine; = sign means antihistamines were not different.
† average
Ast—astemizole; bid—twice daily; C—cetirizine; Chl—chlorpheniramine; Cl—clemastine; F—fexofenadine; L—loratadine; Meq—mequitazine; P—placebo; qd—once daily; T—terfenadine; tid—three times dialy.
Adapted from Monroe et al. [1••].

Structural, functional, and inflammatory responses differ between the skin and nasal mucosa and, as such, a cutaneous histamine-antihistamine interaction may not accurately predict the potency of antihistamines in other tissues and organs or their effect on clinical symptoms of allergic disease.

Epicutaneous histamine injection produces a rapid wheal and flare response that lasts approximately 1 hour [1••]. However, this response mimics only a portion of the early phase reaction—before mast cell degranulation and multiple mediator release—and does not reflect late-phase inflammatory events. Hence, the cellular and mediator mechanisms responsible for producing the full allergic response are not depicted by the histamine-induced wheal and flare response. In the nasal mucosa, histamine activates sensory nerves and increases mucosal blood flow, goblet cell secretion, and vascular permeability [1••]. As in the skin, however, nasal topical histamine challenges do not induce cellular infiltration or a late-phase response.

The appreciation that the effect of antihistamines may differ depending on the target organ and the stimulus was demonstrated in a recent study. Two of the new antihistamines, loratadine (10 mg) and cetirizine (10 mg), were compared using skin tests and nasal provocation tests to histamine and grass pollen. Both antihistamines similarly reduced allergen-induced skin test and nasal challenges whereas cetirizine more profoundly decreased the histamine skin test response [12].

Generally, cetirizine is more effective than other antihistamines in suppressing the cutaneous histamine-induced wheal and flare reaction (Table 14-3). However, results of most comparative trials between first- and second-generation antihistamines reveal that the newer agents are no more effective than their predecessors in relieving symptoms of allergic rhinitis, when patients are compliant with treatment regimens (Table 14-4) [1••]. In fact, Klein et al. [13•] recently reported that the first-generation antihistamine brompheniramine (extended-release formulation) provided better relief of rhinitis symptoms than did terfenadine ($P \leq 0.05$). Not surprisingly, however, somnolence was reported more frequently with brompheniramine (42% versus 9%), causing a number of patients to withdraw from the trial.

Because second-generation antihistamines are largely devoid of the central nervous system (CNS) effects associated with their predecessors, they are preferred in the treatment of patients with allergic rhinitis. As the number of second-generation antihistamines increases, it is difficult to prove the clinical superiority of one drug over another (Table 14-4). At best, 75% to 85% of patients who participate in seasonal allergic rhinitis clinical trials obtained moderate to excellent symptom relief with antihistamine use, whereas patients who receive placebo usually have a 25% to 35% response rate [14]. Clinical trials have shown that symptomatic relief is enhanced only minimally with doses exceeding those recommended by the manufacturer.

The new antihistamines—terfenadine, astemizole, acrivastine, levocabastine, ebastine, desloratadine, loratadine, azelastine, cetirizine, and fexofenadine—relieve symptoms of allergic rhinitis in adults, adolescents, and, the latter four, in children. Recent studies have confirmed personal observations that significant interpatient variability exists with the new antihistamines. Studies comparing fexofenadine and loratadine have revealed each to be superior over the other, depending on the outcome measured (ie, onset of action, relief of ocular symptoms, and quality of life) [15–17]. Furthermore, fexofenadine and cetirizine in patients with seasonal allergic rhinitis showed that both agents significantly ($P<0.001$) improved the 24-hour reflective total symptoms score compared with placebo with no significant differences between active treatments [18]. Cetirizine was, however, associated with a significantly higher incidence of drowsiness versus either fexofenadine or placebo.

Although there are no published comparative studies with other new antihistamines, in placebo-controlled studies desloratadine has been shown to provide significant relief of both non-nasal and nasal symptoms in patients with seasonal allergic rhinitis [19,20].

Studies are emerging that explore the benefit of combining an antihistamine with a leukotriene receptor antagonist in the treatment of seasonal allergic rhinitis. One study in 457 patients showed that the combination of loratadine (10 mg once daily) and montelukast (either 10 mg or 20 mg, once daily) was significantly ($P \leq 0.05$) better in reducing individual daytime nasal symptom scores for nasal congestion, rhinorrhea, nasal itching, and sneezing compared with either agent alone or placebo, with the exception of the comparison between that combination and montelukast 10 mg for nasal congestion [21]. However, a more recent study in 907 patients found loratadine and montelukast given alone and in combination to be more effective than placebo at relieving daytime nasal symptom scores; the combination of loratadine and montelukast did not confer statistically significant additional therapeutic benefit. Considered together, these two studies demonstrate inconsistent findings regarding the effectiveness of combining loratadine and montelukast in the treatment of seasonal allergic rhinitis [22].

ADVERSE EFFECTS OF ANTIHISTAMINES

First-generation antihistamines are well known for their effects on the CNS. Because these drugs are lipophilic, they rapidly cross the blood–brain barrier. Besides their ability to block activation of the H_1 receptor, first-generation antihistamines demonstrate activity in serotonergic, cholinergic, and α-adrenergic receptor pathways, inducing stimulatory, neuropsychiatric, peripheral, and depressive CNS effects. Clinical consequences include CNS stimulatory effects (*ie*, seizures, dyskinesia, dystonia, hallucinations, or psychosis), sedation, and impaired psychomotor performance [6••].

Accordingly, second-generation antihistamines were developed with the goal of alleviating these CNS effects. The new antihistamines are large, relatively lipophobic molecules that possess an electrostatic charge and, as such, do not readily cross the blood–brain barrier. Second-generation antihistamines bind preferentially to peripheral over central H_1 receptors and have minimal serotonergic, cholinergic, or α-

adrenergic blocking activity. Hence, the new antihistamines produce less sedation and other CNS effects than their predecessors, and generally do not potentiate the adverse CNS effects of alcohol and other CNS depressants [23–25].

Garbus *et al.* [2••], Adelsburg [26••], and Nolan [27•] each published comprehensive reviews about the side effects of second-generation antihistamines, emphasizing the sedative, psychomotor, and cognitive effects of these drugs. Table 14-5 summarizes the objective and subjective tests used to evaluate and compare these side effects [26••]. The primary objective measures used to detect CNS effects are reduced sleep latency (greater sleepiness) and performance impairment. The Multiple Sleep Latency test measures daytime

TABLE 14-5. TESTS USED TO ASSESS EFFECTS OF ANTIHISTAMINES ON SEDATION, PSYCHOMOTOR FUNCTION, AND COGNITIVE FUNCTION

Sedation	Psychomotor function	Cognitive function
Multiple Sleep Latency Test	Driving performance	Test of learning ability
Digital Symbol Substitution Test	Piloting performance	Information processing
Symbol copying tasks	Trails B Maze Tracking Test	Critical Flicker Fusion Test
		Pauli Concentration Test
Stanford Sleepiness Scale	Symbol copying tasks	
Patient ratings of sedation on visual analog scale	Critical tracking	
	Dynamic visual activity response time	
	Auditory vigilance tests	

Adapted from *Adelsburg* [26••].

TABLE 14-6. CHARACTERISTICS OF SELECTED FIRST- AND SECOND-GENERATION ANTIHISTAMINES

Generic name	Sedative effects*	Anticholinergic activity	Antihistaminic activity
First generation			
Chlorpheniramine	Yes	Moderate	Moderate
Diphenhydramine	Yes	High	Moderate
Promethazine	Yes	High	High
Second generation			
Astemizole	No	Low to none	Moderate to high
Azelastine	Yes	Low to none	Moderate to high
Cetirizine	Yes	Low to none	Moderate to high
Fexofenadine	No	Low to none	Moderate to high
Loratadine	No	Low to none	Moderate to high
Terfenadine	No	Low to none	Moderate to high
Desloratadine	No	Low to none	Moderate to high

* Significantly different from placebo at recommended doses
Adapted from *Garbus* et al. [2••].

sleepiness and alertness using an electroencephalogram (EEG). Performance tests measure reaction time, visual-motor coordination, memory, and alertness.

Sedation

When referring to the adverse effects of antihistamines, sedation describes a wide range of subjective experiences, including drowsiness, sleepiness, loss of alertness, decreased concentration, and reduced psychomotor performance. Sedation can interfere with a patient's activities of daily living, work and school performance, and safety, especially for individuals who drive, pilot aircraft, or operate machinery.

The sedative effects of first-generation antihistamines are well known, with approximately 25% of patients experiencing sedation [28]. Factors that increase a patient's risk of sedation are age group (children and elderly patients), gender (women), presence of hepatic or renal disease, concomitant use of alcohol or CNS-depressing agents, and CNS impairment.

Sedation appears to be largely avoidable with the use of second-generation antihistamines at recommended dosages. However, not all new antihistamines are without sedative effects (Table 14-6) [29••]. A published review of cetirizine data cited conflicting results from studies evaluating the sedative properties of this drug [30]. One study showed a dose-related increase in self-reported drowsiness with 5-, 10-, and 20-mg doses of cetirizine [31]. The United States Food and Drug Administration (FDA) classifies cetirizine as a sedating antihistamine because, in some clinical trials, the drug is associated with a significantly higher incidence of sedation than placebo.

Similarly, studies have shown that loratadine and acrivastine may cause signs of sedation when given at higher than recommended dosages [32•]. Finally, Hindmarch and Shamsi's extensive review of the literature identified a number of tests which appear to be sensitive to the central effects of antihistamines and concluded that fexofenadine, in doses up to 240 mg, is the only oral antihistamine presently available devoid of sedative activity [33]. To date, clinical studies with desloratadine show no evidence of increased sedation or drowsiness.

Improvement in patient daily functioning and well being is increasingly being viewed as a clinically relevant treatment endpoint. In separate studies, fexofenadine [34] and cetirizine [35] resulted in greater improvement in all quality of life domain scores and in the overall score using the disease-specific Rhinoconjunctivitis Quality of Life Questionnaire (RQLQ) compared to placebo. Similarly, overall activity impairment was significantly decreased from baseline for fexofenadine-treated patients and cetirizine-treated patients compared to placebo, as measured by the Allergy-Specific Work Productivity and Activity Impairment (WPAI-AS) instrument.

Psychomotor and cognitive impairment

In addition to having little or no sedative effects, second-generation antihistamines appear to have a low potential to cause psychomotor and cognitive impairment. Simons *et al.* [29••], using an objective measure of cognitive function (P300 latency) and subjective measure of somnolence (visual analog scale), demonstrated that second-generation antihistamines vary individually with respect

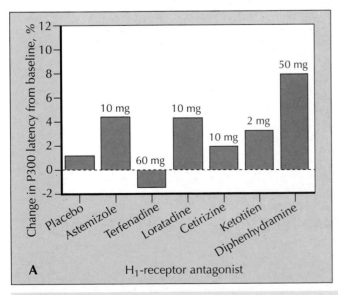
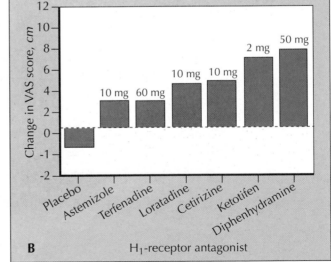

FIGURE 14-2.

A, Percentage change from baseline in P300 event-related potential 2.5 hours after treatment with placebo, terfenadine, cetirizine, ketotifen, loratadine, astemizole, or diphenhydramine. Difference from placebo was significant (*P* < 0.05) for diphenhy-dramine only. **B,** Change in the visual analog scale (VAS) for somnolence 2.5 hours after treatment. Differences from placebo were significant (*P* < 0.05) for cetirizine, ketotifen, and diphenhydramine. *Adapted from* Simons [29••].

to effects on cognitive function and somnolence and that these effects are less than those of the first-generation antihistamine diphenhydramine (Fig. 14-2).

First-generation antihistamines have been and continue to be implicated as a cause of traffic accidents [36,37]. Consequently, 35 states and the District of Columbia have enacted laws against driving under the influence of any agent that impairs performance, including sedating antihistamines (Fig. 14-3) [38].

Investigators in the Netherlands have tested the effects of antihistamines on patients' driving performance under real road and traffic conditions. During these tests, patients drove a specially equipped vehicle over a standardized circuit at a constant speed in normal highway traffic for 1 hour. The primary outcome variable was the standard deviation of lateral position (SDLP) or "weaving index." A clinically relevant change was defined as a difference larger than that demonstrated by "social drinkers" who had blood alcohol concentrations greater than 0.5 mg/mL. These studies revealed that recommended dosages of second-generation antihistamines (acrivastine, cetirizine, ebastine, loratadine, mizolastine, and terfenadine) were significantly less impairing than equivalent dosages of

first-generation agents (clemastine, diphenhydramine, and triprolidine) [39]. Similar results were seen when fexofenadine was compared to diphenhydramine and alcohol on driving performance utilizing the Iowa Driving Simulator [40]. In contrast, two studies found that cetirizine affected patients to a similar degree as alcohol in over-the-road driving tests [41,42]. Moreover, the effects of cetirizine appeared to be additive to that of alcohol. In an over-the-road driving study, desloratadine caused no impairment of driving performance [43]. No potentiation of alcohol effects by desloratadine was observed in a study employing multiple measures of sedation and psychomotor performance [44].

A few studies have evaluated the effects of second-generation antihistamines on piloting skills. In two separate studies, neither terfenadine nor loratadine produced drowsiness or affected piloting skills during flight simulation tests [45,46]. No impairment was observed in flight simulator studies with desloratadine [47]. The United States Federal Aviation Administration (FAA) guidelines now permit the use of only loratadine and fexofenadine before or during flight, provided pilots have a physician's report documenting no side effects

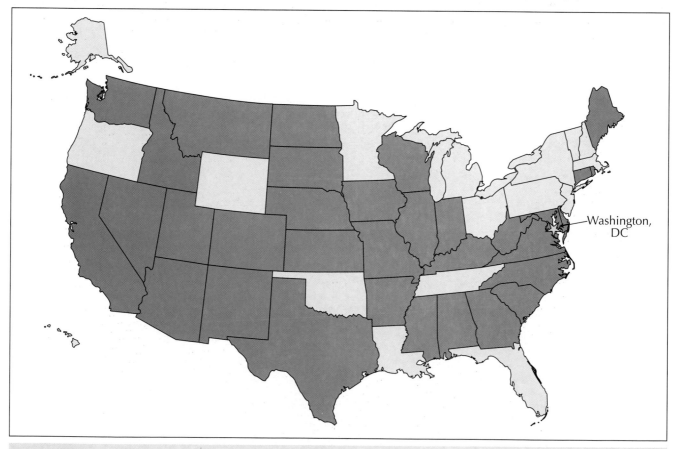

FIGURE 14-3.
United States Department of Transportation statistics on the number of states (shaded) that enacted laws prohibiting operation of a motor vehicle while taking sedating medications. *Adapted from* Nolan [27•].

with treatment. Pilots are prohibited from taking sedating antihistamines within 24 hours before a flight [2••].

Other studies have investigated the psychomotor effects of antihistamines relative to work-related injuries and job performance. A report from the Group Health Cooperative of Puget Sound [48] concluded that the risk of work-related injuries increased among antihistamine users (odds ratio, 1.5; CI, 1.1 to 1.9), and was in fact greater for workers who used sedating antihistamines than for those using sedative hypnotics or narcotics. In one study, researchers evaluated the work performance of normal subjects on a computer-driven simulated assembly line for 8 hours after treatment with cetirizine (10 mg), hydroxyzine (25 mg), or placebo [49]. Subjects who received hydroxyzine made fewer correct responses than did subjects who received cetirizine or placebo ($P < 0.05$); performance was similar for cetirizine and placebo groups.

First-generation antihistamines may also impede the school performance of children with allergic rhinitis, whereas the new antihistamines may ameliorate some of the negative effects of allergic rhinitis on learning. In a study of school children, those with allergic rhinitis did worse on learning tests than did healthy children. Subsequent treatment with the first-generation antihistamine diphenhydramine further impaired their learning, whereas the second-generation antihistamine loratadine improved their performance (although performance was still below the level of healthy children) [50••]. In another study, learning scores of adolescents and young adults improved after concomitant therapy with acrivastine and pseudoephedrine compared with diphenhydramine [51].

Cardiotoxic effects

The second-generation antihistamines terfenadine and astemizole have a propensity to block cardiac muscle potassium channels. High-serum concentrations of both agents have been implicated in causing prolongation of the corrected QT (QT_c) interval and torsades de pointes, a rare but potentially life-threatening ventricular tachyarrhythmia. These cardiotoxic effects occur largely through drug interactions with medications known to inhibit biotransformation of CYP3A4, the isoenzyme responsible for metabolism of terfenadine and astemizole. CYP3A4 is part of the P450 hepatic enzyme system. Studies show that there is no clinically relevant alteration of desloratadine bioavailability when coadministered with drugs that affect the cytochrome P450 system or active drug transporters such as P-glycoprotein or organic anion transporting polypeptide [19].

Medications contraindicated with the use of terfenadine and astemizole include imidazole antifungals (ketoconazole and itraconazole) and macrolide antibiotics (erythromycin and troleandomycin). Other drugs suspected of potential interactions with either agent are nefazodone, a synthetically derived antidepressant;

fluvoxamine, a selective serotonin reuptake inhibitor; and ritonavir, an HIV-specific protease [52]. Concomitant use of terfenadine and cimetidine, another CYP450 enzyme inhibitor, is also implicated in increasing the risk of prolonged QT_c interval and torsades de pointes. Other medications contraindicated for use with terfenadine include those known to block potassium channels, lengthen the cardiac output interval, and increase the risk of torsades de pointes (eg, quinidine, haloperidol, disopyramide, pentamidine, probucol, procainamide, sotalol, and thioridazine). Factors other than concomitant therapies that are linked to an increased risk of adverse cardiac events include drug overdose; coadministration with grapefruit juice; and patients with significant hepatic dysfunction, underlying cardiac abnormalities, or metabolic abnormalities (hypokalemia, hypomagnesemia, or anorexia).

Cardiotoxic effects have not been observed with loratadine, acrivastine, cetirizine, azelastine, or fexofenadine. Fexofenadine, unlike its parent compound terfenadine, has no significant effect on the QT_c interval, even at doses tenfold greater than the recommended dose. Additionally, no significant increase in the QTc interval was observed with fexofenadine when used concomitantly with erythromycin or ketoconazole [53].

In a recent study, Hey et al. [54•] used an experimental guinea pig model predictive of adverse electrocardiogram (ECG) effects in humans to evaluate the arrhythmogenic potential of several second-generation antihistamines. Terfenadine, astemizole, and ebastine produced significant arrhythmogenic effects, including QT_c interval prolongation, bradycardia, and distortion of ECG morphology. Carebastine, cetirizine, loratadine, norastemizole, desloratadine, and fexofenadine were devoid of QT_c prolongation effects.

TOPICAL ANTIHISTAMINES

Topical administration of antihistamines, such as levocabastine and azelastine, provide a new therapeutic option for the treatment of patients with allergic rhinitis. Some comparison studies have shown that these agents are as effective as oral antihistamines and may provide better relief of nasal symptoms. In a double-blind, parallel-group trial comparing levocabastine (0.5 mg/mL eye drops, one drop in each eye twice daily; and nasal spray, two sprays in each nostril twice daily) with terfenadine (60 mg twice daily), levocabastine was more effective than terfenadine in relieving ocular itch ($P = 0.02$) and nasal symptoms [55]. Another double-blind, parallel-group trial comparing intranasal azelastine (0.28 mg twice daily) with terfenadine (60 mg twice daily) revealed no clinically relevant differences between treatments in patients with perennial rhinitis [56]. Azelastine showed trends toward better relief of rhinorrhea and nasal obstruction, whereas terfenadine showed trends toward better control of sneezing and nasal itch.

After intranasal administration, the systemic bioavailability of azelastine hydrochloride is approximately 40%. Maximum plasma concentrations (Cmax) are achieved in 2 to 3 hours. Based on intravenous and oral administrations the elimination half-life, steady-state volume of distribution, and plasma clearance are 22 hours, 14.5 L/kg, and 0.5 L/h/kg, respectively.

In general, antihistamines have not been beneficial in relieving symptoms of vasomotor rhinitis (chronic, perennial nonallergic, noninfectious rhinitis). While the prevalence of nonallergic rhinitis can only be estimated, these estimates range from 17% to 52% of all rhinitis sufferers and may involve tens of millions in the United States alone [57]. Recently, azelastine nasal spray was compared to placebo in patients with well-defined vasomotor rhinitis. In both studies, azelastine nasal spray significantly (study 1, $P=.002$; study 2, $P=.005$) reduced the total vasomotor rhinitis symptom score from the baseline when compared with placebo. Improvements over placebo were observed for all individual symptoms (nasal congestion, rhinorrhea, sneezing, and postnasal drip) of the vasomotor rhinitis symptom complex [58]. Based on its structure, azelastine may possess a far wider range of activities than just antihistaminic activity. It has been shown to have diverse anti-inflammatory activity (see section on anti-inflammatory effects) that may account for its effect in nonallergic rhinits.

The onset of action of topical antihistamines is similar to, if not faster than, oral antihistamines. In one study, 94% of patients experienced relief of ocular symptoms within 15 minutes of using levocabastine eye drops [59]. In another study, 73% of patients who used levocabastine nasal spray reported symptom relief within 30 minutes of application [60]. Similarly, 30 minutes after topical application of azelastine (0.28 mg) to the nasal mucosa, allergen-induced sneezing was attenuated, with effects lasting up to 10 hours [61].

In a study of children with allergic conjunctivitis, combination levocabastine eye drops (0.5 mg/mL solution) and terfenadine syrup (0.6%) increased the conjunctival threshold dose of allergen over that of terfenadine and placebo, suggesting that topical antihistamines can have an additive effect to oral antihistamine therapy [62].

Theoretically, topical antihistamines should offer advantages over oral antihistamines because these agents are not absorbed systemically and, as such, should cause fewer side effects and little or no adverse drug interactions with concomitant medications. For topical levocabastine, the most frequent side effects are nasal and ocular irritation, which occurs in 5% to 10% of patients, respectively (a rate not significantly different from placebo) [59,63]. Side effects of topical azelastine therapy include headache, taste perversion (metallic taste), nasal

irritation, and somnolence. The incidence of somnolence with azelastine is similar to that of cetirizine, due to systemic absorption [64].

ANTI-INFLAMMATORY EFFECTS

The ability of some second-generation antihistamines to inhibit the release of inflammatory mediators after allergen challenge and effect eosinophil migration expands the potential therapeutic application of these drugs beyond simple H_1 receptor antagonism to a contributory role in dampening the entire allergic inflammatory cascade. Subtle differences observed among the newer antihistamines may have important clinical implications.

Recent studies show that cetirizine, loratadine, and fexofenadine reduce expression of the intercellular adhesion molecule-1 (ICAM-1) on epithelial membranes. ICAM-1, a transmembrane glycoprotein, promotes adhesion in immunologic and inflammatory reactions, and is found in increased concentrations on nasal epithelial cells of patients with allergic rhinitis [65,66]. In one study of patients with seasonal allergic rhinitis, both loratadine (10 mg daily) and cetirizine (10 mg daily) significantly ($P < 0.05$) reduced release of soluble ICAM-1 in nasal secretions compared with placebo [67•]. Similarly, 2 weeks of treatment with loratadine (10 mg daily) or cetirizine (10 mg daily) reduced symptoms, eosinophil and metachromatic cell infiltration, eosinophil cationic protein (ECP), eosinophil peroxidase and histamine levels, and ICAM-1 expression on epithelial cells of patients with allergic rhinitis [68]. In children with allergic rhinitis, 4 weeks of cetirizine treatment significantly ($P < 0.05$) improved clinical symptoms compared with placebo, and reduced inflammatory cell infiltrate (neutrophils and eosinophils), ICAM-1 expression on epithelial cells, and soluble ICAM-1 and ECP concentrations in nasal lavage fluid [69]. Fexofenadine may also possess the potential to treat nasal inflammation by modulating nasal epithelial cell function. In a study using nasal epithelial cells cultured from biopsy specimens of patients with seasonal allergic rhinitis (outside of pollen season), fexofenadine attenuated eosinophil-induced release of interleukin-8, granulocyte-macrophage colony-stimulating factor (GM-CSF), and soluble ICAM-1 [70]. The direct beneficial effects of desloratadine on inflammatory mediators have been demonstrated in human basophils [71]. Another intriguing observation, when considering that antihistamines typically have no appreciable effect on nasal congestion, is that cetirizine inhibits leukotriene C_4 and D_4 [72] production in nasal secretions and eosinophil recruitment in the cutaneous late phase [73].

Topical antihistamines levocabastine and azelastine also demonstrate pharmacologic activities beyond H_1 receptor blockade. Levocabastine (0.5 mg/mL solution) significantly reduced nasal symptoms and eosinophil and neutrophil influx after allergen challenge compared with placebo [74]. In double-blind, placebo-controlled trials, pretreatment with levocabastine (one drop in each eye) and azelastine (one spray, 0.14 mg, in each nostril) 30 minutes before an allergen challenge significantly reduced inflammatory cell infiltration and epithelial cell ICAM-1 expression compared with placebo [75].

Azelastine has been shown to reduce levels of leukotrienes and kinins following nasal allergen challenge [76] and to downregulate (ICAM-1) expression on nasal epithelial cells while reducing eosinophil and neutrophil infiltration in both the early- and late-phase of the allergic response [77]. In addition, azelastine caused a dose-dependent inhibition of superoxide free radical production in human neutrophils and eosinophils [78].

ANTIHISTAMINES IN ASTHMA

Researchers now are suggesting that allergic rhinitis and asthma are not separate diseases, but rather a continuum of inflammation involving a common pathway [79•]. Epidemiological studies show that allergic rhinitis and asthma commonly coexist. Interestingly, as many as 78% of patients with asthma report nasal symptoms, and as many as 38% of patients with allergic rhinitis have asthma [80•].

Histamine is recognized as an important mediator in the pathogenesis of asthma; however, first-generation antihistamines were not considered as a treatment for asthma because the high doses required produced intolerable side effects. Moreover, product labels for antihistamines contraindicated their use in patients with asthma, warning that these agents may thicken mucous and cause bronchoconstriction. Later investigations would prove that antihistamines do not cause bronchoconstriction but instead have bronchodilating effects [81].

Concerns about side effects with second-generation antihistamines are less troublesome and not substantiated by studies investigating their effects in patients with asthma. In fact, some nonsedating antihistamines demonstrate mild anti-asthmatic effects. Terfenadine [82,83], loratadine [6], and astemizole [84,85] have exhibited modest bronchodilating effects, reduced bronchial hyperreactivity to histamine, and protected against exercise- and antigen-induced bronchospasm, although most treatment benefits were reported with doses higher than currently recommended. Cetirizine demonstrated some protective effects against bronchial hyperreactivity to methacholine at 6 hours [86], and when used concomitantly with salbutamol provided prolonged relief (over 7 to 8 hours) of lower airway obstruction [87]. In patients with allergic rhinitis and perennial asthma, cetirizine (20 mg) significantly reduced baseline severity of both rhinitis (itchy nose, nasal congestion, watery eyes) and asthma symptoms (chest tightness, wheezing, shortness of breath, and nocturnal asthma) [88].

Some antihistamines also demonstrate treatment effects when used at recommended dosages. In one study, cetirizine (10 mg daily) reduced the severity of seasonal rhinitis and asthma but had no effect on pulmonary function [89]. Combination treatment with loratadine (5 mg twice daily) and pseudoephedrine (120 mg twice daily) improved asthma symptoms, peak expiratory flow rates, spirometry, and quality-of-life measurements for patients with seasonal allergic rhinitis and asthma [80•]. In studies of patients with seasonal allergic rhinitis (SAR) and mild to moderate asthma, desloratadine has been shown to relieve the signs and symptoms of both SAR and asthma, including a significant decrease in the use of inhaled B_2-agonists while maintaining a normal FEV_1 [90]. It is interesting to speculate about the potential effects of fexofenadine in patients with asthma. Unlike other second-generation antihistamines, the dosage of fexofenadine can be increased to maximize anti-inflammatory effects without the risk of sedation and cardiovascular events.

One study also has shown that combination therapy with loratadine (10 mg twice daily) and the leukotriene receptor antagonist zafirlukast (80 mg twice daily) reduced ($P < 0.05$) early and late asthmatic reactions in patients with allergic asthma more than either agent alone, suggesting that this combination therapy may present a new strategy for treating asthma [91••]. Recently, combination therapy was examined in the treatment of chronic asthma in a short 2-week pilot study; montelukast (10 mg every evening) and loratadine (20 mg every evening) in combination was significantly better than montelukast (10 mg every evening) alone in improving FEV_1, AM and PM $PEFR_1$, beta agonist use, daytime asthma scores, nighttime asthma scores, and nocturnal awakenings [92]. What remains to be seen is whether the improvement in chest symptoms was the direct effect of two antimediator drugs on the lower airway or the result of appropriate treatment of allergic rhinitis in the upper airway.

GUIDELINES FOR THE USE OF ANTIHISTAMINES

When prescribing antihistamines for patients, physicians should consider drug action and efficacy as well as safety profile. First- and second-generation antihistamines may show equivalent efficacy but differ in terms of side effects. From a patient's perspective, one of the most important considerations when choosing an appropriate therapy is its impact on quality of life.

Because of the sedation and psychomotor impairment associated with first-generation antihistamines, some physicians recommend the use of these agents only at bedtime so that the sedative effects occur during sleep. Other physicians recommend a combination regimen as a cost-saving measure, prescribing a nonsedating antihistamine in the morning and a sedating antihistamine in the evening. However, until studies confirm the safety of a mixed morning/evening regimen, caution is advised. The side effects of sedating antihistamines can persist into the morning hours, contributing to potential adverse consequences during the day (*eg*, traffic accidents, work-related injuries, and impaired performance).

Kay *et al.* [93••] investigated the carryover effects of a morning/evening treatment regimen with terfenadine (mornings) and the over-the-counter sedating antihistamine chlorpheniramine (evenings). Results of the Multiple Sleep Latency test and Stanford Sleepiness Scale test showed that the morning/evening regimen increased daytime sleepiness, decreased alertness, and caused a carryover sedation effect (*ie*, patients fell asleep more quickly and were less able to concentrate the following day). In an editorial, Simons [94••] summarized the safety concerns of first-generation antihistamines and cautioned that cost containment should not impel health-care providers to prescribe a first-generation antihistamine over a second-generation agent. Moreover, studies have shown that patients may not recognize when perfor-

mance is impaired [95,96]. CNS impairment can exist even when drowsiness is not reported by patients, as demonstrated by discrepancies between subjective reporting and objective measures of sedation [39,97,98].

Compliance may be another issue to consider when prescribing an antihistamine. A number of anecdotal and subjective reports describe tolerance to first-generation antihistamines over time; however, this decrease in clinical response may be related to a gradual decrease in compliance rather than drug tolerance. In one study, the decrease in clinical response to chlorpheniramine over 3 weeks was associated with a decrease in patient compliance [99]. Noncompliance was attributed to side effects, such as drowsiness, lightheadedness, and anticholinergic effects (dry mouth and urinary hesitancy). Hence, the adverse effects of first-generation antihistamines may interfere with their value as long-term treatment.

Second-generation antihistamines, therefore, play a prominent role in a consensus report on the diagnosis and management of rhinitis (Fig. 14-4) [100]. The first step in the medical management of patients with mild to moderate allergic rhinitis begins with an oral nonsedating

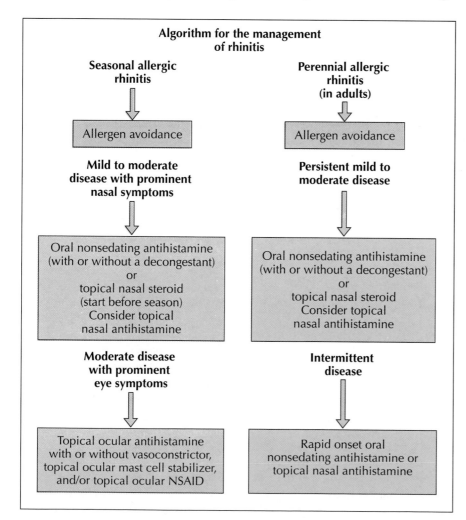

Algorithm for the management of rhinitis

Seasonal allergic rhinitis

↓

Allergen avoidance

Mild to moderate disease with prominent nasal symptoms

↓

Oral nonsedating antihistamine (with or without a decongestant) or topical nasal steroid (start before season) Consider topical nasal antihistamine

Moderate disease with prominent eye symptoms

↓

Topical ocular antihistamine with or without vasoconstrictor, topical ocular mast cell stabilizer, and/or topical ocular NSAID

Perennial allergic rhinitis (in adults)

↓

Allergen avoidance

Persistent mild to moderate disease

↓

Oral nonsedating antihistamine (with or without a decongestant) or topical nasal steroid Consider topical nasal antihistamine

Intermittent disease

↓

Rapid onset oral nonsedating antihistamine or topical nasal antihistamine

FIGURE 14-4.
Guidelines for the stepwise approach to the treatment of patients with rhinitis. NSAID—nonsteroidal anti-inflammatory drug. (*Adapted from* The Task Force on Allergic Disorders [90].)

antihistamine. Patients with more moderate disease fall into two categories: those with predominantly nasal symptoms and those with predominantly ocular symptoms. Patients with eye symptoms should begin therapy with a topical ocular antihistamine daily. If nasal symptoms are not controlled with antihistamines alone or if patients have more prominent nasal blockage, a topical anti-inflammatory medication (ie, an intranasal steroid) should also be prescribed.

CONCLUSIONS

The new, nonsedating antihistamines are the recommended first-line pharmacotherapeutic approach for the management of mild-to-moderate allergic rhinitis, especially when ocular symptoms predominate. Advantages of the new antihistamines include oral or topical administration; a once- or twice-daily treatment regimen (which should improve compliance); specific H_1 receptor antagonism; inhibition of other inflammatory mediators involved in the allergic response; and mild anti-asthmatic effects. Aside from their lack of sedative effects, perhaps the most compelling reason to prescribe second-generation antihistamines is that they do not interfere with performance and learning. Factors that will most likely dictate drug choice among the newer agents are cost, convenience, compliance, and patient preference.

REFERENCES AND RECOMMENDED READING

Recently published papers of particular interest have been highlighted as:
•   Of interest
••   Of outstanding interest

1.•• Monroe EW, Daly AF, Shalhoub RF: Appraisal of the validity of histamine induced wheal and flare to predict the clinical efficacy of antihistamines. *J Allergy Clin Immunol* 1997, 99:S798–S806.
This is a review of comparative studies of antihistamines in the treatment of chronic idiopathic urticaria and seasonal allergic rhinitis, and the lack of predictive value of antihistamine suppression of cutaneous histamine-induced wheal and flare reaction.

2.•• Garbus SB, Moulton BW, Meltzer EO, *et al.*: Considerations in pharmaceutical conversion: focus on antihistamines. *Am J Man Care* 1997, 3:617–630.
This paper discusses issues related to and implications of pharmaceutical conversion using the antihistamine class of drugs as the case situation.

3. Kastrup EK, ed.: *Drug Facts and Comparisons.* St. Louis: Facts and Comparisons; 1997:188–194a.

4. Kreutner W, Hey JA, Anthes J, *et al.*: Preclinical pharmacology of desloratadine, a selective and nonsedating histamine H_1 receptor antagonist. 1st communication: receptor selectivity, antihistamine activity, and antiallergenic effects. *Arzneimittelforschung* 2000, 50:345–352.

5. Kreutner W, Hey JA, Chiu P, Barnett A: Preclinical pharmacology of desloratadine, a selective and nonsedating histamine H_1 receptor antagonist. 2nd communication: Lack of central nervous system and cardiovascular effects. *Arzneimittelforschung* 2000, 50:441–448.

6.•• Du Buske LM: Clinical comparison of histamine H_1 receptor antagonist drugs. *J Allergy Clin Immunol* 1996, 98:S307–S318.
This is a comprehensive review of the second-generation antihistamines, focusing on their pharmacokinetics, adverse effect profiles, antiallergic activities, and antiasthmatic effects.

7.• Day JH, Briscoe MP, Clark RH, *et al.*: Onset of action and efficacy of terfenadine, astemizole, cetirizine, and loratadine for the relief of symptoms of allergic rhinitis. *Ann Allergy Asthma Immunol* 1997, 79:163–172.
This study employs an environmental exposure unit as a model to differentiate the onset of action and efficacy of second-generation antihistamines.

8.• Day JH, Briscoe MP, Welsh A, *et al.*: Onset of action, efficacy, and safety of a single dose of fexofenadine hydrochloride for ragweed allergy using an environmental exposure unit. *Ann Allergy Asthma Immunol* 1997, 79:533–540.
This paper extends findings by Day et al. [5] to include the onset of action and efficacy of fexofenadine hydrochloride without a direct comparison to other antihistamines.

9. Horak F, Stubner UP, Zieglmayer R, *et al.*: Onset and duration of action of desloratadine after controlled pollen challenges in patients with seasonal allergic rhinitis. *Allergy* 2000, 55(Suppl 63):279.

10. Watson WTA, Simons KJ, Chen XY, *et al.*: Cetirizine: a pharmacokinetic and pharmacodynamic evaluation in children with seasonal allergic rhinitis. *J Allergy Clin Immunol* 1989, 84:457–464.

11. Howarth PH, Emmanual MB, Holgate ST, *et al.*: Astemizole, a potent histamine H_1 receptor antagonist: effect in allergic rhinoconjunctivitis, on antigen and histamine induced skin wheal responses and relationship to serum levels. *Br J Clin Pharmacol* 1984, 18:1–8.

12. Laurence P, Pascal B, Harris AG, *et al.*: Comparison between nasal provocation tests and skin tests in patients treated with loratadine and cetirizine. *J Allergy Clin Immunol* 1999, 103:591–594.

13.• Klein GL, Littlejohn T III, Lockhart EA, *et al.*: Brompheniramine, terfenadine, and placebo in allergic rhinitis. *Ann Allergy Asthma Immunol* 1996, 77:365–370.
This is a thought-provoking study comparing a first-generation antihistamine with a second-generation antihistamine.

14. Meltzer EO, Schatz M: Pharmacotherapy of asthma: 1987 and beyond. *Immunol Allergy Clin North Am* 1987, 7:57–91.

15. Van Cauwenberge P, Juniper ER, Meltzer E: Efficacy, safety and quality of life: a comparison between fexofenadine, loratadine and placebo in the treatment of seasonal allergic rhinitis. *Ann Allergy Asthma Immunol*, in press.

16. Prenner B, Caprano D, Harris AG: The safety and efficacy of loratadine (Claritin®) versus fexofenadine HCl (Allegra®) in the treatment of seasonal allergic rhinitis (SAR): a multicenter crossover comparison with treatment of nonresponders. *Allergy* 1999, 54:148.

17. Kaiser H, Harris AG, Capano D: A double-blind placebo-controlled comparison of the safety and efficacy of loratadine (Claritin®), fexofenadine HCl (Allegra®), and placebo in the treatment of subjects with seasonal allergic rhinitis (SAR). *Allergy* 1999, 54:155.

18. Howarth PH, Stern MA, Roi L, *et al.*: Double-blind, placebo-controlled study comparing the efficiency and safety of fexofenadine hydrochloride (120 and 180 mg once daily) and cetirizine in seasonal allergic rhinitis. *J Allergy Clin Immunol* 1999, 104:427–933.

19. Geha RS, Meltzer EO: Desloratadine: a new, nonsedating, oral antihistamine. *J Allergy Clin Immunol* 2001, 107:751–762.

20. Meltzer EO, Prenner BM, Nayak A: Efficacy and safety of once-daily 5 mg desloratadine, a potent H_1 receptor antagonist in patients with seasonal allergic rhinitis. Assessment during the spring and fall allergy season. *Clin Drug Invest* 2001, 21:25–32.

21. Meltzer EO, Malmstrom K, Lu S, et al.: Concomitant montelukast and loratadine as treatment for seasonal allergic rhinitis: a randomized, placebo-controlled clinical trial. *J Allergy Clin Immunol* 2000, 105:917–922.

22. Lis K, Malmstrom K, Nayak AS, et al.: Treatment of fall allergic rhinitis with montelukast alone or in combination with loratadine in a multicenter, double-blind, randomized, placebo-controlled study. *J Allergy Clin Immunol* 2001, 107:S158.

23. Simons FER, Simons KJ: Second-generation H$_1$ receptor antagonists. *Ann Allergy* 1991, 66:5–19.

24. Drouin MA: H$_1$ antihistamines: perspective on the use of the conventional and new agents. *Ann Allergy* 1985, 55:747–752.

25. Kaliner MA, Check WA: Nonsedating antihistamines. *Allergy Proc* 1988, 9:649–661.

26.•• Adelsburg BR: Sedation and performance issues in the treatment of allergic conditions. *Arch Intern Med* 1997, 157:494–500.
This is an excellent review article on CNS effects with particular emphasis on psychomotor and cognitive effects of second-generation antihistamines.

27.• Nolan TM: Sedative effects of antihistamines: safety, performance, learning, and quality of life. *Clin Ther* 1997, 19:39–55.
This is another review article on the side-effect profile of the sedating and nonsedating antihistamines with emphasis on patient satisfaction and quality-of-life parameters.

28. Simons FER, Simons KJ: H$_1$ receptor antagonist treatment of chronic rhinitis. *J Allergy Clin Immunol* 1988, 81:975–980.

29.•• Simons FER, Fraser TG, Reggin JD, et al.: Comparison of the central nervous system effects produced by six H$_1$ receptor antagonists. *Clin Exp Allergy* 1996, 26:1092–1097.
This is a comprehensive comparative study of the newer antihistamines and their effects on cognitive functioning and somnolence.

30. Spencer CM, Faulds D, Peters DH: Cetirizine. *Drugs* 1993, 46:1055–1080.

31. Falliers CJ, Brandon ML, Buchman E, et al.: Double-blind comparison of cetirizine and placebo in the treatment of seasonal rhinitis. *Ann Allergy* 1991, 66:257–262.

32.• Davies RJ, Bagnall AC, McCabe RN, et al.: Antihistamines: topical vs oral administration. *Clin Exp Allergy* 1996, 26(suppl):11–17.
This paper gives supporting evidence that it is logical to administer antihistamines directly to the target organ, the nose.

33.•• Hindmarch I, Shamsi Z: Anithistamines: models to assess sedative properties, assessment of sedation, safety and other side-effects. *Clin Exp Allergy* 1999, 29(suppl):133–142.
An excellent review of various antihistamine-sensitive models of sedation and sedative properties of second-generation antihistamines.

34. Meltzer EO, Casale TB, Nathan RA, Thompson AK: Once-daily fexofenadine HCl improved quality of life and reduced work and activity impairment in patients with seasonal allergic rhinitis. *Ann Allergy Asthma Immunol* 1999, 83:311–317.

35. Murray J, Nathan R, Bronsky E, et al.: Cetirizine in the management of seasonal allergic rhinitis: impact on patient health-related quality of life (HRQL) work productivity and activity impairment (WPAI). *Ann Allergy Asthma Immunol*, in press.

36. Cimbura G, Lucas DM, Bennett RC, et al.: Incidence and toxicological aspects of drugs detected in 484 fatally injured drivers and pedestrians in Ontario. *Forensic Sci* 1982, 27:855–867.

37. Warren R, Simpson H, Hilchie J, et al.: Drugs detected in fatally injured drivers in the province of Ontario. In: *Alcohol, Drugs and Traffic Safety*, vol 1. Edited by Goldburg L. Stockholm: Almquist & Wiskell, 1981:203–217

38. US Department of Transportation: *Digest of the State Alcohol-Highway Safety Related Legislation*, edn 14. Washington, DC: United States Department of Transportation, 1996.

39. O'Hanlon JF: Antihistamines and driving performance: the Netherlands. *J Respir Dis* 1988, 9:12–17.

40. Weiler JM, Bloomfield JR, Grantar, et al.: Effects of fexofenadine, diphenhydramine and alcohol on driving performance: a randomized, placebo-controlled trial in the Iowa Driving Simulator. *Ann Intern Med*, in press.

41. Van Cauwenberge PB: New data on the safety of loratadine. *Drug Invest* 1992, 4:283–291.

42. Ramaekers JG, Uiterwijk MM, O'Hanlon JF: Effects of loratadine and cetirizine on actual driving and psychometric test performance, and EEG during driving. *Eur J Clin Pharmacol* 1992, 42:363–369.

43. Vuurman E, Ramaekers JG, Rikken G, de Halleux F: Desloratadine does not impair actual driving performance: a 3-way crossover comparison with diphenhydramine and placebo. *Allergy* 2000, 55(Suppl 63):263–264.

44. Rikken G, Scharf MB, Danzig MR, Staudinger H: Desloratadine and alcohol co-administration: no increase in impairment of performance over that induced by alcohol alone. *Allergy* 2000, 55(Suppl 63):277.

45. Offenloch K, Zahner G: Rated performance, cardiovascular and quantitative EEG parameters during simulated instrument flight under the effect of terfenadine. *Arzneimittelforschung* 1992, 42:864–868.

46. Neves-Pinto RM, Lima GM, da Mota Teixeira R: A double-blind study of the effects of loratadine versus placebo on the performance of pilots. *Am J Rhinology* 1992, 6:23.

47. Valk P, van Roon D, Simons M, et al.: No impairment of flying ability with desloratadine use in healthy volunteers under conditions of simulated cabin pressure. *Allergy* 2001. In press.

48. Gilmore TM, Alexander BH, Mueller BA, et al.: Occupational injuries and medication use. *Am J Ind Med* 1996, 30:234–239.

49. Walsh JK, Muehlbach MJ, Schweitzer PK: Simulated assembly line performance following ingestion of ceterizine or hydroxyzine. *Ann Allergy* 1992, 69:195–200.

50.•• Vuurman EF, van Veggel L, Uiterwijk MM, et al.: Seasonal allergic rhinits and antihistamine effects on children's learning. *Ann Allergy* 1993, 71:121–126.
Important study that illustrates that first-generation antihistamines further impede school performance in children with allergic rhinitis, whereas second-generation antihistamines may lessen some of the negative effects of the disease.

51. Vuurman EF, van Veggel L, Sanders RL, et al.: Effects of Semprex-D and diphenhydramine on learning in young adults with seasonal allergic rhinitis. *Ann Allergy Asthma Immunol* 1996, 76:247–252.

52. Tatro DS, Olin BR, Hebel SK: *Drug Interaction Facts*. St. Louis: JB Lippincott, 1997.

53. Pratt C, Mason J, Russel T, Ahlbrand R: Cardiovascular safety of fexofenadine HCl. *Am J Cardiol* 1999, 83:1451–1454.

54.• Hey JA, del Prado M, Sherwood J, et al.: Comparative analysis of the cardiotoxicity proclivities of second generation antihistamines in an experimental model predictive of adverse clinical ECG effects. *Arzneimittelforschung* 1996, 46:153–158.
This is an interesting article using a guinea pig model to predict the arrhythmogenic potential of second-generation antihistamines in humans.

55. Bahmer FA, Ruprecht KW: Safety and efficacy of topical levocabastine compared with oral terfenadine. *Ann Allergy* 1994, 72:429–434.

56. Gastpar H, Nolte D, Aurich R, et al.: Comparative efficacy of azelastine nasal spray and terfenadine in seasonal and perennial rhinitis. *Allergy* 1994, 49:152–158.

57. Settipane RA, Settipane GA: Nonallergic rhinitis. In *Current Review of Allergic Diseases*. Edited by Kaliner MA. Philadelphia: Current Medicine; 1999:101–110.

58. Banov C, LaForce C, Lieberman P: Double-blind trial of Astelin® nasal spray in the treatment of vasomotor rhinitis. *Ann Allergy Asthma Immunol*, in press.

59. Janssens MM-L: Levocabastine: A new topical approach for the treatment of paediatric allergic rhinoconjunctivitis. *Rhinology* 1992, 13(suppl):39–49.

60. Janssens MM-L, Vanden Bussche G: Levocabastine: an effective topical treatment of allergic rhinoconjunctivitis. *Clin Exp Allergy* 1991, 21(suppl):29–36.

61. Thomas KE, Ollier S, Ferguson H, *et al.*: The effect of intranasal azelastine, Rhinolast, on nasal airways obstruction and sneezing following provocation testing with histamine and allergen. *Clin Exp Allergy* 1992, 22:642–647.

62. Falconieri P, Monteleone AM, Mancuso T, *et al.*: Effectiveness of levocabastine eye drops in children with allergic conjunctivitis: a double-blind study. *Pediatr Asthma Allergy Immunol* 1994, 8:111–115.

63. Dechant KL, Goa KL: Levocabastine: a review of its pharmacological properties and therapeutic potential as a topical antihistamine in allergic rhinitis and conjunctivitis. *Drugs* 1991, 41:202–224.

64. Grossman J, Halverson PC, Meltzer EO, *et al.*: Double-blind assessment of azelastine in the treatment of perennial allergic rhinitis. *Ann Allergy* 1994, 73:141–146.

65. Canonica GW, Ciprandi G, Buscaglia S, *et al.*: Adhesion molecules of allergic inflammation: recent insights into their functional roles. *Allergy* 1994, 49:135–141.

66. Ciprandi G, Pronzato C, Ricca V, *et al.*: Evidence of intracellular adhesion molecule-1 expression on nasal epithelial cells in acute rhinoconjunctivitis caused by pollen exposure. *J Allergy Clin Immunol* 1994, 94:738–746.

67.• Campbell A, Chanal I, Czarlewski W, *et al.*: Reduction of soluble ICAM-1 levels in nasal secretion by H$_1$ blockers in seasonal allergic rhinitis. *Allergy* 1997, 52:1022–1025.
This study examines the ability of both loratadine and cetirizine to reduce the release of soluble ICAM-1 in nasal secretions supporting an anti-inflammatory effect of second-generation antihistamines.

68. Ciprandi G, Pronzato C, Ricca V, *et al.*: Loratadine treatment of rhinitis due to pollen allergy reduces epithelial ICAM-1 expression. *Clin Exp Allergy* 1997, 27:1175–1183.

69. Ciprandi G, Tosca M, Ricca V, *et al.*: Cetirizine treatment of rhinitis in children with pollen allergy: evidence of its antiallergic activity. *Clin Exp Allergy* 1997, 27:1160–1166.

70. Abdelaziz MM, DeValia JL, Khair OA, *et al.*: Effect of fexofenadine on eosinophil-induced changes in epithelial permeability and cytokine release from nasal epithelial cells of patients with seasonal allergic rhinitis. *J Allergy Clin Immunol* 1998, 101:410–420.

71. Lichtenstein LM, Schroeder JT, Schleimer RP, Kreutner W: Inhibition of cytokine generation and mediator release in human basophils by desloratadine. *J Allergy Clin Immunol* 2001, 107:S162.

72. Naclerio RM, Porud D, Kagey-Sobotka A, *et al.*: The effect of cetirizine on early allergic response. *Laryngoscope* 1989, 99:596–599.

73. Charlesworth EN, Massey WA, Kagey-Sobotka A, *et al.*: Effect of H$_1$ receptor blockade on the early and late response to cutaneous allergen challenge. *J Pharmacol Exp Ther* 1992, 262:964–970.

74. Pazdrak K, Gorski P, Ruta U: Inhibitory effect of levocabastine on allergen-induced increase of nasal reactivity to histamine and cell influx. *Allergy* 1993, 48:598–601.

75. Buscaglia S, Catrullo A, Ciprandi G, *et al.*: Levocabastine eye drops reduce ICAM-1 expression both in vitro and in vivo [abstract]. *Allergy* 1995, 50(suppl):79.

76. Shin MH, Baroody F, Proud D, *et al.*: The effect of azelastine on the early allergic response. *Clin Exp Allergy* 1992, 22:289–295.

77. Ciprandi G, Pronzato C, Passalacqua G, *et al.*: Topical azelastine reduces eosinophil activation and intercellular adhesion molecule-1 expression on nasal epithelial cells: an antiallergic activity. *J Allergy Clin Immunol* 1996, 98:1088–1096.

78. Busse W, Randley B, Sedgwick J, Sofia RD: The effect of azelastine on neutrophil and eosinophil generation of superoxide. *J Allergy Clin Immunol* 1989, 83:400–405.

79.• Grossman J: One airway, one disease. *Chest* 1997, 111:11S–16S.
This paper suggests that allergic rhinitis and asthma are not separate diseases but a continuum of inflammation in a common airway.

80.• Corren J, Harris AG, Aaronson D, *et al.*: Efficacy and safety of loratadine plus pseudoephedrine in patients with seasonal allergic rhinitis. *J Allergy Clin Immunol* 1997, 100:781–788.
This study demonstrates that treating allergic rhinitis with an antihistamine and decongestant can also improve symptoms of asthma, pulmonary function, and quality of life.

81. Popa VT: Bronchodilating activity of an H$_1$ blocker, chlorpheniramine. *J Allergy Clin Immunol* 1977, 59:54–63.

82. Taytard A, Beaumont D, Pujet JC, *et al.*: Treatment of bronchial asthma with terfenadine: a randomized controlled trial. *Br J Clin Pharmacol* 1987, 24:743–746.

83. Raffety P, Jackson L, Smith R, *et al.*: Terfenadine, a potent H$_1$ receptor antagonist in the treatment of grass pollen sensitive asthma. *Br J Clin Pharmacol* 1990, 30:229–235.

84. Clee MD, Ingram CG, Reid PC, *et al.*: The effect of astemizole on exercise-induced asthma. *Br J Dis Chest* 1984, 78:180–183.

85. Cistero A, Abadias M, Lieonaart R: Effect of astemizole on allergic asthma. *Ann Allergy* 1992, 69:123–127.

86. Aubier M, Neukirch C, Melac M: Effect of cetirizine on bronchial hyperresponsiveness in patients with allergic rhinitis [abstract]. *J Allergy Clin Immunol* 1996, 97:316.

87. Spector SL, Nicodemus CF, Corren J, *et al.*: Comparison of the bronchodilatory effects of cetirizine, salbuterol, and both together versus placebo in patients with mild to moderate asthma. *J Allergy Clin Immunol* 1995, 96:174–181.

88. Aaronson DW: Evaluation of cetirizine in patients with allergic rhinitis and perennial asthma. *Ann Allergy Asthma Immunol* 1996, 76:440–446.

89. Grant JA, Nicodemus CF, Findlay SR, *et al.*: Cetirizine in patients with seasonal allergic rhinitis and concomitant asthma: prospective, randomized, placebo-controlled trial. *J Allergy Clin Immunol* 1995, 95:923–932.

90. Baena-Cagnani CE: Desloratadine activity in concurrent seasonal allergic rhinitis and asthma. *Allergy* 2001, 56:21–27.

91.•• Roquet A, Dahlen B, Kumlin M, *et al.*: Combined antagonism of leukotrienes and histamine produces predominant inhibition of allergen-induced early and late phase airway obstruction in asthmatics. *Am J Resp Crit Care Med* 1997, 155:185–186.
This study examines the effects of a second-generation antihistamine, loratadine, alone and in combination with a leukotriene receptor antagonist, zafirlukast, on allergic asthma.

92. Reicin A, White R, Weinstein SE, *et al.*: Montelukast, a leukotriene receptor antagonist, in combination with loratadine, a histamine receptor antagonist, in the treatment of chronic asthma. *Arch Intern Med* 2000, 160:2481–2488.

93.•• Kay GG, Plotkin KE, Quig MB, *et al.*: Sedating effects of AM/PM antihistamine dosing with evening chlorpheniramine and morning terfenadine. *Am J Man Care* 1997, 3:1843–1848.
This study investigates and clearly demonstrates the carryover sedative effects of giving a sedating antihistamine at bedtime.

94.•• Simons FER: The eternal triangle: benefit, risk, and cost of therapeutic agents. *Ann Allergy Asthma Immunol* 1996, 77:337–338.
This editorial criticizes employing a sedating antihistamine only for the purpose of cost containment.

95. Goetz DW, Jacobson JM, Murnane JE, *et al.*: Prolongation of simple and choice reaction times in a double-blind comparison of twice daily hydroxyzine versus terfenadine. *J Allergy Clin Immunol* 1989, 84:316–322.

96. Seidel WF, Cohem S, Bliwise NG, *et al.*: Direct measurement of daytime sleepiness after administration of cetirizine and hydroxyzine with a standardized electroencephalographic assessment. *J Allergy Clin Immunol* 1990, 86:1029–1033.

97. Seidel WF, Cohen S, Bliwise NG, *et al.*: Cetirizine effects on objective measures of daytime sleepiness and performance. *Ann Allergy* 1987, 59:58–62.

98. Goetz DW, Jacobson JM, Apaliski SJ, *et al.*: Objective antihistamine side effects are mitigated by evening dosing of hydroxyzine. *Ann Allergy* 1991, 67:448–454.

99. Bantz EW, Dolan WK, Chadwick EW, *et al.*: Chronic chlorpheniramine therapy: subsensitivity, drug metabolism and compliance. *Ann Allergy* 1987, 59:341–346.

100. The Task Force on Allergic Disorders. Overview of allergic diseases: diagnosis, management, and barriers to care. Milwaukee, WI: American Academy of Allergy, Asthma & Immunology, Inc.; 2000: The Allergy Report; vol.1.

CHAPTER 15

Correlating Rhinitis with Its Treatment

Phillip Lieberman

Since their introduction into clinical use during the 1940s, antihistamines have become the mainstay of pharmacologic therapy for allergic rhinitis. Further refinement of this class of drugs has improved their selectivity for the histamine H_1 receptor and reduced their penetration into the central nervous system (CNS), minimizing many of the side effects that previously limited their use. These benefits have been further enhanced by the recent development of topical antihistamines, the intranasal delivery of which increases local drug concentration and limits systemic distribution, optimizing the efficacy of antihistamines and diminishing their deleterious adverse effects.

ROLE OF HISTAMINE IN ALLERGIC AND NONALLERGIC RHINITIS

The sixth most prevalent chronic condition seen in the outpatient practice of medicine, rhinitis refers to an inflammation of the nasal membranes that manifests as one or more of the following symptoms: rhinorrhea, nasal congestion, nasal itching, postnasal drip, and sneezing [1]. Rhinitis may be either allergic, nonallergic, or mixed. Approximately 40 million people in the United States suffer from the allergic form of rhinitis, which can be provoked by either seasonal or perennial allergens. The National Rhinitis Classification Task Force estimates that roughly 17 million people have chronic nonallergic rhinitis, a heterogeneous group of conditions characterized by similar nasal symptoms without an allergic etiology (negative allergy skin tests and normal serum IgE levels) [2•,3]. Ongoing studies indicate extensive overlap between these two populations, since a considerably larger proportion (at least 34%) of rhinitis patients than was previously realized have mixed rhinitis, a condition that encompasses both allergic and nonallergic components [2•,4].

Allergic rhinitis is a prototypical IgE-mediated disease, manifesting as a biphasic response to allergen inhalation. Symptoms develop within minutes of re-exposure to allergen, after resident mast cells in the nasal mucosa degranulate and release mediators when their surface IgE molecules become crosslinked by bound allergen molecules [5••]. The immediate appearance of acute symptoms that abate within 1 hour is referred to as the early phase reaction (EPR). Approximately half of rhinitis patients also experience a late phase reaction (LPR) in the ensuing 4–8 hours, when the influx of inflammatory cells (eosinophils, basophils, neutrophils, and lymphocytes) to the nasal mucosa causes a recurrence of symptoms, particularly congestion.

While numerous mediators (*eg*, tryptase, leukotrienes, kinins, and prostaglandins) have been detected in the nasal secretions of allergic rhinitis patients, histamine is the most important mediator released from both mast cells and basophils during the EPR and probably plays a prominent role in the LPR as well. Intranasal challenge with histamine reproduces the clinical features of acute allergic rhinitis (Fig. 15-1) [6,7]. Reflex and secretory responses are elicited by histamine binding to H$_1$ receptors located on sensory nerve endings (causing itching and sneezing), on nerves innervating the mucous glands (causing reflex cholinergic stimulation that results in rhinorrhea), and on capacitance vessels in the nose (causing vasodilation and vascular permeability that result in congestion and rhinorrhea) [5••,6–8]. Itching and sneezing may begin as early as 20–30 seconds after allergen exposure, followed closely by increased nasal secretion and then by mucosal swelling, which usually develops within the first 5 minutes of exposure [7–9].

Nonallergic rhinitis (NAR) is an umbrella term for a diverse group of syndromes united by their common symptomatology and negative skin tests. Rather than being elicited by an IgE-mediated reaction, the different NAR syndromes are provoked by a variety of environmental changes such as weather fronts, strong odors, and respiratory irritants including ozone and cigarette smoke [2•,6]. The most prevalent NAR conditions are vasomotor rhinitis (61% of NAR patients), nonallergic rhinitis–eosinophilia syndrome (NARES, 15%–33% of NAR patients), and NAR associated with sinusitis (13%–16% of NAR patients) [2,6,10••]. Less common types of NAR include drug-induced rhinitis (rhinitis medicamentosa), endocrine-induced rhinitis, occupa-tional rhinitis, gustatory rhinitis, and skier's/jogger's nose. Both gustatory rhinitis and skier's/jogger's nose are forms of cholinergic rhinitis characterized by the sudden onset of a profuse, watery rhinorrhea, induced by eating or exposure to cold, dry air. Histamine may play a role in some types of NAR, since the number of mast cells in patients with certain NAR syndromes, such as vasomotor rhinitis, is comparable to that found in patients with allergic rhinitis, and nonimmunologic stimuli such as cold can trigger mast cell degranulation [9,11].

HISTAMINE AND ITS ANTAGONISM

The latter half of the 19th century and the first half of the 20th century were seminal periods in the history of allergy [7,12]. Mast cells were first described in 1863 as being the source of mediators of anaphylaxis and were subsequently characterized by Paul Ehrlich in 1879 [12]. Approximately 20 years later, Ehrlich introduced the receptor theory of immunity, the acceptance of which was delayed for another 25 years. Meanwhile, histamine was identified by Sir Henry Dale in 1907 [13••]. Another 30 years would elapse before the first antihistamines were synthesized by Staub and Bovet, in an effort to counteract the physiological effects of hist-amine [13••,14•]. Although the toxicity of the first antihistamines precluded their clinical use, several anti-histamines, including diphenhydramine, were intro-duced as treatments for allergic disorders during the 1940s [15].

There are 3 different families of histamine receptors, referred to as H$_1$, H$_2$, and H$_3$ [14•]. Both H$_1$ and H$_2$ receptors belong to the large family of G-protein cou-

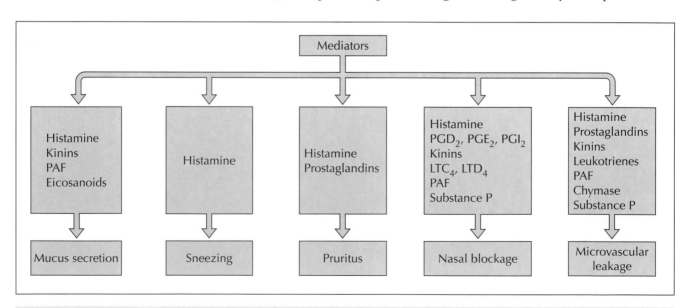

FIGURE 15-1.
Mediators of rhinitis and their effects.

pled receptors involved in cell signal transduction [14•]. Stimulation of the H_1 receptor produces many of the symptoms of rhinitis and asthma including smooth-muscle contraction, increased vascular permeability, increased mucus production, and activation of sensory nerves that cause itching and sneezing. Stimulation of histamine H_2 receptors causes gastric acid secretion and some vascular dilation. Although the H_2 receptor is essentially nonfunctioning in the nose, its role in the gastrointestinal tract has been the focus of numerous anti-ulcer H_2 antihistaminic drugs (eg, cimetidine, ranitidine) [14•]. Even though the H_1 and H_2 receptors have not been purified, cloning and characterization of their respective genes has revealed only faint similarity between them [16]. Instead, the H_1 receptor appears to more closely resemble the family of muscarinic acetylcholine receptors, another type of G-protein coupled receptor [16]. The third histamine receptor, H_3, which was discovered more recently, appears to be localized exclusively to nerve endings in the brain where it has an autoregulatory role in histamine secretion [11,14•].

Antihistamines that effectively reduce the symptoms of rhinitis are competitive antagonists of the histamine H_1-receptor. By occupying H_1-receptor sites on effector cells without activating the cells, antihistamines block H_1-receptor binding and activation by histamine [6,13••,15]. Some of the newer antihistamines, such as the topical agent azelastine, also exhibit noncompetitive inhibition of the receptor, although in some instances noncompetitive inhibition may only occur at high drug concentrations that exceed those achieved physiologically, as in the case of loratadine [11]. A recent notion that may dramatically change the way antihistamines are perceived to function is that of constitutive signaling of G-protein coupled receptors, whereby continual activation of the H_1-receptor is believed to be down-regulated, rather than blocked, by antihistamines [17]. While the clinical implications of constitutive receptor activity have not been clarified as yet, recent studies have reclassified several H_1-receptor antagonists (eg, cetirizine, loratadine) as inverse agonists, as a consequence of their ability to stabilize the inactive conformation of the H_1-receptor [17].

Structurally, antihistamines closely resemble histamine, since both contain nitrogenous bases with an aliphatic side chain that includes a core ethylamine group (see Fig. 15-2), structures also present in anticholinergic and local anesthetic agents [14•]. It is this core ethylamine moiety that confers the blocking capacity of H_1-receptor antagonists, while the aliphatic side chain that adjoins the core determines the unique absorption, distribution, elimination, and other pharmacokinetic properties of each antihistamine [18]. Among the classic first-generation antihistamines, core amine-group hydrogens are frequently substituted by methyl groups, as in the case of chlorpheniramine and diphenhydramine. Additionally, due to their relatively small size and the presence of several aromatic rings, first-generation antihistamines are lipophilic molecules that readily cross the blood-brain barrier.

First-generation antihistamines can be subdivided into six structural classes, based on the substitution of their aliphatic side chain (see Table 15-1) [6]. Among the antihistamine classes most suited for treating allergic rhinitis, the alkylamines (eg, chlorpheniramine) are used frequently because they cause less sedation, and they are often combined with decongestants. The ethanolamines (eg, diphenhydramine, clemastine) and most of the other classes are strongly sedating. Four second-generation antihistamines, introduced since the 1980s, are available in the United States for use in patients with rhinitis. These include the oral agents cetirizine, loratadine, fexofenadine, and the topical agent azelastine. As a group, the second-generation antihistamines are less lipophilic and have considerably larger molecules than the first-generation agents, reducing their sedative and cholinergic actions. Most second-generation antihistamines also can be classified into one of the six standard classes, particularly fexofenadine and cetirizine, which are metabolic products of terfenadine and hydroxyzine, respectively. Other second-generation antihistamines, including the phthalazinone derivative azelastine, are structurally unique [19].

Intranasal sprays containing combinations of an antihistamine and a decongestant were originally introduced into the clinic during the 1950s; however, their use was short-lived because they were no more effective than decongestants alone. There has been a resurgence of interest in topical antihistamines, in an effort to avoid the sedative and anticholinergic side effects of these drugs. While chlorpheniramine has been applied topically and can reduce the itching, sneezing, and secretions that follow histamine challenge, the effectiveness of topical antihistamines awaited the development of more potent agents. For example, azelastine is a second-generation topical antihistamine with a potency approximately 10-fold higher than chlorpheniramine [20]. Although use of the oral formulation of azelastine in asthma and rhinitis was associated with some sedation, subsequent trials of the intranasal spray demonstrated its efficacy in both allergic and nonallergic rhinitis, with minimal sedation [19–21].

CLINICAL CHARACTERISTICS OF ANTIHISTAMINES
The unique pharmacokinetic and pharmacodynamic profiles of each antihistamine influence its clinical utility. For example, all of the second-generation antihistamines have a rapid onset of action that allows them to be taken as needed, and all are eliminated within 24

hours. Within this range, there is extensive variation between the different agents, depending upon the structure of their side chains. The onset of action can vary from 15–30 minutes for topical azelastine to 1–3 hours for oral loratadine (see Table 15-2) [22]. Peak plasma concentrations (C_{max}) are generally attained within 1–3 hours of oral administration, cetirizine being the most rapidly absorbed (0.5 hours) and azelastine being absorbed more slowly (5 hours), with the C_{max} of most first-generation antihistamines occurring somewhere in between. However, since most antihistamines remain present in tissues after they cease being detectable in the serum and some antihistamines have an active metabolite with a longer half-life, their therapeutic effects can extend beyond their serum levels of detectability [10••]. This is particularly evident in the skin, where peak suppression of histamine-induced wheal and flare by antihistamines occurs several hours (5–8 hours after oral administration) after the C_{max}, and persists for several additional hours

after serum drug levels have declined to their lowest limits of detection. The clinical efficacy of a particular antihistamine in rhinitis parallels its cutaneous effect on the size of the wheal, which reflects its ability to decrease vascular permeability and leakage of plasma protein [10••]. In contrast, topical azelastine does not suppress the histamine-induced wheal and flare, suggesting minimal systemic absorption [23]. The clinical implications of the delay in reaching maximal tissue levels relative to peak serum concentrations suggest that antihistamines are optimally effective when administered before exposure to allergen, rather than when used as rescue medications [10••]. Prophylactic use of antihistamines prior to allergen exposure also facilitates effective blocking of H_1-receptor sites before histamine release [24].

Most antihistamines are metabolized by the liver via the cytochrome P_{450} CYP3A4 system, including all first-generation and most second-generation agents [6]. As a result, antihistamine half-life is prolonged in patients

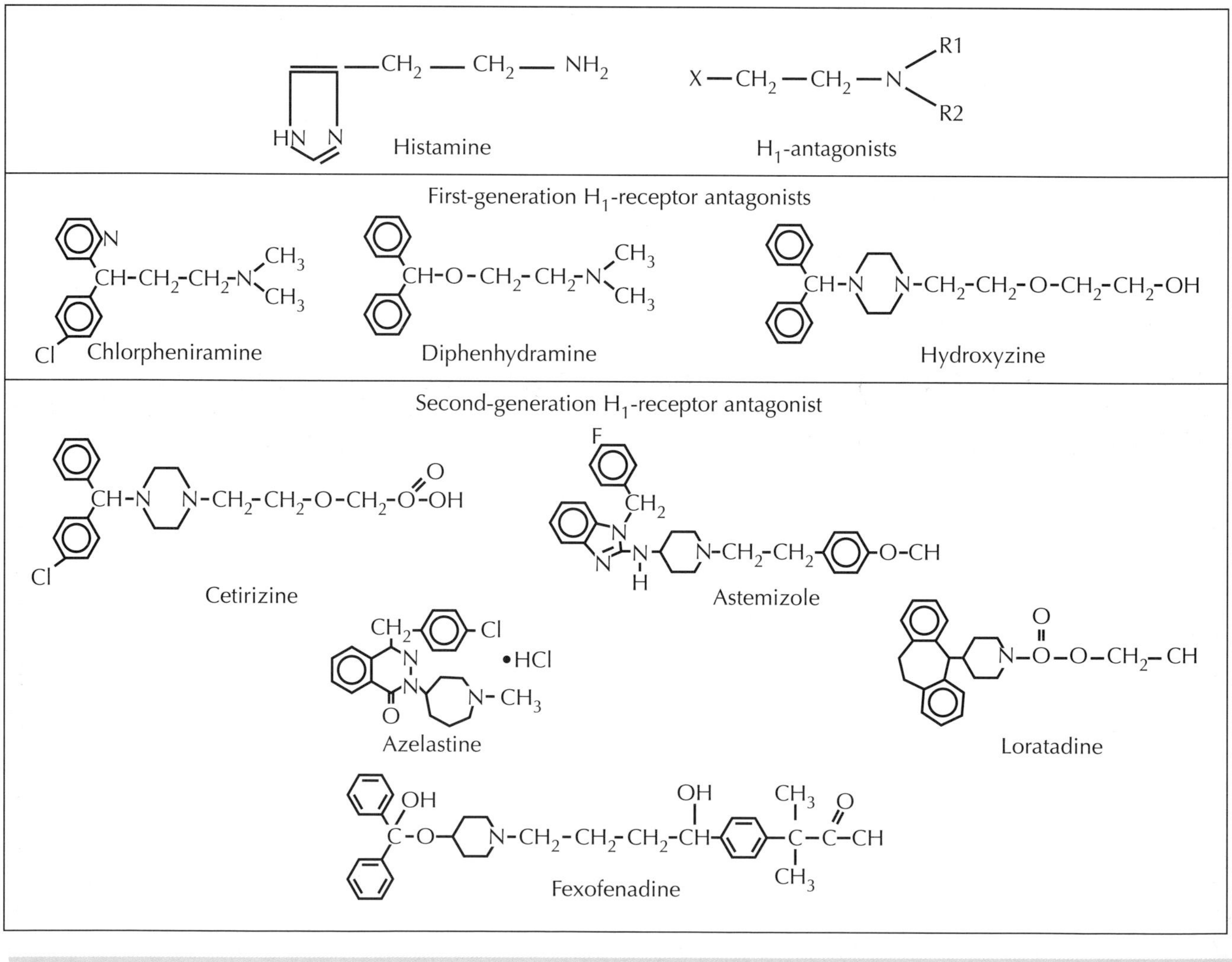

FIGURE 15-2.
Chemical structure of antihistamines.

with hepatic dysfunction and in those taking other drugs that interfere with the cytochrome P_{450} CYP3A4 system, such as macrolide antibiotics or imidazole antifungals [23]. The two exceptions are cetirizine, which is excreted via the kidney, and fexofenadine, which is found unmetabolized in the feces and urine. Thus, dosages of cetirizine and fexofenadine should be lowered in the presence of renal disease, and the dosage of most other antihistamines should be lowered in patients with hepatic dysfunction [10••]. Azelastine is unusual in that despite its metabolism by the P_{450} system, its elimination is not altered in patients with hepatic dysfunction, although renal elimination is slightly lower in those with renal impairment [20]. Another feature unique to azelastine is its systemic bioavailability, which is 40% after intranasal administration.

Clearance rates and terminal elimination half-life values differ for each antihistamine depending upon the structure of the side chain, the terminal elimination half-life ranging from 6.5 to 10 hours for cetirizine to 22 hours for azelastine. Fexofenadine, loratadine, and the first-generation agent diphenhydramine have relatively short half-lives whereas the half-life of azelastine more closely resembles those of the first-generation agents chlorpheniramine and hydroxyzine.

Together, the pharmacokinetic and pharmacodynamic properties help determine the dosage and frequency of administration for each antihistamine, as well as the need for adjustment in special populations. Whereas the first-generation antihistamines generally reach their peak plasma concentrations in 4–6 hours, several sustained-release formulations are available that extend the duration of action to 12 hours. Agents such as chlorpheniramine cause minimal sedation and may be less expensive than second-generation agents, have a rapid onset of action, and may provide additional beneficial anticholinergic drying properties. These factors are important in selecting the appropriate agent for each patient.

TABLE 15-1. CLASSIFICATION OF FIRST- AND SECOND-GENERATION ANTIHISTAMINES

Chemical class	Examples
Ethanolamine	Diphenhydramine
	Clemastine
Alkylamine	Chlorpheniramine
Ethylenediamines	Tripelennamine
	Pyrilamine
Piperazines	Hydroxyzine
	Meclizine
	Cetirizine
Piperadines	Cyproheptadine
	Azatadine
	Loratadine
Phenothiazines	Promethazine
	Trimeprazine
Miscellaneous	
Phthalazinone	Azelastine

TABLE 15-2. PHARMACOKINETIC AND PHARMACODYNAMIC PROPERTIES OF ANTIHISTAMINES

Antihistamine	Time to C_{max}, t_{max}, hr	Terminal half-life, $t_{1/2\beta}$, hr	Wheal ↓ activity, hr	Sedative potential	Time to onset, hr	Route of Metabolism	Population needing dose adjustment	Drug interaction with P450 CYP
First-generation								
Diphenhydramine	.75–2.5	8–9	6–10	Yes		Liver		
Chlorpheniramine	1.5–2.5	20–24	24	Moderate		Liver		
Hydroxyzine	1–2.5	20	36	Yes		Liver		
Brompheniramine	2–3	24	9	Moderate		Liver		
Oral second-generation								
Loratadine	1.2	7.8–11	24	None	1–3	Liver	Hepatic/renal dysfunction	Unlikely
Cetirizine	1	6.5–10	≥ 24	Reduced	.5–1	Kidney	Hepatic/renal dysfunction/ geriatric	Unlikely
Fexofenadine	2.6	11–15	24	None	2	Unmetabolized	Renal dysfunction	Unlikely
Topical second-generation								
Azelastine	2.5	22		Reduced	2–3	Liver		

Caution must be used in oversimplifying the choice of antihistamine, because several additional factors also must be taken into consideration. H_1 antagonists have significantly different side effect profiles, and these vary with the delivery route. More importantly, many of the second-generation antihistamines have additional anti-inflammatory activities that dramatically improve their effectiveness in reducing the symptoms of rhinitis.

ANTI-INFLAMMATORY PROPERTIES

Azatadine, a first-generation antihistamine, was the first agent shown to possess anti-inflammatory activities. These included reducing leukotriene (LT) C_4 production and inhibiting the elevations in histamine and kinin levels following nasal allergen challenge [14•]. The spectrum of anti-inflammatory properties in the oral second-generation antihistamines is far more extensive, although it varies with the specific agent. The ability to not only antagonize histamine binding but to block its production or release from mast cells or basophils would confer obvious clinical advantages on an antihistamine. Several of the second-generation antihistamines, including cetirizine, loratadine, and azelastine, have some of these abilities. Loratadine has been shown to inhibit histamine release from basophils, as well as the production of LTC_4 and histamine from human lung mast cells after either IgE-mediated or non–IgE-mediated stimulation [14•,26]. Loratadine also is able to alter cellular levels of calcium, which is integral to the mediator release process, by inhibiting both the influx of extracellular calcium and the release of calcium from intracellular storage sites. However, some of these effects are only achieved at concentrations that vastly exceed those achievable in vivo, rendering their clinical relevance uncertain [27]. More poignant are the anti-inflammatory effects of loratadine that have been observed after treatment of patients with allergic rhinitis. In parallel with significant reductions in nasal symptoms, loratadine has been shown to abrogate histamine release from basophils, attenuate the influx of eosinophils and metachromatic cells, decrease levels of mediators of inflammation (eosinophil cationic protein [ECP], prostaglandin D_2, and histamine) in nasal secretions, and diminish both soluble ICAM-1 levels and ICAM-1 expression on nasal epithelial cells [14•,25,27]. Allergic inflammation is characterized by the enhanced endothelial/epithelial expression of adhesion molecules, such as ICAM-1, leading to the migration of inflammatory cells into the nasal mucosa [7,28]. The ability of an antihistamine to diminish the expression of adhesion molecules undoubtedly has widespread impact on its anti-inflammatory properties.

Cetirizine is also notable for its extensive anti-inflammatory activities. Cetirizine's ability to reduce ICAM-1 expression on epithelial cells likely facilitates its capacity to prevent the migration of inflammatory cells (eg, eosinophils, neutrophils, and metachromatic cells) into the nasal mucosa and to diminish the presence of nasal inflammatory mediators (eg, LTC_4, ECP), activities that have been demonstrated both in vitro and in patients with allergic rhinitis [11,14•,18,29]. Cetirizine also has been shown to inhibit histamine release from basophils, to prevent LTB_4 production, and to reduce the migration of monocytes and T-lymphocytes that have been stimulated by IgE-independent agents [14•,24,25]. Although cetirizine is unable to inhibit mast cell activation and the resultant levels of histamine, it inhibits the pathophysiologic consequences of the released histamine. Many of the effects of cetirizine have been demonstrated in atopic clinical situations. However, it is unclear whether the anti-inflammatory properties of cetirizine extend its clinical effectiveness to the NAR population.

Fexofenadine is the most recent second-generation antihistamine to become available, and has been the subject of fewer studies than the other antihistamines. Investigations of the anti-inflammatory effects of fexofenadine are restricted to cell culture and have not yet been conducted in allergic or nonallergic rhinitis patients [30–32]. In in vitro analyses, fexofenadine has been shown to inhibit the release of inflammatory mediators (eg, histamine and LTC_4) from human basophils and mast cells [30–33]. In epithelial cells derived from nasal biopsy specimens of patients with allergic rhinitis, fexofenadine decreased eosinophil chemotaxis and adherence to endothelial cells, due to the fexofenadine-induced reduction of soluble ICAM-1 and cytokine levels (eg, GM-CSF, IL-8, and regulated upon activation, normal T-cell expressed and secreted [RANTES]) [14•,34].

Numerous anti-inflammatory activities have been demonstrated for the topical agent azelastine, some of which also have been demonstrated for the oral second-generation antihistamines and some of which are unique to azelastine. Azelastine's ability to antagonize the H_1 receptor is complemented by its ability to inhibit the release of histamine from mast cells and basophils induced by a variety of allergic and nonallergic secretagogues, an activity that is more potent in azelastine than in other antihistamines and that is likely facilitated by its inhibitory effect on cellular degranulation and its interference with calcium influx [14•,25,35]. Perhaps the most illustrative clinical example of the mast cell stabilizing activity of azelastine is its ability to prevent the release of clinically significant levels of histamine in response to high blood acetaldehyde concentrations after consumption of ethanol by individuals who have alcohol-induced bronchial asthma [36].

Several studies have demonstrated the inhibitory effects of azelastine on the IgE-mediated and non-IgE-mediated synthesis of LTC$_4$ by virtue of its interference with a key enzyme in arachidonic acid metabolism, 5-lipoxygenase [20]. In vivo azelastine has been shown to diminish the synthesis of multiple inflammatory mediators after allergen challenge. These include leukotrienes, kinins, ECP, TAME-esterase activity, and the neurokinins substance P and vasointestinal peptide [14•,20].

Some of the anti-inflammatory properties of azelastine stem from its ability to inhibit the activation and activity of cells involved in the inflammatory response. Some of these effects have been identified in human cells in vitro, including mast cells, basophils, eosinophils, and T-lymphocytes. Azelastine also inhibits the influx of neutrophils and eosinophils in vivo during the EPR and LPR in patients with allergic rhinitis, and diminishes eosinophil activation [14•,20,25].

Due to its ability to interrupt a variety of intracellular processes, azelastine has been shown to exert many of the same anti-inflammatory properties that have been observed with glucocorticosteroids. This includes reducing the in vitro synthesis of several cytokines (IL-2, IL-3, IL-4, IL-5, IL-6, and GM-CSF) as a consequence of its inhibition of cytokine transcription [14•]. Azelastine also interferes with tyrosine phosphorylation, a ubiquitous process that mediates numerous cellular functions via signal transduction, inhibits the generation of superoxide free radicals, prevents activation of protein kinase C, and decreases the expression of various oncogenes, including c-myc [19]. One of the most important functions of azelastine is its ability to diminish expression of the transcriptional activator nuclear factor NF5-β, which can depress or activate genes and thereby initiate the synthesis of new proteins, including adhesion molecules, in a manner similar to steroids [19,37].

SIDE EFFECT PROFILES OF ANTIHISTAMINES

Side effects of the different antihistamines vary considerably and are most pronounced in the first-generation agents. These agents can induce dopaminergic, serotonergic, and cholinergic responses that manifest as four types of adverse reactions (stimulatory, neuropsychiatric, peripheral neurologic, and depressive) as a consequence of their ability to cross the blood-brain barrier and their lack of selectivity for the H$_1$-receptor site [14•]. Side effects are most pronounced in the elderly. Stimulatory reactions due to antiserotonin activities can include increased appetite with weight gain. Peripheral neurologic effects result from muscarinic cholinergic blockage, and range from dilated pupils and blurred vision to dry mouth, urinary retention, constipation, and impotence [6]. Depressive reactions manifest as sedation, drowsiness, and impaired alertness and cognition, particularly impairment of the ability to drive and

operate machinery [6,24,39]. The individual may not be aware of having reduced cognitive ability, since it can occur independently of sedation [6,24,38–40].

By comparison, second-generation oral antihistamines show markedly improved side effect profiles. Since most show greater affinity for peripheral H$_1$ receptors, they exert few cholinergic, serotonergic, or dopaminergic effects [6,24]. However, as mentioned, some first- and second-generation antihistamines, especially those metabolized by the hepatic cytochrome P$_{450}$ CYP3A4 enzyme system, may interact with other medications that inhibit biotransformation by this enzyme system. Two second-generation antihistamines that are metabolized minimally by the liver are cetirizine and fexofenadine, although cetirizine metabolism can be prolonged in patients with renal impairment. Cetirizine is also reported to cause minimal sedation, in contrast to loratadine and fexofenadine, which have sedative effects comparable to placebo [6,13••,38–42]. Azelastine also causes some sedation when taken orally, although this is reduced after topical delivery [13••,19]. Additionally, bioavailability appears to obviate the need for dose adjustment of azelastine, despite its metabolism by the liver. Azelastine can cause a bitter taste in some individuals [6,19].

The absence of sedative effects in antihistamines is particularly critical for children, since rhinitis itself can impair cognition [6,13••,43]. As demonstrated in a recent study comparing the first-generation agent diphenhydramine with the nonsedating second-generation agent loratadine and placebo in 52 primary schoool children with allergic rhinitis, and a group of age-matched nonatopic controls, cognition in all the atopic children was considerably poorer than in their nonatopic peers [44]. Rhinitic children who were treated with loratadine or placebo performed considerably better than those treated with diphenhydramine, indicating that rhinitis itself can impair cognition, and this effect can be exacerbated by sedating antihistamines [14•,45••].

Large doses of some of the first-generation antihistamines, such as diphenhydramine, also are reported to cause polymorphic ventricular tachycardia or torsades de pointes. Populations that require caution are those taking more than one antihistamine, patients with hypertension who require a diuretic, patients with hypokalemia or hypomagnesemia, and patients taking antiarrhythmic agents [46,50]. While it is not possible to predict which individuals will develop cardiotoxic complications, symptoms of antihistamine-associated arrhythmias induced by QT prolongation include dizziness, lightheadedness, palpitations, and irregular heartbeat. These can be detected by electrocardiogram, which can reveal the presence of a prolonged QT$_c$ interval, a precursor for the development of torsades de pointes in most patients [51,52]. Cardiotoxicity has not

PATIENT RHINITIS SCREEN

This form will help determine the kind of rhinitis you have.
Please check the box next to your symptoms.

Date: _____

Patient Name: _____

Patient Age: _____

Age when you first started having symptoms? _____
When do you have symptoms?

What symptoms do you have?	All year?	Spring	Summer	Fall	Winter
Sneezing					
Stuffy nose/congestion					
Runny nose					
Postnasal drainage					
Itchy eyes/itchy nose					

What medication(s) do you take for your symptoms? _____

Are your symptoms: ☐ completely controlled?   ☐ somewhat controlled?   ☐ uncontrolled?

Patient: Please check all the things you think make your symptoms worse:

Allergens		**Inhaled/Strong Odor Triggers**
Freshly mowed grass		Smoke (tobacco/burning items)
Dead grass		Perfumes/colognes/fragrances
Hay		Cosmetics
Dead leaves		Cleaning products/detergents/soaps
Pollen		Paint fumes or paint products
Trees/tree pollen		Hairspray
Weeds (ragweed)		Outside dust
Molds		Exhaust (cars, trucks, buses)
House dust		Gasoline fumes
Cats/cat hair		
Dogs/dog hair		**Weather Change Triggers**
Feathers		Windy days
		Cold days
		Damp days
		Humidity/temperature changes
		Ingestant Triggers
		Alcoholic beverages (beer, wine)
		Spicy foods
TOTAL		TOTAL

Consider Allergic Rhinitis if ONLY boxes on this side are checked.

Consider Vasomotor (Nonallergic) Rhinitis* if ONLY boxes on this side are checked.

Consider Coexisting Disease if boxes on BOTH sides are checked.

FIGURE 15-3.
Rhinitis patient screening tool. *Vasomotor rhinitis is the major type of nonallergic rhinitis. Other types of nonallergic rhinitis include: infectious, hormonal-, exercise-, drug-, or reflex-induced etiologies, NARES and ciliary dyskinesia syndromes, and atrophic rhinitis. (*Adapted from* Dykewicz et al. [6].)

been reported after the use of loratadine, cetirizine, or azelastine [19,47–49].

SELECTING THE APPROPRIATE ANTIHISTAMINE

First- and second-generation antihistamines are equally effective against the symptoms of sneezing, itching, and rhinorrhea, and many also relieve conjunctival symptoms, although most antihistamines are comparatively ineffective against congestion [6,11,13••]. As a result, they are often combined with oral decongestants, usually pseudoephedrine. What distinguishes antihistamines is their profile of side effects and their unique pharmacokinetic properties [53]. Some second-generation H_1 antagonists also possess additional anti-inflammatory properties that render them more potent, such as cetirizine, and capable of relieving congestion and postnasal drip, as is the case with azelastine. Thus, numerous factors must be considered when selecting the appropriate antihistamine for a patient, including their particular spectrum of symptoms.

Two different approaches can be taken to selecting the appropriate agent. The first approach requires a definitive diagnosis that distinguishes between allergic, nonallergic, and mixed rhinitis, and selection of treatment based on this determination. A definitive diagnosis is extremely important because treatment of allergic rhinitis is a 3-pronged approached that emphasizes

environmental control—the identification and removal of allergens—as the most important step. When prophylactic removal of allergens is impossible or incomplete, pharmacotherapy and immunotherapy play more prominent roles [6,54]. In the primary care setting, use of the Rhinitis Screening Tool (Fig. 15-3) can be helpful in establishing a definitive diagnosis based on symptomatology, without the use of ancillary tests [4]. The patient questionnaire identifies rhinitis triggers and their patterns of appearance, categorizing them as being either allergic or nonallergic in origin. The presence of allergic triggers is indicative of allergic rhinitis, while the presence of three or more nonallergic triggers is indicative of nonallergic rhinitis, and triggers from both categories is indicative of mixed rhinitis.

Another approach that is commonly taken in the primary care setting is empiric treatment based on symptoms. Although this approach is more vague, the choice of a second-generation agent with broader effects, including additional anti-inflammatory properties, can ensure that the entire range of symptoms will be addressed with minimal sedation. The ideal therapeutic agent for managing seasonal allergic rhinitis has been described as one that effectively addresses the pathophysiology of both the EPR and the LPR; that antagonizes histamine at the H_1 receptor of effector cells; that relieves nasal pruritus, sneezing, rhinorrhea, and nasal congestion; that is fast-acting with first-dose effective-

TABLE 15-3. DOSAGE AND ADMINISTRATION OF SELECTED ANTIHISTAMINES

Generic name	Trade name	Dosage
Diphenhydramine HCL	Benadryl*	Adults: 25–50 mg tid Children: 6–11 y: 5 mg/kg/d
Chlorpheniramine maleate	Chlor-Trimeton†	Adults: 8–12 mg bid Children: 6–11 y: 0.35 mg/kg/d 2–5 y: 1.25 mg bid/tid
Hydroxyzine HCL	Atarax‡	Adults: 25–50 mg bid Children: 2 mg/kg/d
Loratadine	Claritin†	Adults: 10 mg qd Children: 6–11 y: 10 mg qd
Cetirizine HCL	Zyrtec‡	Adults: 5–10 mg qd Children: 6–11 y: 5–10 mg qd 2–5 y: 5 mg qd
Fexofenadine	Allegra§	Adults: 60 mg bid or 180 mg qd
Azelastine	Astelin¶	Adults: 2 sprays/nostril bid (0.1% solution) Children: 5–11 y: 1 spray/nostril bid

*Warner-Lambert, Morris Plains, NJ.
†Schering, Kenilworth, NJ.
‡Pfizer, New York, NY.
§Aventis Pharmaceuticals, Parsippany, NJ.
¶Wallace Laboratories, Cranbury, NJ.

ness; that has a dosing schedule of once or twice daily; that has a favorable side effect profile; and that is delivered directly to the nasal mucosa to concentrate the drug and minimize systemic effects [55]. Azelastine conforms to many of these specifications and is considered first-line treatment for nonallergic vasomotor and seasonal allergic rhinitis, due to its potency, rapid onset of action, low side effect profile, and its ability to relieve many of the symptoms of rhinitis including nasal congestion, rhinorrhea, sneezing, itching, conjunctivitis, and postnasal drainage [2,6,19,20]. Azelastine produces significant reductions in nasal resistance and increases in nasal peak flow. It also has been approved for use in vasomotor rhinitis and in the pediatric population for seasonal allergic rhinitis. In nonallergic vasomotor rhinitis patients, azelastine treatment was associated with significant decreases in mean total symptom scores, with 82%–85% of patients reporting significant improvement [2,6].

Some patients may prefer an oral formulation to intranasal delivery. In this case, loratadine, fexofenadine, or cetirizine would be appropriate choices for mild-to-moderate allergic rhinitis [22,56,57]. Of these choices only loratadine and fexofenadine are classified as nonsedating by the Food and Drug Administration and, therefore, their use may be mandatory in certain situations (eg, airline pilots). Although corticosteroids are considered first-line treatment for severe allergic rhinitis, they do not relieve conjunctival symptoms, their onset of action can be delayed for up to 2 weeks, and they can slow bone growth during the first year of therapy, a side effect of concern in the pediatric population [6,13••,22].

A recent survey revealed that a total of $2.4 billion was spent annually on medications for allergic rhinitis in the United States. In the interest of saving money, some practitioners combine first- and second-generation agents, prescribing the first-generation agent at bedtime and the second-generation agent in the morning, in the mistaken belief that this regimen will minimize sedation. However, even when first-generation antihistamines are only dosed at bedtime they can cause daytime sedation in some individuals, and consequently this approach has been questioned [6,43].

Another important clinical consideration is the presence of concomitant asthma, since asthma and rhinitis have a high incidence of comorbidity, particularly in the pediatric population [58,59]. This link between disorders of the upper and lower airways is more common in atopic individuals, as up to 38% of patients with allergic rhinitis have coexisting asthma compared to a prevalence of 3%–5% for asthma in the general population [60]. Rhinitis is considered to be a risk factor for developing asthma, and treating rhinitis can improve asthma outcomes. Treatment of rhinitis in patients with coex-

isting asthma improves both conditions when they are mild to moderate in severity [5••,6]. Treatment of rhinitis patients with cetirizine, loratadine, and azelastine significantly lowers total asthma symptom scores.

CONCLUSIONS

Whereas all antihistamines act as competitive antagonists of the H_1 receptor, the newer second-generation agents exhibit fewer side effects and most have additional anti-inflammatory activities that render them of greater benefit to patients with rhinitis. The development of potent topical agents that exert even fewer systemic effects provides more treatment options, expanding the breadth of effectiveness to patients with NAR. Ideally, the appropriate treatment will be selected after determining a definitive diagnosis of the type of rhinitis present, since allergic rhinitis is best treated by eliminating identified triggers from the environment. In the primary care setting, azelastine is considered first-line treatment for both nonallergic vasomotor and seasonal allergic rhinitis.

REFERENCES AND RECOMMENDED READING
Papers of particular interest, published recently, have been highlighted as:
- Of importance
- •• Of major importance

1. Urval KR: Overview of diagnosis and management of allergic rhinitis. *Prim Care* 1998, 25:649–662.
2.• Settipane R, Lieberman PL: Update on nonallergic rhinitis. *Ann Allergy Asthma Immunol* 2001, 86:494-507.
Excellent review of the types of nonallergic rhinitis, their epidemiology, and how to distinguish between them. Includes detailed description of management options for many types of nonallergic rhinitis.
3. Settipane R: The broad spectrum of rhinitis: etiology, diagnosis, and advances in treatment. Data presented at: National Allergy Advisory Council Meeting; October 16, 1999; St. Thomas, US Virgin Islands.
4. Use of a New Screening Tool to Aid in the Differential Diagnosis of Allergic, Nonallergic, and Mixed Rhinitis. Data on file at Wallace Laboratories, Cranbury, NJ.
5.•• Togias A: Unique mechanistic features of allergic rhinitis. *J Allergy Clin Immunol* 2000, 105:S599–S604.
The paper reviews the pathophysiologic process of allergic rhinitis. It describes the inflammatory cells and mediators that orchestrate the development of nasal hyperreactivity, and the role of the mast cell.
6. Dykewicz MS, Fineman S: Diagnosis and management of rhinitis: complete guidelines of the Joint Task Force on Practice Parameters in Allergy, Asthma, and Immunology. *Ann Allergy Asthma Immunol* 1998, 81:478–518.
7. Bachert C: Histamine: a major role in allergy? *Clin Exp Allergy* 1998, 28:15–19.
8. Naclerio RM, Baroody F: Understanding the inflammatory processes in upper allergic airway disease and asthma. *J Allergy Clin Immunol* 1998, 101:S345–351.
9. Hurwitz ME: Treatment of allergic rhinitis with antihistamines and decongestants and their effects on the lower airway. *Ped Annals* 2000, 29:411–420.

10.•• Lieberman PL: Rhinitis. In *Current Practice of Medicine.* Philadelphia: Current Medicine; 1999: 295–310.
This text gives an excellent clinical overview of the different types of rhinitis, their diagnosis, and management options.

11. Busse WW, Holgate ST: *Asthma and Rhinitis.* Boston: Blackwell Scientific Publications; 2000.

12. Emanuel MB: Histamine and the antiallergic antihistamines: a history of their discoveries. *Clin Exp Allergy* 1999, 29:1–11.

13.•• Slater JW, Zechnich AD, Haxby DG: Second-generation antihistamines: a comparative review. *Drugs* 1999, 57:31–47.
This paper provides an excellent review of the second-generation antihistamines. It includes comprehensive descriptions of their side effects and compares their role in rhinitis therapy.

14.• Day J: Pros and cons of the use of antihistamines in managing allergic rhinitis. *J Allergy Clin Immunol* 1999, 103:S395–S399.
This is a comprehensive review of the activity of H_1-receptor antagonists, including a detailed description of their anti-inflammatory properties.

15. Howarth PH: Assessment of antihistamine efficacy and potency. *Clin Exp Allergy* 1999, 29:87–97.

16. Smit MJ, Hoffmann M, Timmerman H, *et al.*: Molecular properties and signaling pathways of the histamine H_1 receptor. *Clin Exp Allergy* 1999, 29:19–28.

17. Bakker RA, Wieland K, Timmerman H, *et al.*: Constitutive activity of the histamine H_1 receptor reveals inverse agonism of histamine H_1 receptor antagonists. *Eur J Pharmacol* 2000, 387:R5–R7.

18. Meltzer EO: Pharmacological treatment options for allergic rhinitis and asthma. *Clin Exp Allergy* 1998, 28:27–36.

19. McNeely W, Wiseman LR: Intranasal azelastine: a review of its efficacy in the management of allergic rhinitis. *Drugs* 1998, 56:91–114.

20. Lieberman P: Management of allergic rhinitis with a combination antihistamine/anti-inflammatory agent. *J Allergy Clin Immunol* 1999, 103:S400–S404.

21. Banov C, Lieberman P: Efficacy of Azelastine nasal spray in the treatment of vasomotor (perennial nonallergic) rhinitis. *Ann Allergy Asthma Immunol* 2001, 86:28–35.

22. Scadding GK: Clinical assessment of antihistamines in rhinitis. *Clin Exp Allergy* 1999, 29:77–81.

23. Simons FER, Simons KJ: Clinical pharmacology of new histamine H_1 receptor antagonists. *Clin Pharmacokinet* 1999, 36:329–352.

24. Rachelefsky GS: Pharmacologic management of allergic rhinitis. *J Allergy Clin Immunol* 1998, 101:S367–S369.

25. Cuss FM: Beyond the histamine receptor: effect of antihistamines on mast cells. *Clin Exp Allergy* 1999, 29:54–59.

26. Weldon D: Diagnosis and management of rhinitis. *Prim Care* 1998, 25:831–848.

27. Miadonna A, Cottini M, Milazzo N, *et al.*: In vivo and ex vivo inhibitory effects of loratadine on histamine release in patients with allergic rhinitis. *Allergy* 1998, 53:1183–1188.

28. Ciprandi G, Passalacqua G, Canonica GW: Effects of H_1 antihistamines on adhesion molecules: a possible rationale for long-term treatment. *Clin Exp Allergy* 1999, 29:49–53.

29. Canonica GW, Ciprandi G: Minimal persistent inflammation may be controlled by cetirizine. *Ann Allergy Asthma Immunol* 1999, 83:445–448.

30. Simpson K, Jarvis B: Fexofenadine: a review of its use in the management of seasonal allergic rhinitis and chronic idiopathic urticaria. *Drugs* 2000, 59:301–321.

31. Markham A, Wagstaff AJ: Fexofenadine. *Drugs* 1998, 55:269–274.

32. Howarth PH, Stern MA, Roi L, *et al.*: Double-blind, placebo-controlled study comparing the efficacy and safety of fexofenadine hydrochloride (120 and 180 mg once daily) and cetirizine in seasonal allergic rhinitis. *J Allergy Clin Immunol* 1999, 104:927–933.

33. Simons FER, Johnston L, Gu X, *et al.*: Suppression of the early and late cutaneous allergic responses using the H_1-receptor antagonist fexofenadine and the cysteinyl leukotriene 1-antagonist montelukast. *J Allergy Clin Immunol* 2000.

34. Abdelaziz MM, Devalia JI, Khair OA, *et al.*: Effect of fexofenadine on eosinophil-induced changes in epithelial permeability and cytokine release from nasal epithelial cells of patients with seasonal allergic rhinitis. *J Allergy Clin Immunol* 1998, 101:410–420.

35. Shichijo M, Inagaki N, Nakai N, *et al.*: The effects of anti-asthma drugs on mediator release from cultured human mast cells. *Clin Exp Allergy* 1998, 28:1228–1236.

36. Takao A, Shimoda T, Matsuse H, *et al.*: Inhibitory effects of azelastine hydrochloride in alcohol-induced asthma. *Ann Allergy Asthma Immunol* 1999, 82:390–394.

37. Howarth PH: A comparison of the anti-inflammatory properties of intranasal corticosteroids and antihistamines in allergic rhinitis. *Allergy* 2000, 62:6–11.

38. Kay GG, Harris AG: Loratadine: a non-sedating antihistamine. Review of its effects on cognition, psychomotor performance, mood and sedation. *Clin Exp Allergy* 1999, 29:147–150.

39. Weiler JM, Bloomfield JR, Woodworth GG, *et al.*: Effects of fexofenadine, diphenhydramine, and alcohol on driving performance. *Ann Intern Med* 2000, 132:354–363.

40. Simons FER: Non-cardiac adverse effects of antihistamines (H_1-receptor antagonists). *Clin Exp Allergy* 1999, 29:125–132.

41. Salmun LM, Gates D, Scharf M, *et al.*: Loratadine versus cetirizine: assessment of somnolence and motivation during the workday. *Clin Ther* 2000, 22:573–582.

42. Mason J, Reynolds R, Rao N: The systemic safety of fexofenadine HCl. *Clin Exp Allergy* 1999, 29:163–170.

43. Kay GG: The effects of antihistamines on cognition and performance. *J Allergy Clin Immunol* 2000, 105:S622–S627.

44. Rihoux JP, Donnelly F: CNS effects of histamine H_1 antagonists. *Clin Exp Allergy* 1999, 29:143–146.

45.•• Fireman P: Therapeutic approaches to allergic rhinitis: treating the child. *J Allergy Clin Immunol* 2000, 105:S616–S621.
This article provides a clinically-oriented description of diagnosis and management of allergic rhinitis in the pediatric population. It includes descriptions of how to recognize allergic rhinitis in children, the consequences of untreated rhinitis, its coexistence with asthma, and treatment options.

46. Taglialatela M, Annunziato L: Evaluation of the cardiac safety of second-generation antihistamines. *Allergy* 2000, 55:22–30.

47. Renwick AG: The metabolism of antihistamines and drug interactions: the role of cytochrome P450 enzymes. *Clin Exp Allergy* 1999, 29:116–124.

48. DuBuske LM: Second-generation antihistamines: the risk of ventricular arrhythmias. *Clin Ther* 1999, 21:281–295.

49. Hey JA, Affrime B, Cobert B, *et al.*: Cardiovascular profile of loratadine. *Clin Exp Allergy* 1999, 29:197–199.

50. Pratt C, Brown AM, Rampe D, *et al.*: Cardiovascular safety of fexofenadine HCl. *Clin Exp Allergy* 1999, 29:212–216.

51. Pinto YM, van Gelder IC, Heeringa M, *et al.*: QT lengthening and life-threatening arrhythmias associated with fexofenadine. *Lancet* 1999, 353:980.

52. Taglialatela M, Castaldo P, Pannaccione A, *et al.*: Cardiac ion channels and antihistamines: possible mechanisms of cardiotoxicity. *Clin Exp Allergy* 1999, 29:182–189.

53. Nicolas JM: The metabolic profile of second-generation antihistamines. *Allergy* 2000, 55:46–52.

54. Bagenstose SE, Bernstein JA: Treatment of chronic rhinitis by an allergy specialist improves quality of life outcomes. *Ann Allergy Asthma Immunol* 1999, 83:524–528.

55. Spector S: Ideal pharmacotherapy for allergic rhinitis. *J Allergy Clin Immunol* 1999, 103:S386–S387.

56. Day JH, Briscoe M, Widlitz MD: Cetirizine, loratadine, or placebo in subjects with seasonal allergic rhinitis: effects after controlled ragweed pollen challenge in an environmental exposure unit. *J Allergy Clin Immunol* 1998, 101:638–645.

57. Persi L, Demoly P, Harris AG, *et al.*: Comparison between nasal provocation tests and skin tests in patients treated with loratadine and cetirizine. *J Allergy Clin Immunol* 1999, 103:591–594.

58. Simons FER: Is antihistamine (H_1-receptor antagonist) therapy useful in clinical asthma? *Clin Exp Allergy* 1999, 29:98–104.

59. Knol K: Clinical use of antihistamines in infants and children at risk of asthma development. *Allergy* 2000, 55:31–34.

60. Hurwitz ME: Treatment of allergic rhinitis with antihistamines and decongestants and their effects on the lower airway. *Pediatr Ann* 2000, 29:411–420.

CHAPTER **16**

Immunotherapy for Allergic Rhinitis

J. Andrew Grant
Muhammad Rais
Jaime Castillo

Modulation of the immune system was first attempted during the last century with protocols designed to achieve protection against microorganisms and toxins. The smallpox vaccination of Jenner is an obvious example. Allergen injection therapy for alleviation of allergic diseases is a natural extension of this concept, and this new form of treatment can be traced directly to the pioneering report by Noon [1] in 1911 from England. Soon thereafter, its use became popular, especially in the United States. However, controlled studies demonstrating the efficacy of allergen injections were not performed until the second half of this century. The term *immunotherapy* has been applied to this procedure, although it is also referred to as *desensitization* or *hyposensitization*. Other forms of immunotherapy are discussed at the end of this chapter.

Allergen injection immunotherapy is a slow immunizing process consisting of the administration of increasing doses of allergenic extract to an allergic individual. The ultimate goal is to develop increased tolerance to the injected antigens and to subsequent exposure to the causative allergen. The purpose is to reduce the symptoms caused by specific allergens and the accompanying tissue inflammatory response. Consequential development of tolerance with effective immunotherapy is associated with modulation of specific IgG and IgE antibodies, reduced cellular responses including the release of mediators, and changes in the pattern of cytokines generated. Immunotherapy is clearly indicated for alleviation of allergic rhinitis, allergic asthma, and prevention of anaphylaxis from future Hymenoptera stings in sensitive individuals.

Practice parameters for the safe use of allergen immunotherapy recently have been developed [2•]. In addition, the World Health Organization, in conjunction with several national and international allergy societies, has revised guidelines for immunotherapy [3••], and both of these documents are of interest. The latter monograph has proposed that the proper term for this form of treatment should be *therapeutic vaccines for allergic diseases* [3••]. A recent issue of the *Journal of the American Medical Association* [4•] also includes an excellent chapter on immunotherapy.

BIOLOGY AND STANDARDIZATION OF AEROALLERGENS

Major advances have recently been made in the characterization of allergens and the immunologic response to them. Allergenic extracts are derived from multiple sources, including pollens, fungi, acarids, insects, mammals, and foods, and care must be taken to ensure a quality product. The value of an extract depends on the presence of most relevant allergens and preservation of allergenicity. Successful immunotherapy requires high-quality allergenic extracts, standardized for lot-to-lot and manufacturer-to-manufacturer consistency [3••].

The naming of allergens is based on a convention using the first three letters of the genus, the first letter of the species, and numeration of distinct allergens. For example, the most important allergen thought to derive from cats is Fel d 1. Similarly, the predominant allergens for sensitivity to the dust mite species growing in humid climates are Der p 1 and 2. Finally, the principle allergen in short ragweed is Amb a 1.

Standardization of allergens is a vital requisite for safe and effective immunotherapy. To ensure consistency, the prescribing physician must know the most relevant allergens present and their concentration. Comparisons are often made to standardized preparations, and recombinant sources of several allergens should improve the reliability of standards [3••]. Current methods for standardization include detection of IgE antibodies to allergens both in vivo and in vitro. Skin testing remains a popular technique for comparison of the total allergenic potency of extracts; end point titration is a standard of the United States Food and Drug Administration (FDA) [5,6]. Other biologic techniques include bronchial or nasal inhalation challenge and histamine release from basophils. The most commonly used in vitro techniques are radioallergosorbent test (RAST) inhibition and direct immunoassays. The availability of recombinant allergens has increased the precision of standardization. One major breakthrough in standardization is the ability to measure the concentration of major allergens in an extract. Examples include determining the amounts of Der p 1 in house dust-mite extracts, Fel d 1 in cat dander extracts, and Amb a 1 in ragweed pollen extracts.

MECHANISMS OF IMMUNOTHERAPY

Many investigations have evaluated mechanisms for immunotherapy. Initially, modulation of circulating antibodies and changes in effector cells were thought the most important changes. However, recent studies have emphasized the modulation of cytokines and T-cell response.

The T-cell response in allergic rhinitis is predominantly driven by chemicals induced by a specialized population called T_H2 cells, whose function is regulated by another group called T_H1 cells. A potential goal of immunotherapy is the induction of T_H1 cellular activity with a concomitant reduction in T_H2 cellular activity. Clinically, effective immunotherapy is correlated with a reduction in both mucosal and cutaneous responses to allergen challenge [7–9]. Both the immediate and late-phase response to allergen skin testing is dramatically reduced (Fig. 16-1).

EFFICACY OF IMMUNOTHERAPY

Since 1980, numerous studies have verified the efficacy of immunotherapy in allergic rhinitis not adequately responsive to avoidance and pharmacotherapy. The allergens that have been evaluated in controlled studies are outlined in Table 16-1, as well as investigations of both allergic rhinitis and asthma. Immunotherapy is the only procedure that anticipates significant reduction in target-organ sensitivity over time. Many double-blind controlled trials have shown the efficacy of immunotherapy in allergic rhinitis and conjunctivitis secondary to grass and ragweed [3••,8–10•,11–15]. A limited number of investigations have been conducted for alleviation of rhinitis due to other pollen, fungal, and mite allergens [3••,16–17].

The predominant technique for allergen immunotherapy currently in use is administration of allergens through periodic subcutaneous injections. In the United States, the frequency of injections is usually once or twice weekly during the build-up stage to a maintenance dosage after which injections may be given at longer intervals [2•].

Parenteral immunotherapy necessitates frequent visits for injections that may be uncomfortable and associated with other adverse reactions. Thus, other routes have been evaluated. A considerable amount of literature exists regarding topical immunotherapy with allergens delivered intranasally, orally, sublingually, and by inhalation modalities. The sublingual route appears to be the most promising alternative to parenteral immunotherapy. Larger studies are needed, however, to verify the most appropriate population, the optimal doses, and efficacy of this route [18]. This subject has been reviewed recently [3••], but because it is not currently practiced to any extent in the United States, it is not considered further in this chapter.

PRACTICAL ISSUES IN IMMUNOTHERAPY
Selection of patients

Immunotherapy has definite value to patients with significant upper respiratory symptoms related to aeroallergens. This is the only treatment offering a significant long-term reduction in symptoms and the need for time-consuming avoidance procedures and expensive pharmacotherapy. Special care is necessary with patients who have coexistent bronchial asthma [19].

Selection of allergenic extracts

The extracts most frequently used in the United States are prepared by aqueous extraction of appropriate source materials. Standardized extracts are highly desirable to ensure reduced variation among lots and manufacturers. Lyophilized extracts can be stored for extended periods before reconstitution. Moreover, commercial extracts are prepared in glycerin to extend potency. Addition of albumin to aqueous solutions also fosters preservation of potency by reducing protein-binding to glass. In all circumstances, extracts should be kept refrigerated to reduce losses. Highly concentrated extracts have increased stability. When highly diluted preparations are made for initiating immunotherapy, strict labeling with short periods before expiration is essential. Finally, care must be taken in mixing certain extracts, because preliminary description of proteases has been found in certain allergens.

A variety of modified extracts has been developed with the anticipation of reducing immediate reactions without reducing the long-term efficacy [3••]. Several of these products are popular in other countries, but the most frequently used extracts in the United States are unmodified aqueous extracts. One technique for modification is the absorption of allergens to carriers such as aluminum and tyrosine [20]. Another procedure involves the cross-linking of allergens with formaldehyde [14,15] or glutaraldehyde [13].

As emphasized previously, most of the controlled trials of immunotherapy have been conducted with only a single or limited number of aeroallergens. In this manner, the therapeutic dose can be optimized. Unfortunately, it is more common in the United States to use a multiplicity of allergens, and this may seriously limit the effectiveness of the dose reached for individual allergens. For this reason, the allergist should carefully select the most critical allergens for inclusion in immunotherapy based on clinical history, knowledge of local allergens, and positive testing for sensitivity.

Risks versus benefits

The chief benefits anticipated from immunotherapy are reductions in the frequency and severity of reactions and the need for avoidance and pharmacotherapy. Dust mite immunotherapy in children may help prevent new sensitizations [21]. An ongoing study also has demonstrated that progression of rhinitis to asthma may be prevented by immunotherapy [22]. The most frequent side effect is local reactions at the site of injection, but this does not predict the likelihood of systemic reactions. Most systemic reactions occur within 20 minutes after injection; therefore, patients must be carefully monitored for at least this time period [23,24]. The risk of fatal reactions is low and has been estimated at about one in every two million injections [25,26]. No data suggest the likelihood of immunotherapy inducing autoimmune disorders. Risk factors for systemic reactions include patients with symptomatic asthma, highly sensitive patients, introduction of a new vaccine vial, dosing errors, injections during the pollen season, short stay after injection, and use of concomitant medications such as β-blockers [2•,3••,4•,23–28].

Guidelines for optimal immunotherapy

Recommended guidelines for improving the benefit of immunotherapy and reducing the risk are given in Table 16-2. Although self-administration of allergens has been used in some practices, this procedure is rarely warranted [24]. It is not possible for the prescribing allergist to administer all injections, so a close relationship with the medical facility where injections will be given is essential. The physician supervising the administration of extracts

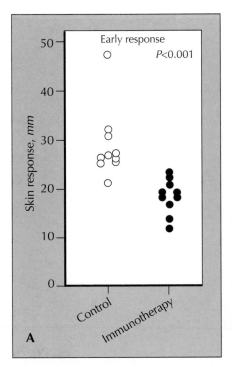

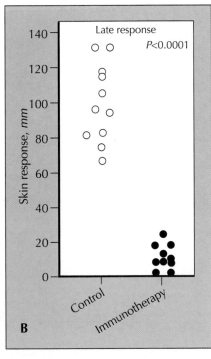

FIGURE 16-1.
Size of early (15 minute, **A**) and late (24 hour, **B**) skin responses after intradermal allergen in control and immunotherapy-treated patients. (*Adapted from* Hamid *et al.* [10].)

TABLE 16-1. CONTROLLED STUDIES SHOWING
EFFICACY OF ALLERGEN
IMMUNOTHERAPY

	Rhinitis	Asthma
Allergen		
Grasses	X	X
Ragweed	X	X
Mountain cedar	X	X
Parietaria	X	
Fungi		
Cladosporium	X	X
Alternaria	X	X
Mites	X	X
Animals		
Dog		X
Cat		X

Adapted from *Bousquet* et al. *[3••] and Weber [4•].*

TABLE 16-2. GUIDELINES FOR OPTIMAL
ALLERGEN INJECTION
IMMUNOTHERAPY

1. Follow strict criteria for selecting candidates for immunotherapy
2. Obtain written informed consent
3. Maintain close cooperation between the allergist and the physician who is administering injections, with actual administration only under medical supervision
4. Select allergens based on demonstrated sensitivity (usually positive skin tests) and clinical relevance
5. Carefully prepare and store extracts with conservative expiration dates
6. Carefully monitor side effects from immunotherapy, drug usage, and clinical response; ask patients at each visit about reactions to previous injection and use of new drugs since last visit
7. Follow established protocols for adjustment of dosage when systemic reactions occur
8. Make certain that drugs and equipment for treatment of anaphylaxis are available and that personnel know how to treat anaphylaxis
9. Prescribe epinephrine and antihistamines to be carried by patients receiving immunotherapy
10. Measure peak flow routinely before injections in patients with asthma and omit injections if values are less than 70% of personal best
11. Require patients to remain at medical facility for at least 20 minutes
12. Increase dosage to a maintenance dose of 5 to 20 μg of each relevant allergen
13. Obtain commitment of patient to continue maintenance immunotherapy for at least 3 to 5 years

and the office personnel involved must be familiar with the risks of immunotherapy and be able to recognize anaphylaxis and respond appropriately. Patients should be interviewed carefully before each injection for prior systemic symptoms, allergic symptoms, and changes in medications, especially institution of β-blockers. Dosing regimens must be modified when patients experience systemic reactions. The necessary equipment and drugs have been recommended by the American Academy of Asthma Allergy and Immunology [24]. The waiting time of at least 20 minutes must be carefully monitored. In our practice, all patients receive a routine prescription for injectable epinephrine and antihistamines for self-administration if a systemic reaction occurs after leaving the clinic. All patients with asthma have peak flow monitored before each visit, and the injection is withheld if values fall below 70% of personal best.

Several studies with standardized allergens show the optimal maintenance dose should be between 5 and 20 μg of the major allergen in each injection [3••,7,29–31]. This dose is associated with significant clinical improvement, although systemic reactions would require a lower dose. Lower doses do not improve clinical symptoms or reduce sensitivity to allergen challenge in experimental protocols [7].

The length of time for which patients should receive immunotherapy has been evaluated in several controlled studies. A recent report by Durham *et al.* [32] of grass immunotherapy for rhinitis has shown evidence of prolonged clinical remission coupled with persistently altered immunoreactivity after 3 to 5 years of desensitization [32]. Similar studies support the same recommendations for other allergens [7,20,33,34•,35].

REFERENCES AND RECOMMENDED READING

Recently published papers of particular interest have been highlighted as:

• Of interest

•• Of outstanding interest

1. Noon L: Prophylactic inoculation against hay fever. *Lancet* 1911, 1:1572–1573.

2.• Nicklas RA, Bernstein LI, Blessing-Moore J: Practice parameters for allergen immunotherapy. *J Allergy Clin Immunol* 1996, 98:1–11.
This review gives the consensus of the two American allergy societies for immunotherapy.

3.•• Bousquet J, Lockey R, Malling HJ: Allergen immunotherapy: therapeutic vaccines for allergic diseases: WHO position paper. *Allergy* 1998, 53:1–42.
This comprehensive review and update gives the most complete review of current literature and international consensus for management of immunotherapy.

4.• Weber RW: Immunotherapy with allergens. *JAMA* 1997, 278:1881–1887.
This is an excellent chapter on immunotherapy appearing in the recently revised Primer on Allergic and Immunologic Diseases.

5. Turkeltaub PC, Campbell G, Mosimann JE: Comparative safety and efficacy of short ragweed extracts differing in potency and composition in the treatment of fall hay fever: use of allergenically bioequivalent doses by parallel line bioassay to evaluate comparative safety and efficacy. *Allergy* 1990, 45:528–546.

6. Van Metre TE Jr, Adkinson NF Jr, Kagey-Sobotka A, *et al.*: How should we use skin testing to quantify IgE sensitivity?. *J Allergy Clin Immunol* 1990, 86:583–586.

7. Furin MJ, Norman PS, Creticos PS, *et al.*: Immunotherapy decreases antigen-induced eosinophil migration into the nasal cavity. *J Allergy Clin Immunol* 1991, 88:27–32.

8. Hedlin G, Silber G, Naclerio R, *et al.*: Comparison of the in vivo and in vitro response to ragweed immunotherapy in children and adults with ragweed-induced rhinitis. *Clin Exp Allergy* 1990, 20:491–500.

9. Varney VA, Hamid QA, Gaga M, *et al.*: Influence of grass pollen immunotherapy on cellular infiltration and cytokine mRNA expression during allergen-induced late-phase cutaneous responses. *J Clin Invest* 1993, 92:644–651.

10.• Hamid QA, Schotman E, Jacobson MR, *et al.*: Increases in IL-12 messenger RNA+ cells accompany inhibition of allergen-induced late skin responses after successful grass pollen immunotherapy. *J Allergy Clin Immunol* 1997, 9:254–260.
This paper reviews the changes in lymphocytes and cytokines with effective immunotherapy.

11. Durham SR, Ying S, Veronica A, *et al.*: Grass pollen immunotherapy inhibits allergen-induced infiltration of CD4+ T lymphocytes and eosinophils in the nasal mucosa and increases the number cells expressing messenger RNA for interferon gamma. *J Allergy Clin Immunol* 1996, 97:1356–1365.

12. Bousquet J, Becker WM, Hejjaoui A, *et al.*: Differences in clinical and immunologic reactivity of patients allergic to grass pollens and to multiple-pollen species. II. Efficacy of a double-blind, placebo-controlled, specific immunotherapy with standardized extracts. *J Allergy Clin Immunol* 1991, 88:43–53.

13. Grammer LC, Zeiss CR, Suszko IM, *et al.*: A double-blind, placebo-controlled trial of polymerized whole ragweed for immunotherapy of ragweed allergy. *J Allergy Clin Immunol* 1982, 69:494–499.

14. Meriney DK, Kothari H, Chinoy P, *et al.*: The clinical and immunologic efficacy of immunotherapy with modified ragweed extract (allergoid) for ragweed hay fever. *Ann Allergy* 1986, 56:34–38.

15. Norman PS, Lichtenstein LM, Kagey-Sobotka A, *et al.*: Controlled evaluation of allergoid in the immunotherapy of ragweed hay fever. *J Allergy Clin Immunol* 1982, 70:248–260.

16. Ortolani C, Pastorello EA, Incorvaia C, *et al.*: A double-blind, placebo-controlled study of immunotherapy with an alginate-conjugated extract of Parietaria judaica in patients with Parietaria hay fever. *Allergy* 1994, 49:13–21.

17. McHugh SM, Lavelle B, Kemeny DM, *et al.*: A placebo-controlled trial of immunotherapy with two extracts of Dermatophagoides pteronyssinus in allergic rhinitis, comparing clinical outcome with changes in antigen-specific IgE, IgG, and IgG subclasses. *J Allergy Clin Immunol* 1990, 86:521–531.

18. Frew A, White PJ, Smith HE: Sublingual immunotherapy. *J Allergy Clin Immunol* 1999, 104:267–270.

19. Hejjaqui A, Ferrando R, Dhivert H, *et al.*: Systemic reactions occurring during immunotherapy with standardized extracts. *J Allergy Clin Immunol* 1992; 89:925–933.

20. Price JF, Warner JO, Hey EN, *et al.*: A controlled trial of hyposensitization with adsorbed tyrosine *Dermatophagoides pteronyssinus* antigen in childhood asthma: in vivo aspects. *Clin Allergy* 1984, 14:209–219.

21. Bousquet J, Des Roches A, Paradis L, *et al.*: Immunotherapy with standardized *Dermatophagoides pteronyssinus* extract. VI. Specific immunotherapy prevents the onset of new sensitizations in children. *J Allergy Clin Immunol* 1997, 99: 450–453.

22. Jacobsen L, Dreborg S, Ferduosi A, *et al.*: Prevention of asthma by specific immunotherapy (the PAT study): five year follow up. *Allergy* 1998, 53:169.

23. Stewart GD, Lockey RF: Systemic reactions from allergen immunotherapy. *J Allergy Clin Immunol* 1992, 90:567–578.

24. American Academy of Allergy and Immunology Board of Directors: Guidelines to minimize the risk from systemic reactions caused by immunotherapy with allergenic extracts. *J Allergy Clin Immunol* 1994, 93:811–812.

25. Lockey RF, Benedict LM, Turkeltaub PC, Bukantz SC: Fatalities from immunotherapy (IT) and skin testing (ST). *J Allergy Clin Immunol* 1987, 79:660–677.

26. Reid MJ, Lockey RF, Turkeltaub PC, Platts-Mills TA: Survey of fatalities from skin testing and immunotherapy 1985–1989. *J Allergy Clin Immunol* 1993, 92:6–15.

27. Norman PS: Safety of allergen immunotherapy. *J Allergy Clin Immunol* 1989, 84:438–439.

28. Hepner MJ, Ownby DR, Anderson JA, *et al.*: Risk of systemic reactions in patients taking beta-blocker drugs receiving allergen immunotherapy injections. *J Allergy Clin Immunol* 1990, 86:407–411.

29. Creticos PS, Marsh DG, Proud D, *et al.*: Responses to ragweed-pollen nasal challenge before and after immunotherapy. *J Allergy Clin Immunol* 1989, 84:197–205.

30. Haugaard L, Dahl R, Jacobsen L: A controlled dose-response study of immunotherapy with standardized, partially purified extract of house dust mite: clinical efficacy and side effects. *J Allergy Clin Immunol* 1993, 91:709–722.

31. Bousquet J, Hejjaoui A, Clauzel AM, *et al.*: Specific immunotherapy with a standardized *Dermatophagoides pteronyssinus* extract, II: prediction of efficacy of immunotherapy. *J Allergy Clin Immunol* 1988, 82:971–977.

32.• Durham S, Walker S, Varga E, *et al.*: Long-term clinical efficacy of grass-pollen immunotherapy. *N Engl J Med* 1999, 341:468–475.
This study showed that clinical improvement from pollen immunotherapy is persistent for years after discontinuation of therapy.

33. Hedlin G, Heilborn H, Lilja G, *et al.*: Long-term follow-up of patients treated with a three-year course of cat or dog immunotherapy. *J Allergy Clin Immunol* 1995, 96:879–885.

34.• Naclerio RM, Proud D, Moylan B, *et al.*: A double-blind study of the discontinuation of ragweed immunotherapy. *J Allergy Clin Immunol* 1997, 100:293–300.
This is a careful evaluation of the response to stopping pollen immunotherapy.

35. Jacobsen L, Nuchel Petersen B, Wihl JA, *et al.*: Immunotherapy with partially purified and standardized tree pollen extracts, IV: results from long-term (6-year) follow-up. *Allergy* 1997, 52:914–920.

CHAPTER 17

Corticosteroids and Their Use in Rhinitis

Kerry L. Drain
James T.C. Li

Intranasal corticosteroids have been available for treatment of rhinitis since 1974 and are an important component in the treatment of allergic rhinitis, nonallergic rhinitis, and nasal polyps. Studying the local anti-inflammatory and immunologic effects of topical nasal corticosteroids has furthered the understanding of the immunologic nasal reactions that occur in patients with rhinitis.

PHARMACOLOGY

Corticosteroids secreted from the adrenal cortex are divided into glucocorticoids and mineralocorticoids. The main glucocorticoid in humans is hydrocortisone (cortisol); aldosterone is the main mineralocorticoid. The human body produces about 10 mg of cortisol and 0.125 mg of aldosterone per day under normal conditions. Corticosteroids have diverse effects including metabolism of carbohydrates, lipids and proteins, fluid and electrolyte balance, and preservation of normal function of the cardiovascular, renal, muscular, endocrine, nervous, and immune systems. The discovery of the anti-inflammatory, immunosuppressive actions of corticosteroids spurred on their use as medications used at times at levels much higher than those normally secreted by the body.

Hydrocortisone, like all corticosteroids, has 21-carbon structure (Fig. 17-1). Corticosteroids are rapidly absorbed either orally or systemically from sites of local injection. Certain water-soluble esters of hydrocortisone and its synthetic analogs can be administered intravenously to achieve high drug concentrations rapidly. Minor changes in chemical structure alter the rate of absorption, onset of effect, and duration of action. Following absorption, over 90% of cortisone in the plasma becomes reversibly bound to proteins in normal circumstances; only the unbound fraction can enter cells. When administered in supraphysiologic doses, the capacity of this binding is exceeded; thus the amount of free corticosteroid is increased, leading to more transmembrane movement and receptor activation. Corticosteroids are metabolized both by the liver and the kidney and are excreted in urine.

PHARMACOLOGIC MECHANISMS

Corticosteroids are lipophilic and cross the cell membrane rapidly to bind to the corticosteroid receptor complex (Fig. 17-2). Once bound, the heat shock protein that held the receptor in an inactive state dissociates, allowing the corticosteroid complex to enter the cell nucle-

FIGURE 17-1.

The structure of hydrocortisone, represented in two dimensions. The steroid ring system is not completely planar and the orientation of the two groups attached to the steroid rings is an important determinant of the biologic activity. (*Adapted from Schimmer et al.* [1].)

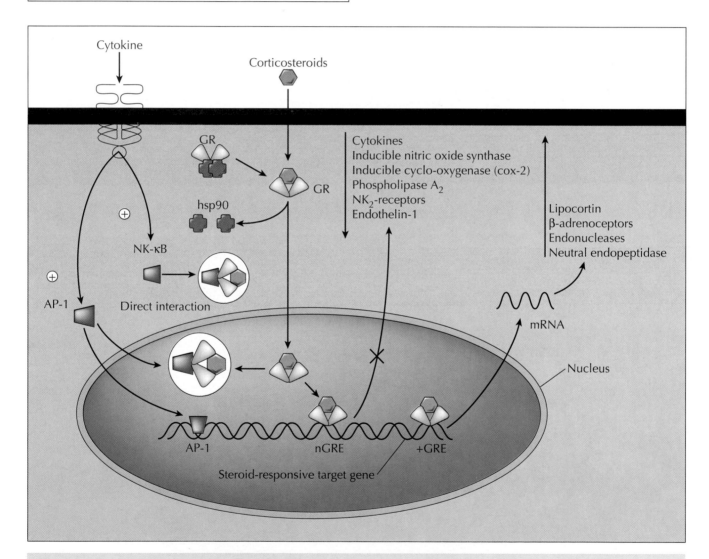

FIGURE 17-2.

The molecular mechanism of action of corticosteroids. Corticosteroids are lipophilic and cross the cell membrane to bind to the glucocorticosteroid receptor (GR) and dissociate the heat shock protein (hsp90) that has held the receptor in an inactive state. The GR complex then enters the cell nucleus and acts as a transcription factor, binding to specific recognition sequences on the DNA in the promotor region of the corticosteroid-responsive elements (GRE). Corticosteroids may either activate or suppress target genes by increasing or decreasing the specific mRNA. (*Adapted from Bachert et al.* [2].)

us. There the corticosteroid complex acts as a transcription factor binding to specific recognition sequences on the DNA in the promotor region of corticosteroid receptive elements. Corticosteroids can cause either activation or suppression of target genes by increasing or decreasing specific messenger ribonucleic acid (mRNA) production. This interaction causes a decrease in the transcription of inflammatory mediators such as cytokines. The production of anti-inflammatory mediators and other proteins such as lipocortin-1 and beta-adrenergic receptors is increased. Corticosteroid complex can interact directly on transcription factors that are activated by cytokine binding its receptor, inactivating the effects of the cytokine on the cell, and preventing further cytokine production [2]. Due to the intricate interactions of corticosteroid, the onset of action of corticosteroids is measured in hours and days instead of seconds to minutes as seen with other medications.

MECHANISMS OF ACTION OF INTRANASAL CORTICOSTEROIDS IN RHINITIS

Immunologic mechanisms

Intranasal corticosteroids act at multiple sites in the inflammatory process (Table 17-1). The inflammatory response is promoted by the activated T-lymphocytes and the cytokines produced by T-helper cells (T_H2). The cytokines produced by the T_H2 cells cause IgE secretion by B lymphocytes and production of other cytokines that promote the maturation and activation of eosinophils. Intranasal corticosteroids have been shown to inhibit T-lymphocyte activation, prevent increases in cytokine production, and inhibit eosinophil recruitment and activation. There is also a reduction in the number of lymphocytes due to corticosteroid induction of apoptosis. Intranasal corticosteroids act by decreasing the infiltration of mast cells, eosinophils, and lymphocytes into the nasal mucosa and thus decrease the release of their proinflammatory mediators [4].

Eosinophils are thought to play a key role in inflammation and hyperresponsiveness of airway tissues in affected patients. Eosinophils act by releasing preformed cytotoxic proteins, synthesizing leukotrienes, and producing superoxide radicals that are directly toxic to the respiratory epithelium. Corticosteroids, in general, are known to affect eosinophils in many ways, eg, direct induction of eosinophil apoptosis. With the decreased production of certain cytokines there is less eosinophil recruitment, and migration is affected by a decreased expression of adhesion molecules on endothelial cells [5]. Cytologic studies done on nasal secretions of patients with perennial allergic rhinitis treated with intranasal corticosteroid resulted in a reduction not only in the number of eosinophils but in the amount of cytotoxic proteins such as eosinophil cationic protein [6].

Finally, airway epithelial cells act as a primary defense against irritants providing a direct barrier as well as an effector cell secreting inflammatory mediators and cytokines. These cells metabolize arachidonic acid via the cyclo-oxygenase pathway, resulting in production of leukotrienes, prostaglandins, thromboxane, and platelet-activating factor. These metabolites regulate vascular tone and permeability, stimulate mucus secretion, chemotaxis, and regulate inflammatory cell proliferation. Corticosteroids generally produce an anti-inflammatory protein, lipocortin, that inhibits phospholipase A2, an important enzyme in the arachidonic acid cascade. Blockage of this inflammatory cascade affects not only the epithelial cells but also blood vessels. Without these mediators, the increase in blood flow and vascular permeability is blunted. Plasma proteins and inflammatory cells are not as readily transported to affected sites [4]. Intranasal steroids used in patients with seasonal allergic rhinitis have been shown to reduce nasal lavage levels of bradykinin and fibrinogen, markers of plasma exudation [7].

Clinical mechanisms

Intranasal corticosteroids are currently the mainstay of treatment for moderate to severe cases of seasonal and perennial allergic rhinitis, nonallergic rhinitis, and nasal polyps. Many studies have shown that intranasal corticosteroids inhibit both the early (within minutes) and late (3 to 11 hours) phase of inflammation after an experimental allergen challenge in patients with seasonal and perennial rhinitis [8]. Treatment with intranasal corticosteroids for as little as 48 hours to 1 week shows inhibition of acute phase response such as nasal pruritus, sneezing, and discharge as measured by symptom scores and the appearance of mediators within nasal lavage fluid. Late-phase symptoms such as nasal obstruction are inhibited after 1 week of use [9].

INTRANASAL CORTICOSTEROID PREPARATIONS

Six intranasal corticosteroids are currently in use in the United States: beclomethasone, budesonide, flunisolide, fluticasone, mometasone, and triamcinolone (Table 17-2). All of the available preparations have been found to be effective in the treatment of seasonal and perennial rhinitis. Potency, lipophilicity, and systemic bioavailability of these intranasal corticosteroids may differ.

Pharmacologic profiles

Topical potency of corticosteroids can be compared by use of the McKenzie assay (Table 17-3). Skin-blanching response, a gauge of cutaneous vasoconstriction, is measured; this test is relevant to the vasoconstrictive effects of corticosteroids but it is unknown whether this assay correlates to the anti-inflammatory properties of the drug. A newer method of determining potency centers on the binding of the drug to the corticosteroid receptor and the strength of the binding affinity. Smith *et al.* compared the binding affinities of several topical corticosteroids and determined that the ranked order of binding affinity from highest to lowest was mometasone furoate, fluticasone, budesonide, triamcinolone acetonide, and dexamethasone [11]. In the same study the drug with the highest affinity was found to be the most potent stimulator of receptor-mediated transcription of gene expression.

Lipophilicity is defined as the index of lipid-partitioning potential of glucocorticoid compounds. The highly lipophilic drug is taken up into the nasal tissue at a faster rate and a higher level of retention within the tissue. This is thought to enhance the ability of the drug to reach the glucocorticoid receptor. The ranked order of lipophilicity from highest to lowest was mometasone furoate, fluticasone propionate, beclomethasone dipropionate, budesonide, triamcinolone acetonide, and flunisolide [12].

The systemic bioavailability is the sum of the portion of the drug that is swallowed plus the portion that is absorbed by the nasal mucosa. Systemic bioavailability of intranasal corticosteroid is thought to be mainly comprised by the amount that is swallowed and absorbed by the gastrointestinal tract [13]. The oral bioavailability of the flunisolide and budesonide, considering a significant first pass metabolism by the liver, is between 20% and 50%. In contrast, the newer agents mometasone and fluticasone are not readily absorbed via the GI tract and have a very low oral bioavailability of <0.1% and <0.2%, respectively. Intranasal corticosteroid is absorbed by the nose without first pass effect so the unchanged drug will be absorbed directly into the systemic circulation [14]. Plasma drug levels of mometasone and fluticasone are extremely low.

Intranasal corticosteroids are formulated as a dry powder inhalation, an aerosol propellant, and as an aqueous spray. These products are considered equally effective. Some aqueous sprays have a floral scent and a tendency to drip. Dry powder inhalants do not drip but may be overly forceful or irritating.

SYSTEMIC CORTICOSTEROIDS

There have been five placebo-controlled studies of systemic corticosteroids and their use in seasonal allergic rhinitis. All showed that systemic corticosteroids are highly effective in relieving nasal blockage and decreasing sneezing and rhinorrhea. One study used oral prednisolone and found that a daily dose of 7.5 mg was marginally effective, while 30 mg daily for 5 days was effective for all symptoms. Single injectable doses of tri-

TABLE 17-1. INFLAMMATORY MEDIATORS IN ALLERGIC RHINITIS AND ASSOCIATED SYMPTOMATOLOGY

Cells affected	Corticosteroid effect
T-lymphocytes	Reduction of circulating cell number, apoptosis
	Inhibition of:
	T-lymphocyte activation
	IL-2 production
	IL-2 receptor generation
	IL-4 production
	Antigen-driven proliferation
Eosinophils	Reduction of circulating cell number, apoptosis
	Reduction of epithelial and mucosal cell counts
	Reduction of cell influx in late-phase response
	Inhibition of IL-4– and IL-5–mediated cell survival
Mast cells/basophils	Reduction of circulating cell counts
	Reduction of cell influx in late-phase response
	Reduction of mast cell–derived mediators after challenge
	Reduction of histamine content and release
Neutrophils	Reduction of cell influx after challenge
Macrophages/monocytes	Reduction of circulating cell counts
	Inhibition of release of IL-1, interferon-γ, TNF-α, GM-CSF

Adapted from Meltzer [4].

amcinolone acetonide, 80 mg, methylprednisolone acetate, 80 mg, or betamethasone dipropionate, 5 mg, plus betamethasone phosphate, 2 mg, were effective in reducing symptoms of allergic rhinitis. In one study all patients given systemic corticosteroids showed suppression of plasma cortisol for up to 21 days after administration [3]. Intramuscular injections may cause fat necrosis at the injection site.

Clinical efficacy

Assessment of efficacy of intranasal preparations includes several different measures. Clinicians and patients rate improvement in symptomatology in individual and total symptom scores, number of symptom-free days, use of rescue medication, and global evaluation of efficacy. Most studies ask subjects to record nasal symptoms such as congestion, rhinorrhea, itching, and

TABLE 17-2. INTRANASAL STEROID PREPARATIONS

Chemical name	Trade name	Formulation	Dose/actuation, µg	Age, y	Recommended dosage
Beclomethasone dipropionate	Beconase* inhalation aerosol or	Propellant	42	≥12	1 spray/nostril bid to quid (168–336 µg/d)
	Vancenase PocketHaler†			6–12	1 spray/nostril tid (252 µg/d)
	Beconase AQ* nasal spray	Aqueous, 0.042%	42	≥12	1–2 sprays/nostril bid (168–336 µg/d)
				6–12	1–2 sprays/nostril bid (168–336 µg/d)
	Vancenase AQ†	Aqueous, 0.042%	42	≥6	1–2 sprays/nostril bid (168–336 µg/d)
	Vancenase AQ† 84 µg	Aqueous, 0.084%	84	≥6	1–2 sprays/nostril qd (168–336 µg/d)
Triamcinolone acetonide	Nasacort‡, Nasacort AQ	Propellant, aqueous	55	≥12	2 sprays/nostril qd (220 µg/d)
				6–11**	2 sprays/nostril qd (110–220 µg/d)
Budesonide	Rhinocort§, Rhinocort AQ	Propellant, aqueous	32	≥6	2 sprays/nostril bid or 4 sprays/nostril in AM (256 µg/d)
Flunisolide	Nasalide¶	0.025% solution	25	>14	2 sprays/nostril bid to tid (200–300 µg/d)
	Nasarel¶			6–14	1 spray/nostril tid (150 µg/d) 2 sprays/nostril bid (200 µg/d)
Fluticasone propionate	Flonase*	0.05% nasal spray (aqueous)	50	4 y to adolescent	1 spray/nostril qd (100 µg/d)
				Adults	2 sprays/nostril qd (200 µg/d)
Mometasone furoate	Nasonex†	Aqueous	50	≥12	2 sprays/nostril qd (200 µg/d)
				3–11	1 spray/nostril qd (100 µg/d)

*Glaxo Wellcome, Research Triangle Park, NC
†Schering, Kenilworth, NJ
‡Aventis Pharmaceuticals, Parsippany, NJ
§AstraZenenca, Wilmington, DE
¶Dura Pharmaceuticals, San Diego, CA
**Not FDA approved for children younger than 12 years.
qd–once daily; bid–twice daily; tid–three times daily.
Adapted from Baroody [10].

sneezing in a diary. Non-nasal symptoms and signs such as itching or burning eyes, tearing, ocular injection, and pruritus of the ears and palate are also noted. Symptoms and signs are graded by severity on a scale for a number of days before study and for the duration of the study. Symptom-free days and use of rescue medications are at times also recorded. Objective measures include nasal airflow, cytological investigations, mucociliary clearance, and olfactory function. Nasal airway resistance (NAR) is measured by rhinomanometric analysis.

Intranasal corticosteroids versus placebo

When intranasal steroids are compared with placebo, the active treatment group shows improvement in all parameters examined. In a randomized, double-blind, 3-week study of 429 patients (adults and children 12 years and older) with allergic rhinitis, triamcinolone acetonide, 220 μg/d, significantly decreased symptoms of nasal congestion, discharge, and sneezing ($P < 0.03$) [15]. In placebo-controlled double-blind studies of fluticasone propionate, 100 μg twice daily or 200 μg/d, fluticasone was significantly more effective than placebo in increasing the number of symptom-free days and improving nasal and ocular symptom scores [16]. Studies of mometasone versus placebo in a double-blind, randomized control study of patients with allergic rhinitis again demonstrated a significantly greater decrease in subjective and objective measures in the active treatment group. Total symptom scores ($P < 0.05$), total nasal scores ($P < 0.024$), and individual nasal symptoms decreased in the mometasone group versus placebo. The overall therapeutic response was significantly greater with active treatment. The measurement of eosinophil, basophil, and neutrophil counts as well as mucociliary clearance was significantly improved in mometasone-treated patients compared with those using placebo. Measures of cellular activity including levels of eosinophilic cationic protein, tryptase, and albumin (as an indicator of vascular permeability) were lower within the mometasone group at day 15 compared to baseline [17].

A comparison of agents

Comparisons between intranasal corticosteroids have been studied. Welsh *et al.* compared beclomethasone dipropionate, 168 μg twice daily, versus flunisolide, 100 μg twice daily, in patients with seasonal allergic rhinitis and found the two drugs to be equally effective [18]. Trials comparing beclomethasone, budesonide, flunisolide, and triamcinolone found them to be equally effective [19].

Multiple studies have compared beclomethasone dipropionate with fluticasone propionate. In a 2-week study of seasonal allergic rhinitis beclomethasone was as effective as fluticasone. In perennial allergic rhinitis both a 3-month and a 6-month study found that beclomethasone and fluticasone were equally effective [20,21]. However, a 12-month study found fluticasone superior to beclomethasone [22].

Budesonide and fluticasone have been compared in a number of trials involving patients with seasonal or perennial rhinitis. A 6-week study comparing budesonide with fluticasone in subjects with seasonal allergic rhinitis found budesonide more effective than fluticasone in reducing sneezing [23]. In two separate studies budesonide was equally effective as fluticasone in all studied parameters [24]. Triamcinolone was compared to fluticasone in seasonal rhinitis and both were found to be equivalent in all studied parameters [25]. Studies of mometasone and fluticasone found no advantage of one medication over another.

It appears that there is no clinically significant difference in the efficacy of various inhaled corticosteroids; however, onset of action may differ. Package inserts for beclomethasone and flunisolide recommend 2 weeks of use before clinical improvement is expected. More recent studies suggest that budesonide, fluticasone, mometasone, and triamcinolone demonstrate clinical improvement within 1 to 2 days of use. Jen *et al.* demonstrated that fluticasone nasal spray was more effective than placebo within 12 hours of initiation of treatment, although peak efficacy took several days to obtain. Their study also showed not only subjective improvement as seen by decreased symptom score in the

Table 17-3. Effects of Corticosteroids on Inflammatory Cells

Corticosteroid	Receptor binding affinity*	Skin blanching potency*
Flunisolide	1.8	330
Triamcinolone acetonide	3.6	330
Beclomethasone dipropionate	0.4	600
Budesonide	9.4	980
Fluticasone propionate	18.0	1200

*Relative to dexamethasone (where dexamethasone = 1).
Adapted from Meltzer [4].

active treatment group as compared to placebo (4.5 versus 8.5, respectively, $P=0.0001$), but objective reduction in the number of eosinophils seen in nasal lavage fluid in the active medication group versus placebo ($P=0.007$) [26]. After an initial dose of triamcinolone acetonide, symptom relief was noted as soon as 12 to 16 hours post dose [18]. Mometasone furoate was found to provide symptom relief with 12 hours in 28% of patients as compared to 13% of patients using placebo; the median time to symptom relief was 36 hours versus 72 hours with placebo [27].

Comparison with antihistamines

A total of 2267 subjects identified in 16 studies (mean age 32 years ranging 12 to 75 years, with 55% being men) were identified and evaluated by meta-analysis [28••]. A study would be excluded if it was not randomized, was single-blind, combined intranasal corticosteroids and oral antihistamine in the comparison arm, used topical antihistamines in a comparison arm, or a decongestant in a comparison arm, used nonclinical challenge or outcomes, or if findings were published only in abstract form without reporting clinical details. Intranasal corticosteroids produced significantly greater relief of nasal blockage and decreased nasal discharge than did oral antihistamines. Intranasal corticosteroids produced significantly greater relief of nasal pruritus as compared to oral histamine. Two studies showed a modest but significant decrease in postnasal drip in the intranasal corticosteroid-treated subjects versus oral antihistamine. Intranasal corticosteroids showed greater relief of total nasal symptoms than did oral antihistamines. There was no difference in ocular symptoms comparing the intranasal corticosteroids versus oral antihistamine in 11 studies, but in two others oral antihistamines were found to be superior. The meta-analysis showed that intranasal corticosteroids are more effective than oral antihistamine in treating patients with allergic rhinitis. The authors recommended intranasal corticosteroids as first-line treatment of allergic rhinitis.

Combination with antihistamines

Benincasa *et al.* investigated the effectiveness of monotherapy with fluticasone, 200 µg/d, for 8 weeks versus fluticasone at the same dose along with antihistamine cetirizine, 10 mg/d. Mean symptoms scores, including nasal and ocular symptoms and headache, and the number of symptom-free days were similar in each group. Eighty-eight per cent of the monotherapy group ($n=227$) reported control of their nasal symptoms compared with 89% of the combined treatment group ($n=227$). Interestingly, eye drops were used by all patients as a rescue treatment 20% of study days [29].

INTRANASAL CORTICOSTEROIDS IN NONALLERGIC RHINOSINUSITIS WITH EOSINOPHILIA SYNDROME

Patients with nonallergic rhinosinusitis with eosinophilia syndrome (NARES) have eosinophil-dominated inflammation of the mucous membrane of the nose and paranasal sinuses, at times in association with nasal polyps. Most of the experience with intranasal corticosteroids in NARES is from studies of patients with nasal polyps without allergic trigger. Some limited studies have shown efficacy in the majority of patients with NARES [30]. A double-blind, three-week study divided thirty patients with NARES into two treatment groups. One group received flunisolide and loratadine while the other received flunisolide and placebo. The combination group had less sneezing and rhinorrhea compared with the monotherapy group [31].

INTRANASAL CORTICOSTEROIDS IN NASAL POLYPOSIS

Many studies have looked at the effectiveness of intranasal corticosteroids in nasal polyposis. Studies of beclomethasone dipropionate compared with placebo showed a reduction in severity of nasal symptoms. Long-term studies show continued efficacy of beclomethasone over a 1-year period with slow recurrence of symptoms after treatment is discontinued [32]. A 16-week study comparing budesonide and placebo showed significantly increased nasal peak flow over the treatment period [33]. Fluticasone, 200 µg/d, was effective in the treatment of nasal polyps in randomized studies, and it was found to be at least as effective as beclomethasone, 200 µg twice daily, and significantly better than placebo in improving nasal blockage and overall symptoms [15]. Polyp size was significantly reduced by intranasal corticosteroids as compared to placebo [34]. It is unclear if this represents action on the polyp itself or the nasal mucosa. Several studies demonstrate a significant reduction in recurrence of polyposis when intranasal corticosteroid is introduced after surgery. Intranasal budesonide reduced the recurrence of symptoms and the need for further polypectomy for over 30 months [35]. Similar findings have been noted in beclomethasone, 100 µg twice daily, and fluticasone, 100 µg/d [15].

INTRANASAL CORTICOSTEROIDS AND NONEOSINOPHILIC, NONALLERGIC RHINITIS

Patients with noneosinophilic, nonallergic rhinitis are thought to have an abnormality of the response to autonomic stimuli. When tested in this group, intranasal corticosteroids demonstrated little efficacy. There was no difference in nasal resistance before and after intranasal corticosteroid administration [34].

SAFETY AND SIDE EFFECTS

The risk of systemic glucocorticoid effects with intranasal corticosteroids is very low. Intranasal corticosteroids have a 30-year track record of safety with no reports of serious side effects. The introduction of more potent lipophilic intranasal corticosteroids to younger patient populations has renewed the interest in potential adverse effects. Evaluation of the hypothalamic pituitary adrenal (HPA) axis function is one measure of the systemic effects of intranasal corticosteroids. There have been no reports of acute adrenal crisis or chronic adrenal insufficiency with intranasal corticosteroids. Other parameters that are studied when evaluating systemic side effects include indicators of bone metabolism, growth in children, formation of cataracts, and increased intraocular pressure.

The use of intranasal corticosteroids may result in nasal dryness, stinging, and burning in 5% to 10% of patients. Septal perforation and nasal mucosa atrophy are other possible local complications.

Hypothalamic pituitary adrenal axis

Edelman et al. reviewed 30 years of available literature on beclomethasone dipropionate, which showed that intranasal doses of up to 400 μg/d did not suppress the hypothalamic pituitary adrenal (HPA) axis when administered for up to 6 months [36]. In one study intranasal fluticasone, 200 μg/d, did not interfere with morning plasma cortisol concentration [37]. Once-daily administration of intranasal fluticasone in children with allergic rhinitis did not affect 24-hour urinary excretion of free cortisol and 17-ketogenic steroids when compared to placebo [38]. Overnight urinary cortisol levels were decreased in healthy volunteers on a 4-day course of fluticasone, 200 μg/d, but no effect was seen when the volunteers took triamcinolone, 220 μg/d, or beclomethasone, 336 μg/d. Serum cortisol and ACTH response were not affected by the use of these intranasal corticosteroids [39]. Wihl et al. found that intranasal budesonide, 400 and 800 μg, administered as single dose, decreased urinary cortisol [40].

A recent review that summarized more than twenty clinical trials involving more than 6000 patients found that mometasone had no detectable effect on the HPA axis [41]. Brannan et al. found a single dose of intranasal mometasone, 4000 μg, did not affect adrenal function [42]. There was no effect seen on the HPA axis in children given mometasone at either 50, 100, or 200 μg/d in a 7-day course of therapy [43]. Thus, intranasal corticosteroids have a minimal effect on the HPA axis.

Bone mineralization

Beclomethasone, 400 μg/d or less, was not associated with osteoporosis nor risk of fracture. One study in children did not show any effect of beclomethasone on bone metabolism [44]. Fluticasone, 200 μg/d, for one year did not affect bone mineral density nor biochemical markers of bone turnover [45]. Budesonide, 200 μg /d, mometasone, 200 μg/d, and triamcinolone, 220 μg/d, showed no effect on the biochemical marker of bone metabolism, osteocalcin [46•].

Growth in children

Skoner et al. studied the effect of beclomethasone, 168 μg twice daily, on the growth of children aged 6 to 9 years. The mean change in standing height after one year in the active treatment group was 5.0 cm, while the subjects treated with placebo grew 5.9 cm in the same time frame. The difference in growth rates was evident after as little as one month of treatment. The change in growth was seen across all age and gender subgroups and among subjects with or without prior corticosteroid use. There was no noted suppression noted on HPA axis [47••]. Schenkel et al. in a study of children aged 3 to 9 years of age taking mometasone, 100 μg/d, found no difference in mean height attained by either group at 1 year. Cosyntropin stimulation testing showed no effect on the HPA axis [48•]. Thus, intranasal beclomethasone can reduce growth velocity in children.

Posterior subcapsular cataract /increased intraocular pressure

Case reports have linked intranasal beclomethasone and the development of posterior subcapsular cataracts [44]. The majority of reported patients had been on beclomethasone for more than 5 years, often exceeding the recommended dosages or simultaneously taking systemic corticosteroids. In a case control study involving 10,000 subjects, there was no increased risk of ocular hypertension or open angle glaucoma even after high doses of fluticasone, beclomethasone, budesonide, and triamcinolone [49].

Local side effects

The localized symptoms of dryness, stinging, and burning occur in 5% to 10% of treated patients irrespective of compound or formulation. Epistaxis occurs in an estimated 5% of patients using intranasal corticosteroids and its incidence is not increased with the use of more potent agents. Septal perforations are reported rarely and can be averted by directing spray toward the inferior turbinate rather than toward the septum [19]. Mucosal biopsies from patients treated with beclomethasone showed no effect on the nasal mucosa [44]. Triamcinolone, 220 μg/d, and mometasone, 200 μg/d, were shown to have no deleterious effect on the nasal mucosa [15,50].

Safety in pregnancy and lactation

There are no controlled studies on the use of intranasal corticosteroids and pregnancy. Recommendations are extrapolated from the data available on orally inhaled corticosteroids in asthma and pregnancy. Teratogenicity in animal models manifested as cleft palates in rats was seen with beclomethasone and triamcinolone. Because data available for pregnant asthmatic women showed no effect on fetal outcome or risk to the fetus with the use of beclomethasone, this drug has been proposed as the corticosteroid of first choice for pregnant asthmatics. There are no studies available on inhaled corticosteroids and lactation. Beclomethasone can be excreted in milk, but therapeutic doses do not result in high concentrations in breast milk [44].

RECOMMENDATIONS

The Joint Task Force on Practice Parameters in Allergy, Asthma and Immunology, co-sponsored by the American Academy of Allergy, Asthma and Immunology and the American College of Allergy, Asthma and Immunology, published guidelines for the diagnosis and management of rhinitis [51•]. Their recommendation is as follows: "Nasally inhaled corticosteroids are the most effective medication in controlling symptoms of allergic rhinitis. They are particularly useful for treatment of more severe allergic rhinitis and may be useful in some other forms of rhinitis. Except for intranasal dexamethasone, these agents are generally not associated with significant systemic side effects in adults. Although local side effects are minimal if the patient is carefully instructed in the use of this class of drugs, nasal irritation and bleeding may occur, and nasal septal perforations are rarely reported. Intranasal corticosteroids should be considered before initiating treatment with systemic corticosteroids for the treatment of severe rhinitis." Their opinion on the use of oral and parenteral corticosteroids is as follows: "A short (3- to 7-day) course of oral corticosteroids may be appropriate for the treatment of very severe or intractable nasal symptoms or to treat significant nasal polyposis. However, the use of parenteral corticosteroids, particularly if administered recurrently, is discouraged because of greater potential for long-term corticosteroid side effects." The Joint Task Force stated that oral antihistamines are the first line of treatment in allergic rhinitis. They noted that antihistamines have limited effects on nasal congestion and NARES.

The Antiallergic Drug Subcommittee of the European Academy of Allergology and Clinical Immunology stated that intranasal corticosteroids are a first choice treatment for rhinitis [44]. They recommended use at the lowest clinically effective dose and careful evaluation of patients after initiation of therapy. They advise that special caution be exercised when using intranasal corticosteroids in children.

Patients with mild allergic rhinitis may benefit from an initial trial of a nonsedating antihistamine.

Intranasal corticosteroids should be prescribed if the antihistamine treatment is not effective. Intranasal corticosteroids are first-line treatment for patients with more severe allergic rhinitis, especially if nasal congestion is a major symptom. Those with significant nasal congestion may require topical decongestants for the first few days of therapy. For severely refractory cases a short "burst" of oral steroid may be employed.

Once symptoms are controlled by the intranasal corticosteroid, the dose should be titrated so that administration of the lowest possible but clinically effect dose is used. Using the lowest dose tolerated may decrease side effects and defray the cost of the therapy.

Intranasal corticosteroids are first-line agents for NARES or nasal polyposis. In noneosinophilic, nonallergic rhinitis, intranasal corticosteroids have not been shown to be effective.

Epidemiologic surveys have demonstrated that allergic rhinitis and asthma frequently coexist. Allergic rhinitis is a risk factor for asymptomatic bronchial hyperresponsiveness. Intranasal corticosteroids and antihistamines reduce asthma symptoms in patients with both rhinitis and asthma and may improve pulmonary function and bronchial hyperresponsiveness [52]. These findings support using intranasal and orally inhaled corticosteroids in patients with both allergic rhinitis and asthma.

Special consideration must be made when considering the use of intranasal corticosteroids in children. Growth suppression must be considered when prescribing intranasal corticosteroids, especially beclomethasone, in growing children. Parents should be told of the small but real risk that intranasal corticosteroids may decrease their child's growth. However, not all intranasal corticosteroids have the same effect on growth velocity. Intranasal beclomethasone should not be used in growing children.

Most patients with allergic rhinitis should use intranasal corticosteroids once daily on a regularly scheduled basis. Initiating treatment with intranasal corticosteroids early in the allergy season can avoid the severe nasal congestion that can compromise intranasal administration of corticosteroid.

Patients have opinions about formulations of their nasal steroid. Studies have not shown one nasal steroid superior to others in the class based on symptoms, so patients need to discover a preparation that is right for them. Choosing an intranasal steroid with once daily dosing may improve compliance. Patients should be allowed to try the different types in the office and leave with a prescription for their favorite. This would also be the optimal time for teaching of technique followed by a demonstration by the patient. Proper technique can aid in compliance by minimizing the chance of local side effects. Patients using intranasal corticosteroids should be evaluated periodically, at least once yearly for most patients. At the periodic visit, the physician can assess the patient for symptom control, compliance, and adverse effects.

CONCLUSIONS

Intranasal corticosteroids are the most effective medications in the treatment of allergic rhinitis. These agents should be considered first-line therapy for patients with allergic rhinitis. There is a very small risk of systemic corticosteroid adverse effects with intranasal corticosteroids. Mometasone may be the preferred intranasal corticosteroid for use in children.

REFERENCES AND RECOMMENDED READING

Papers of particular interest, published recently, have been highlighted as:
• Of importance
•• Of major importance

1. Schimmer BP, Parker KL: Adrenocorticotropic hormone; adrenocortical steroids and their synthetic analogs; inhibitors of the synthesis and actions of adrenoncortical hormones. In *Goodman & Gilman's The Pharmacological Basis of Therapeutics*. Edited by Hardman JG, Limbird LE. New York: McGraw-Hill; 1996:1459–1485.

2. Bachert C, Geveart P: Effect of intranasal corticosteroid on release of cytokines and inflammatory mediators. *Allergy* 1999, 57:116–123.

3. Mygind N: Systemic corticosteroid treatment for seasonal allergic rhinitis: a common but poorly documented therapy. *J Allergy Clin Immunol* 2000, 55:11–15.

4. Meltzer EO: The pharmacological basis for the treatment of perennial allergic rhinitis and non-allergic rhinitis with topical corticosteroids. *Allergy* 1997, 36(Suppl):33–40.

5. Stellato C, Beck LA, Gorgone GA, *et al*.: Expression of the chemokine RANTES by a human bronchial epithelial cell line: modulation by cytokines and glucocorticoids. *J Immunol* 1995, 155:410–418.

6. Konno A, Yamakoshi T, Terada N, Fujita Y: Mode of action of a topical steroid on immediate phase reaction after antigen challenge and nonspecific nasal hyperreactivity in nasal allergy. *Int Arch Allergy Immunol* 1994, 103:79–87.

7. Svensson C, Klementsson H, Andersson M, *et al*.: Glucocorticoid-induced attenuation of mucosal exudation of fibrinogen and bradykinins in seasonal allergic rhinitis. *Allergy* 1994, 49:177–183.

8. Levenson T, Greenberger P: Immunologic effects of intranasal corticosteroids. *Allergy Asthma Proc* 1996, 17:157–159.

9. Pipkorn U, Proud D, Lichtenstein LM, *et al*.: Inhibition of mediator release in allergic rhinitis by pretreatment with topical glucocorticoids. *N Engl J Med* 1987, 316:1506–1510.

10. Baroody FM: Allergic rhinitis caused by inhalant factors. In *Conn's Current Therapy, 2001*. Edited by Rakel RE, Bope ET. Philadelphia: WB Saunders; 2001:787-793.

11. Smith CL, Kreutner W: In vitro glucocorticoid receptor binding and transcriptional activation by topically active glucocorticoids. *Arzneimittelforschung* 1998, 48:956–960.

12. Johnson M: Development of fluticasone propionate and comparison with other inhaled corticosteroids. *J Allergy Clin Immunol* 1998, 101(Suppl):S434–S439.

13. Lipworth BJ: New perspectives on inhaled drug delivery and systemic bioactivity. *Thorax* 1995, 50:105–110.

14. Lipworth BJ: Pharmacokinetics of inhaled drugs. *Br J Clin Pharmacol* 1996, 42:697–705.

15. Settipane G, Korenblat PE, Winder J, *et al*.: Triamcinolone acetonide aqueous nasal spray in patients with seasonal ragweed allergic rhinitis: a placebo contolled trial. *Clin Ther* 1995, 17:252–263.

16. Wiseman L, Benfield P: Intranasal fluticasone propionate: a reappraisal of its pharmacology and clinical efficacy in the treatment of rhinitis. *Drugs* 1997, 53:885–907.

17. Meltzer EO, Jalowayski AA, Orgel AH, *et al*.: Subjective and objective assessments in patients with seasonal allergic rhinitis: effects of therapy with mometasone furoate nasal spray. *J Allergy Clin Immunol* 1998, 102:39–49.

18. Welsh PW, Stricker WE, Chu CP, *et al*.: Efficacy of beclomethasone nasal solution, flunisolide and cromolyn in relieving symptoms of ragweed allergy. *Mayo Clin Proc* 1987, 62:125–134.

19. Corren J: Intranasal corticosteroids for allergic rhinitis: how do the different agents compare? *J Allergy Clin Immunol* 1999, 104:S144–S149.

20. Scadding GK, Lund VJ, Jacques LA, *et al*.: A placebo controlled study of fluticasone propionate aqueous nasal spray and beclomethasone dipropionate in perennial rhinitis: efficacy in allergic and non-allergic perennial rhinitis. *Clin Exp Allergy* 1995, 25:737–743.

21. Van As A, Bronsky EG, Dockhorn RJ, *et al*.: Once daily fluticasone propionate is as effective for seasonal allergic rhinitis as twice daily beclomethasone dipropionate. *J Allergy Clin Immunol* 1993, 91:1146–1154.

22. Haye R, Gomez EG: A multicentre study to assess long-term use of fluticasone propionate aqueous nasal spray in comparison with beclomethasone dipropionate aqueous nasal spray in the treatment of perennial rhinitis. *Rhinology* 1993, 31:169–174.

23. Stern MA, Dahl R, Nielsen LP, *et al*.: A comparison of aqueous suspensions of budenoside nasal spray (128 µg and 256 µg once daily) and fluticasone propionate (200 µg once daily) in the treatment of adult patients with seasonal allergic rhinitis. *Am J Rhinol* 1997, 11:323–330.

24. Day J, Carrillo T: Comparison of the efficacy of budesonide and fluticasone propionate aqueous nasal spray for once daily treatment of perenial allergic rhinitis. *J Allergy Clin Immunol* 1998, 102:902–908.

25. Small P, Houle PA, Day JH, *et al*.: A comparison of triamcinolone acetonide nasal aerosol spray and fluticasone propionate aqueous solution in the treatment of spring allergic rhinitis. *J Allergy Clin Immunol* 1997, 100:592–595.

26. Jen A, Baroody F, de Tineo M, *et al*.: As needed use of fluticasone propionate nasal spray reduces symptoms of seasonal allergic rhinitis. *J Allergy Clin Immunol* 2000, 105:732–738.

27. Berkowitz RB, Nolop RB, Mesarina-Wicki BE, C93-184 Study Group: Onset of action of mometasone furoate (Nasonex) nasal spray in seasonal allergic rhinitis [abstract 1790]. *J Allergy Clin Immunol* 1997, 99(suppl): S441.

28.•• Weiner JM, Abramson MJ, Puy RM: Intranasal corticosteroids versus oral H$_1$ receptor antagonists in allergic rhinitis: systemic review of randomized controlled trials. *Br Med J* 1998, 317:1624–1629.
This paper provides a good review of why intranasal corticosteroids may be considered first-line agents.

29. Benincasa C, Lloyd RS: Evaluation of fluticasone propionate aqueous nasal spray taken alone and in combination with ceti-rizine in the prophylactic treatment of seasonal allergic rhinitis. *Drug Investigation* 1994, 8:225–233.

30. Mygind N: Effects of corticosteroid therapy on non-allergic rhinosinusitis. *Acta Otolaryngol* 1996, 116:164–166.

31. Purello-d'Ambrosio F, Isola S, Ricciardi L, *et al.*: A controlled study on the effectiveness of loratadine in combination with flunisolide in the treatment of nonallergic rhinitis with eosinophilia (NARES). *Clin Exp Allergy* 1999, 29:1143–1147.

32. Mygind N, Pederson CB, Prytz S, *et al.*: Treatment of nasal polyps with intranasal beclomethasone dipropionate aerosol. *Clin Allergy* 1975, 5:159–164.

33. Holopainen E, Grahne B, Malmberg H, *et al.*: Budesonide in the treatment of nasal polyposis. *Eur J Resp Dis* 1982, 122(suppl):221–228.

34. Jones AS: Autonomic reflexes and non-allergic rhinitis. *Allergy* 1997, 36(suppl):14–19.

35. Karlsson G, Rundcrantz H: A randomized trial of intranasal beclomethasone dipropionate after polypectomy. *Rhinology* 1982, 20:144–148.

36. Edelman DA, van Os WAA: Safety of intranasal becolmetha-sone dipropionate: a review. *Respir Care* 1996, 11:1025–1030.

37. Bronsky EA, Dockhorn RJ, Meltzer EO, *et al.*: Fluticasone propionate aqueous nasal spray compared with terfenadine tablets in the treatment of seasonal allergic rhinitis. *J Allergy Clin Immunol* 1996, 97:915–921.

38. Gulant SP, Ahrens RC, Dockhorn RJ, *et al.*: Treatment of sea-sonal allergic rhinitis with once daily intranasal fluticasone propionate therapy in children. *J Pediatr* 1994, 125:628–634.

39. Wilson AM, McFarlane LC, Lipworth BJ: Effects of repeated once daily dosing of three intranasal corticosteroids on basal and dynamic measures of hypothalamic-pituitary adrenal axis activity. *J Allergy Clin Immunol* 1998, 101:470–474.

40. Wihl JA, Andersson KE, Johansson SA: Systemic effects of two nasally administered glucocorticosteroids. *Allergy* 1997, 52:620–626.

41. Davies RJ, Nelson HS: Once daily mometasone furoate nasal spray: efficacy and safety of a new intranasal glucocortico-steroid for allergic rhinitis. *Clin Ther* 1997, 19:27–38.

42. Brannan MD, Herron JM, Reidenberg P, *et al.*: Lack of HPA suppression following 36 days of intranasal mometasone furoate. *Ann Allergy Asthma Immunol* 1997, 78:154.

43. Brannan MD, Herron JM, Affrime MB: Safety and tolerability of once daily mometasone furoate aqueous nasal spray in children. *Clin Therap* 1997, 19:1330–1339.

44. Passalacqua G, Albano M, Canonica GW, *et al.*: Inhaled and nasal corticosteroids: safety aspects. *Allergy* 2000, 55:16–33.

45. Howland WC III: Fluticasone propionate: topical or systemic effects. *Clin Exp Allergy* 1996, 26:18–22.

46.• Wilson AM, Sims EJ, McFarlane, *et al.*: Effects of intranasal corticosteroids on adrenal, bone and blood markers of sys-temic activity in allergic rhinitis. *J Allergy Clin Immunol* 1998, 102:598–604.
This paper gives an excellent review of the safety considerations when prescribing inhaled corticosteroids.

47.•• Skoner DP, Rachelefsky GS, Meltzer EO, *et al.*: Detection of growth suppression during treatment with intranasal beclomethasone dipropionate. *Pediatrics* 2000, 105:415–416.
This study changed the way physicians think when prescribing intranasal glucocorticosteroids to children.

48.• Schenkel EJ, Skoner DP, Bronsky EA, *et al.*: Absence of growth retardation in children with perennial allergic rhinitis after one year treatment with mometasone furoate aqueous nasal spray. *Pediatrics* 2000, 150:415.
This articule helps allay fears of using intranasal corticosteroids in children.

49. Abuektish FJ, Kirkpatrick N, Russel G: Posterior subcapsular cataracts and inhaled corticosteroid therapy. *Thorax* 1995, 50:674–676.

50. Minshall E, Ghaffar O, O'Brien F, *et al.*: Assessment by nasal biopsy of long term use of mometasone furoate aqueous nasal spray (Nasonex) in the treatment of perennial rhinitis. *Otolaryngol Head Neck Surg* 1998, 118:648–654.

51.•• Dykewicz MS, Fineman S, Nicklas R, *et al.*: Joint task force algorithm and annotations for diagnosis and management of rhinitis. *Ann Allergy Asthma Immunol* 1998, 81:469–518.
This article provides a concise review of which agent to use under what circumstances, supported by clinical and pharmacological data.

52. Corren J: Allergic rhinitis and asthma: how important is the link? *J Allergy Clin Immunol* 1997, 99:781–786.

CHAPTER 18

Anticholinergic Agents, Guaifenesin, and Decongestants in the Treatment of Rhinitis

Richard J. Sveum
William F. Schoenwetter

Rhinitis affects more than 20% of the United States population, many of whom suffer year-round symptoms [1]. Patients with perennial rhinitis are divided into those with and without an allergic cause. Some patients have a mixed-type rhinitis, with both allergic and non-allergic factors contributing to their symptom complex. In our allergy referral practice, 30% of referred patients have symptoms caused by seasonal allergens (pollen or mold), whereas 70% experience perennial rhinitis. Of these perennial patients, only 50% have an allergic etiology. The most recent population studies done in the 1980s found 5% of the adult population had chronic rhinitis in the absence of demonstrated IgE-mediated hypersensitivity [2]. Patients with nonallergic perennial rhinitis pose a more difficult treatment challenge because they are unable to avoid causative allergens and certainly are not candidates for immunotherapy injections.

The treatment approach is to target relief of symptoms using agents that act on the pathophysiologic mechanisms, although little is actually understood about these mechanisms. A prominent symptom in some patients with nonallergic rhinitis is profuse rhinorrhea; it is not surprising for these individuals to describe their tissue usage as more than 30 per day. Some who suffer seasonal allergic rhinitis also have mucus gland hypersecretion. Postnasal drainage may also be present in these patients.

CHOLINERGIC MECHANISMS IN RHINITIS

Rhinorrhea is related to cholinergic-mediated hypersecretion from both goblet cells and submucosal seromucous glands in the nasal airway. The nasal mucosa and upper airway are innervated by parasympathetic nerves of the autonomic nervous system. The action of acetylcholine on end organs is regulated by specific muscarinic receptor subtypes. Four receptors have been defined using pharmacologic ligand-binding studies (M_1-M_4). Autoradiographic radioligand studies indicate that muscarinic receptors are located on airway smooth muscle, submucosal glands, parasympathetic ganglia, and nerve bundles. In nasal mucosa, M_3 and M_1 receptors are found on glands with lower levels of epithelial cells and endothelial cells [3,4••]. M_3 receptors predominate by a 2:1 ratio.

Clinical studies

Atropine methonitrate was the first drug used for nasal gland hypersecretion and resulted in decreased rhinorrhea [5]. However, atropine applied intranasally is absorbed systemically and produces anticholinergic side effects, including drowsiness, dryness of mouth, and urinary retention. It is therefore not clinically useful.

The pharmacologic development of ipratropium bromide produced a drug with very limited systemic absorption and good tolerability. Ipratropium is poorly absorbed by the oral and nasal mucosa, and the swallowed drug is poorly absorbed from the gastrointestinal tract. It is marketed in the United States as an aqueous intranasal preparation. The most common dosage based on clinical studies is two sprays of a 0.03% aqueous-based ipratropium bromide 42 μg administered 2 or 3 times daily per nostril.

Both allergic and nonallergic rhinitis patients were studied for periods of 4 to 8 weeks. Each of the multicenter studies found a decrease in both the severity and duration of rhinorrhea with ipratropium compared to placebo [6–8]. Two other studies assessed quality of life issues and found improvement in those patients treated with ipratropium bromide [6,9]. The drug was tolerated; adverse effects compared to saline placebo were epistaxis in 9% versus 5% and nasal dryness in 5% versus 1%. The same preparation was studied in children aged 6 to 18; rhinorrhea improved during the one-month clinical trial and was tolerated [10,11]. Two studies investigating whether combining 0.03% ipratropium nasal spray with either an antihistamine (terfenadine) or intranasal steroid spray (beclomethasone) improved control of rhinorrhea in allergic and nonallergic perennial rhinitis showed a modest additional benefit [12,13].

Tiotriopium, a selective M_3 receptor antagonist with a unique mechanism of subtype selectivity, may have pharmacologic advantages with therapeutic implications and is being researched.

Other uses

Ipratropium, 400 μg 4 times daily during the first 2 days of a cold, improved symptom scores by 56% and reduced nasal secretion rates by 58%, but produced excessive dryness of nose and mouth [14]. Later similar studies found that doses of 42 to 168 μg per nostril 3 to 4 times daily to patients with colds reduced rhinorrhea [13,15]. As expected, adverse effects were dose-related, with excessive nasal dryness and blood-spotted mucus occurring in up to 70% of patients. A clinical trial of 410 patients, aged 15 to 50, found a significant reduction of rhinorrhea and sneezing with ipratropium, two 42 μg sprays per nostril 3 to 4 times daily. The most frequent side effect was blood-tinged mucus in 17% of patients versus 4% in the control group receiving saline placebo [16].

Pretreatment with ipratropium may be useful for patients with paroxysmal rhinorrhea caused by hot or spicy foods (gustatory rhinitis) and cold air (skier's nose) [14,17].

Adverse effects

In the recommended intranasal doses, ipratropium is generally well tolerated but may produce dryness of the nasal mucosa, particularly in elderly patients. Higher doses are more drying. It causes no rebound effect, does not decrease olfaction, and does not impair mucociliary transport. If mistakenly administered into the eye, it may cause mydriasis or aggravate glaucoma [18]. Ipratropium nasal spray is classified as category B for use in pregnancy.

Summary

Ipratropium bromide is a topically active anticholinergic. Unlike atropine, it does not cross the blood-brain barrier or cause systemic side effects. Its effects on the nasal mucosa are due to its local effect on the many submucosal glands that have a rich parasympathetic innervation. Ipratropium blocks rhinorrhea by parasympathetic transmission to the submucosal glands. It has no important effect on nasal itching, sneezing, or congestion. Side effects of dryness of nasal mucosa and blood-tinged mucus are dose-related. It is effective within minutes and has a duration of action of at least four hours. The usual dose is 42 μg in each nostril 3 to 4 times daily and is approved for use in children older than 6 years. Ipratropium is used primarily in patients suffering perennial allergic rhinitis manifested by prominent rhinorrhea. It may be useful for cold air-induced rhinorrhea and early symptoms of the common cold.

GUAIFENESIN

Guaifenesin, also known as glycerol guaiacolate, is derived from guaiacol, a component of creosote [19]. The Food and Drug Administration (FDA) has approved the use of guaifenesin as an expectorant, has classified it as safe and effective, and has also granted it over-the-counter (OTC) status. Its effectiveness has been debated. Although there are subjective improvements, there is only partial evidence that the improvement is associated with changes in the characteristics and volume of the sputum. When given in high doses, guaifenesin acts as an emetic, but when given in subemetic doses, it has a theoretic possibility of gastric irritation which promotes an increase in mucus secretion by a cholinergic reflex mechanism. It is also thought to stimulate the secretion of more watery mucus by reducing the surface tension of the mucus.

Guaifenesin is relatively nontoxic with few side effects. Nausea and vomiting have been reported, and if used in excess may cause drowsiness. Guaifenesin has also been known to interfere with clinical laboratory determinations of urinary 5-hydroxyindoleacetic acid and urinary vanillylmandelic acid.

Guaifenesin is included in over 100 products, mostly OTC cold remedies. The recommended adult dose is 200–400 mg every 4 to 6 hours or 600–1200 mg every 12 hours in the sustained-acting preparation, not to exceed 2400 mg daily. For children 6 to 12 years of age, the oral dose is 100–200 mg every 4 hours, not to exceed 1200 mg daily, and in children 2 to 6 years of age 50–100 mg every 4 hours, not to exceed 600 mg daily. Guaifenesin is classified as category C for use in pregnancy and should be given to a pregnant woman only if clearly needed.

There have been no recent studies on the use of guaifenesin [20]. The previously reported studies have not been conclusive, and the effectiveness of guaifenesin continues to be debated in the absence of additional data.

DECONGESTANTS

Decongestants are commonly used in the treatment of rhinitis [21]. They are often used in combination with expectorants and antihistamines because antihistamines alone do not relieve the nasal congestion associated with rhinitis. They can be delivered either orally or topically. The only currently available oral agent is pseudoephedrine hydrochloride, a stereoisomer of ephedrine, that acts as an alpha-adrenergic receptor antagonist (sympathomimetic). Topical decongestants can be administered as vapors, sprays, or drops and are known to be more effective than the oral route. Topical decongestants include phenylephrine hydrochloride, which is found in Dristan (Whitehall-Robins, Madison, NJ) and Neo-Synephrine (Sanofi-Synthelabo, New York, NY) OTC nasal sprays and is considered short-acting. Imidazolines, including naphazoline hydrochloride, oxymetazoline hydrochloride, tetrahydrozoline hydrochloride, and xylometazoline hydrochloride provide longer duration of action. These can be found in OTC medications like Afrin (Schering-Plough, Kenilworth, NJ) and Dristan 12-Hour Nasal Spray (Whitehall-Robins, Madison, NJ).

The alpha-adrenergic agonists are sympathomimetic agents that work through receptor excitatory functions. These agents cause the constriction of smooth muscles of arteries, veins, bronchi, urinary bladder trigone sphincter, and relaxation of the intestinal smooth muscles. The drugs decrease resistance to airflow by decreasing the volume of the nasal mucosa. The venous capacitance vessels in the nasal tissue that have erectile characteristics are most affected by the alpha-adrenergic agents. A major limitation of the topical decongestants is rebound hyperemia and worsening of the symptoms that occur with chronic use (rhinitis medicamentosa). Therefore, topical decongestants generally are used on a short-term basis for less than five days. If long-term therapy is needed, oral agents are recommended. The

recommended dose for pseudoephedrine is 60 mg every 4-6 hours and in the sustained-release form, 120 mg every 12 hours. Pseudoephedrine is classified as category C and should be given to a pregnant woman only if clearly needed.

Phenylpropanolamine

The Center for Drug Evaluation and Research in the FDA recently issued a public health advisory and took steps to remove phenylpropanolamine (PPA) from all drug products [22]. PPA had been marketed for several years, and in 1970 the FDA initiated a scientific review of OTC drug products to determine safety and effectiveness. In 1976, an expert panel recommended that PPA be recognized generally as safe and effective as a nasal decongestant. In 1982, another expert panel recommended that it also be recognized as generally safe and effective for weight control. The FDA did not finalize the status because of concerns about occasional reports of hemorrhagic stroke associated with PPA. A case control study of men and women aged 18 to 49 hospitalized with subarachnoid or intracerebral hemorrhage reported an association between PPA use and hemorrhagic stroke in women. The increased risk of hemorrhagic stroke was detected among women using the drug for weight control in the 3 days after starting use of PPA and for nasal decongestion in the first day of use. The study clearly demonstrated the risk of stroke in women; however, researchers concluded that men may also be at risk. In October 2000, the FDA Nonprescription Drug Advisory Committee determined there was an association between PPA and hemorrhagic stroke and recommended that PPA not be considered generally safe for OTC use. Although the risk of hemorrhagic stroke is very low, even with PPA use, the conditions for which these products are used do not appear to warrant an increased risk of this serious event from using PPA.

REFERENCES AND RECOMMENDED READING

Papers of particular interest, published recently, have been highlighted as:
•   Of importance
••   Of major importance

1. Turkeltaub PC, Gergen PJ: The prevalence of allergic and non-allergic respiratory symptoms in the U.S. population: Data from the Second National Health and Nutrition Examination Survey 1976-80. *J Allergy Clin Immunol* 1998, 81:305–315.

2. Mullarkey MF, Hill JS, Webb DR: Allergic and nonallergic rhinitis: their characterization with attention to the meaning of eosinophilia. *J Allergy Clin Immunol* 1980, 65:112–116.

3. Okayama M, Baraniuk JN, Merida M, Kaliner M: Autoradiographic localization of muscarinic receptor subtypes in human nasal mucosa. *J Allergy Clin Immunol* 1992, 89:1144–1151.

4.•• Barnes PJ: Airway muscarinic receptors. In *Anticholinergic Agents in the Upper and Lower Airways*. Edited by Spector SL. New York: Marcel Dekker; 1999:31–55.
This paper provides a comprehensive review of receptor location and function.

5. Raphael G, Hauptschein-Raphael M, Kaliner M: Gustatory rhinitis: a syndrome of food-induced rhinorrhea. *J Allergy Clin Immunol* 1989, 83:110–115.

6. Meltzer E, Orgel A, Bronsky E, *et al.*: Ipratropium bromide aqueous nasal spray for patients with perennial allergic rhinitis: a study of its effect on their symptoms, quality of life and nasal cytology. *J Allergy Clin Immunol* 1992, 90(2):242–249.

7. Druse HM, Spector SL, Fireman P, *et al.*: Double-blind study of intranasal ipratropium bromide in nonallergic perennial rhinitis. *Ann Allergy* 1992, 69:53–60.

8. Bronsky EAE, Druse H, Findley S, *et al.*: A clinical trial of ipratropium bromide nasal spray in patients with perennial rhinitis. *J Allergy Clin Immunol* 1995, 95(2):1117–1122.

9. Georgitis JW, Banov C, Boggs P, *et al.*: Ipratropium bromide nasal spray in nonallergic rhinitis: efficacy, nasal cytology, and patient evaluation on quality of life. *Clin Exp Allergy* 1993, 24:1049–1055.

10. Meltzer EO, Orgel HA, Biondi R, *et al.*: Ipratropium nasal spray in children with perennial rhinitis. *Ann Allergy Asthma Immunol* 1997, 78:485–491.

11. Milgrom H, Biondi R, Georgitis J, *et al.*: Comparison of ipratropium bromide to beclomethasone dipropionate in the treatment of perennial rhinitis in children. *Ann Allergy Asthma Immunol* 1997, 78:125.

12. Finn A, Korenblat P, Lumry W, *et al.*: A randomized double-blind comparison of combined use of Atrovent nasal spray 0.03% plus Seldane vs. Seldane plus vehicle in patients with allergic and nonallergic perennial rhinitis. *Am J Respir Crit Care Med* 1996, 153(4):A525.

13. Dockhorn R, Bronsky E, Chervinsky P, *et al.*: A randomized, double-blind, six-week, placebo-controlled parallel comparison of Atrovent nasal spray .03% alone, Beconase AQ alone, and the combined use in patients with allergic and nonallergic rhinitis. *Am J Respir Crit Care Med* 1996, 153(4):A525.

14. Ostberg B, Winther B, Mygind N: Cold air-induced rhinorrhea in high-dose ipratropium. *Arch Otolaryngol Head Neck Surg* 1987, 113:160–162.

15. Diamond L, Dockhorn RJ, Grossman J, *et al.*: A dose-response study of the efficacy and safety of ipratropium bromide nasal spray in the treatment of the common cold. *J Allergy Clin Immunol* 1995, 95:1139–1146.

16. Hayden FG, Diamond L, Wood PB, *et al.*: Effectiveness and safety of intranasal ipratropium bromide in common colds. *Ann Intern Med* 1996, 125:89–97.

17. Malmberg H, Grahne B, Holopaine NE: Ipratropium in the treatment of vasomotor rhinitis in the elderly. *Clin Otolaryngol* 1983, 8:273–276.

18. Meltzer EO: Anticholinergic treatment of nasal disorders. *Immunol Allergy Clin North Am* 1991, 11:35–44.

19. Ziment I: Agents That Affect Mucus and Cough. In *Pharmacology and Therapeutics in Respiratory Care*. Edited by Witek TJ Jr, Schachter EN. Philadelphia: W.B. Saunders; 1994:239–257.

20. Sisson JH, Yonkers AJ, Waldman RH: Effects of guaifenesin on nasal mucociliary clearance and ciliary beat frequency in healthy volunteers. *Chest* 1995, 107:747–751.

21. Empey DW, Medder KT: Nasal decongestants. *Drugs* 1981, 21:438–443.

22. FDA/Center for Drug Evaluation and Research page. Phenylpropanolamine (PPA) Information Page. Available at: http://www.fda.gov/cder/drug/infopage/ppa/default.htm. Accessed May 7, 2001.

CHAPTER 19

Nasal Saline Washing

G. Paul Digoy
Terence M. Davidson

Nasal irrigation is practiced around the world. Because irrigating the nose provides improved nasal hygiene, health, and function, nasal irrigation has become as much a daily ritual as tooth brushing for many people. Clinical study in nasal irrigation has not been funded by the National Institutes of Health and there is not enough profit for the private sector to invest in product development and research. Progress is made by trial and error, and nasal irrigation is relegated to the field of complementary medicine. However, many people practice nasal irrigation and claim substantial improvement in nasal hygiene and, as a result, improved well-being and qualify of life. Several rhinologic illnesses can be ameliorated by nasal irrigation with virtually no side effects or downside risks.

Nasal diseases like allergic rhinitis, chronic rhinosinusitis, atrophic rhinitis, and aging rhinitis are common illnesses that are difficult to treat but can improve with nasal irrigation. It is an important addition to the armamentarium of those who treat rhinologic illness.

HISTORY OF NASAL IRRIGATION

Nasal lavage was a documented practice in the nineteenth century. In the 1870s, nasal irrigation was advertised for routine "cleansing and medicating of the nasal passages" [1]. In 1926, Proetz wrote a classic work on nasal sinus lavage. His studies on the physiology of the nasal cilia challenged the validity of some traditional therapies, particularly the use of the caustic silver nitrate compound argerol in the nose. Instead he recommended isotonic saline nasal irrigation, a practice that continues today.

Nasal irrigation has become a daily practice in preventing, treating, and diagnosing many sinonasal diseases. Until the late 1980s, the majority of reports validating the practice of nasal lavage were anecdotal. However, advances in the ability to measure ciliary motility, including the saccharin test of nasal mucociliary function [2], have allowed for reproducible studies showing an increase in the rate of mucociliary clearance (MCC) after nasal lavage.

Any process that increases the viscosity of nasal mucus will directly slow the ciliary beat frequency and MCC [3]. Some of these disease processes include upper respiratory tract infections, rhinosinusitis, allergic rhinitis, aging rhinitis, and cystic fibrosis. Furthermore, any disease that causes nasal obstruction, crusting, and mucosal apposition may also lead to worsening MCC. Certain drugs, most notably antihistamines, have also been shown to cause a decrease in MCC (Table 19-1) [4].

Supported in part by an educational grant from the complementary medicine project at UCSD School of Medicine.

ANATOMY AND PHYSIOLOGY

The internal nose is divided into two sections by the nasal septum, a thin structure composed of cartilage anteriorly and two bones (the perpendicular plate of the ethmoid and the vomer) posteriorly. Mucosal lining covers the entire septum and is continuous with the nasal floor and lateral nasal walls.

Each lateral wall of the nose contains three bony protrusions known as turbinates or conchae. These folds increase the surface area of the nasal cavity and create turbulence in the stream of passing air, facilitating the conditioning, warming, cooling, and filtration of the air. The inferior turbinate is the largest and has a thick mucosa, rich in blood vessels and semierectile tissue. The middle turbinate is rich in mucous glands. Below each turbinate lies a corresponding meatus (ie, passage). The inferior meatus contains the opening of the nasolacrimal duct and makes up part of the nasal floor. The middle meatus contains the drainage sites for the maxillary, frontal, and anterior ethmoid sinuses, commonly called the osteomeatal complex. Anatomical or inflammatory obstruction in the osteomeatal complex is a common cause of sinusitis. The posterior ethmoid cells and sphenoid sinuses drain into the superior meatus, in the sphenoethmoid recess.

The paranasal sinuses are four mucosa-lined air-filled spaces located on each side of the head. The largest of these is the maxillary sinus, located beneath the orbit and within the maxilla. In the adult, each maxillary sinus has a volume of approximately 15 ml. The 18 to 20 ethmoid sinuses per side are small and are found just medial to the orbit. Above the ethmoid sinuses are the frontal sinuses, which sit on the superior and medial aspect of the orbital rim. The sphenoid sinuses lie posterior to the ethmoid sinuses. These are variable in size and unequally divided by a bony septum. Important structures that lie near the sphenoid sinus include the internal carotid artery and the optic nerve.

The pseudostratified respiratory mucosa lining the nasal cavities and paranasal sinuses consists of ciliated columnar cells, intermediate cells, basal cells, and mucus-producing goblet cells. Mucous and serous glands in the lamina propria supplement the secretion of the goblet cells. Veins in the lamina propria form thin-walled cavernous sinusoids, also called cavernous bodies.

Tall (15 to 20 μm) ciliated columnar cells predominate, extending from the basement membrane to the luminal surface. The cilia sit within fluid on the luminal side (Fig. 19-1). On top of the fluid layer floats a layer of mucus, which is slightly acidic and is composed of approximately 95% water, 2.5%–3% glycoproteins, and 1%–2% salt. Immunoglobulins comprise 70% of its protein content. The tenacious and sticky consistency of this mucous blanket traps foreign particles and bacteria. Healthy cilia constantly beat back and forth (Fig. 19-2) in the fluid layer and propel the mucous blanket along, out of the sinuses, into the nose, and down the nasopharynx where it is eventually swallowed. Cilia move the mucous blanket at a rate of a few millimeters per minute, allowing it to be replaced every 20 to 25 minutes. Approximately a quart or more of fluid is generated daily in a normal functioning nose. This mucociliary clearance system is the key to good nasal health.

Physiologic features such as age, sex, posture, sleep, and exercise influence mucociliary clearance due to a change in the cilia, mucus, periciliary layer, or a combination of these factors [6]. Environmental pollutants are known to have a depressant effect on mucociliary clearance, varied by pollutant concentration and duration of exposure. Nasal and sinus secretions stagnate as the mucociliary clearance becomes impaired. The bacteria then remain within the nasal cavity, multiplying and creating a propensity towards infection.

As the nose ages there are changes both in nasal structure and secretions. During aging there is a

---

TABLE 19-1. EFFECTS OF DRUGS ON MUCUS CLEARANCE

Drugs depressing the mucociliary transport system	Drugs increasing the mucociliary transport system	Drugs that either increase or do not affect the mucociliary transport system	Drugs reported not to alter mucociliary transport significantly
Anticholinergics	Cholinergics	Amiloride	Adrenergic antagonists
Aspirin	Methylxanthines	UTP	Guaifenesin
Anesthetic agents	Sodium cromoglycate	Quaternary ammonium compounds	s-Carboxymethylcysteine
Benzodiazepines	Hypertonic saline	Adrenergic agonists	Furosemide
	Saline	Corticosteroids	
	Water aerosol	RhDNase	
		n-Acetylcysteine	
		Bromhexine	
		Ambroxol	

decrease in the water content of the secreted mucus as well as the water content of the mucosa itself. The mucosa subsequently shrinks and the secretions become more viscous and difficult to manage. This is usually perceived as a tenacious postnasal drip. Hormonal changes play an important role in these physiological changes. Although the ratio of these changes is more dramatic in women than in men, they occur in both sexes and cause more symptoms, *ie*, postnasal drip, hoarseness, and coughing.

OVERVIEW

The nose and mucociliary system trap particles and other noxious materials upon inspiration, thereby protecting the respiratory tract. The trapped material and mucus are transported by the cilia to the back of the nose and are deposited into the pharynx and then swallowed. Although this system functions well, it can be assisted or complemented by nasal irrigation. When particulate material are collected in the nasal mucus, especially in patients working in a dirty and dusty environment, nasal irrigation simply washes the mucus and debris out of the nose. Twice daily nasal irrigation appears to provide substantial benefit.

Several conditions in which the mucociliary system no longer functions include atrophic rhinitis, empty nose syndrome (a consequence of overzealous nasal surgery), aging rhinitis, septal perforation, and conditions where

the nose has been radiated, burned, or chemically injured. In all these conditions, thickened inspissated secretions accumulate. This accumulation crusts, obstructs breathing, and causes a feeling of congestion; it can predispose to bleeding and infection.

Nasal irrigation has been shown to increase mucociliary clearance [7•,8••,9•,10•]. Its worldwide use as an adjunctive treatment modality has been recommended in individuals of all ages for the treatment of rhinosinusitis [11,12], allergic rhinitis [13,14], and other sinonasal diseases [15,16]. However, there has been little consensus regarding a uniform protocol for nasal irrigation. Recommendations include saline of varying pH and tonicity, a multitude of delivery vehicles, and several additives.

Hypertonic saline has been reported to be superior to osmotic saline washings in increasing mucociliary clearance [3,7•,16]. This may be due to an actual decrease in edema through the diffusion of osmolar gradients. The improvement in mucociliary clearance is evident despite a recent finding suggesting a decrease in ciliary activity with hyperosmolar solutions [17]. Nonionic douching solutions may be superior to ionic solutions because they avoid ciliary stasis, although this has not been studied.

The alkalinity of the solution does not appear to affect mucociliary function in asymptomatic adults

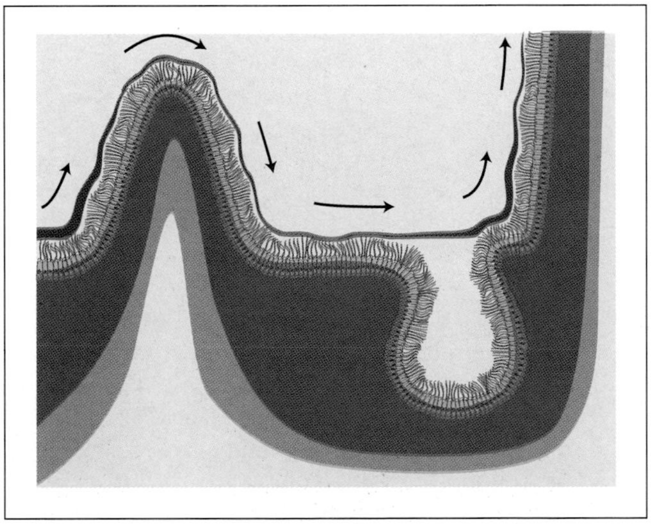

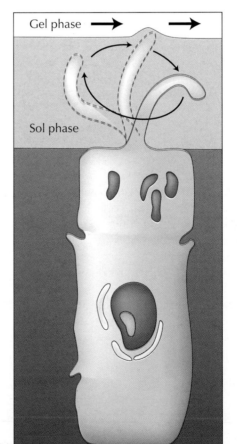

FIGURE 19-2.
A beating cilium. Note how the cilium moves primarily in the sol phase and touches the gel phase only briefly during its fast active beat, pushing the gel and the mucus blanket in the direction of the active beat to the right. The slower recovery beat takes the cilium to the extreme left without touching the gel layer during this movement. (*Adapted from* Stammberger [5].)

FIGURE 19-1.
Mucus transport. When mucosal surfaces come close to each other, the cohesive forces within the mucus blanket of the gel phase can bridge the gap, leaving the recess between the opposing mucosal surfaces filled with the more serous sol phase. This bridging phenomenon allows normal mucus transport to continue. (*Adapted from* Stammberger [5].)

[10•]. Although a benefit has been reported from adding sodium bicarbonate to normal saline solutions, this result is probably due to an increased osmolar gradient and not because of increased pH [3,18]. Because rhinitis itself causes an increase in nasal pH and a subsequent decrease in mucociliary clearance, there may not be much benefit from increasing the pH of the irrigant [18,19]. The authors prefer using slightly acidic solutions and have avoided solutions with a higher pH.

Other additives to saline include aminoglycosides and vasoconstrictors. Aminoglycosides have been used mainly in the management of chronic rhinosinusitis in patients with cystic fibrosis to prevent the colonization of Pseudomonas organisms. The effect of vasoconstrictors was studied by comparing patients with allergic rhinitis who were treated with normal saline nasal irrigation with and without added 1% ephedrine [20]. The addition of ephedrine to the saline nasal wash resulted in significant improvement as measured by symptom scores and nasal inspiratory flow rates. Other additives that have been mentioned include white corn syrup [21] and alkalol [22], although the effects of such additives have not been reported.

PRACTICAL APPLICATION OF NASAL IRRIGATION

The authors' recommendation is to irrigate with tap water, with approximately 5 ml of table salt added to each 500 ml of water. The final solution will be approximately 1.6% NaCl, slightly hypertonic to normal saline (0.9% NaCl). This solution is used even for those who are severely immunocompromised. As tap water is generally sterile, one could question whether the chemicals used to sterilize the water provide some benefit. The authors have always used tap water instead of sterile water or sterile saline and have demonstrated good results [8••].

The majority of current nasal irrigation formulas offer a hypertonic solution. Patients will generally experiment with the amount of salt added and they do quite well over a broad range of saline concentrations. Plain tap water seems to be irritating and too much salt also seems to be irritating.

In special circumstances, additives to the nasal irrigation solution are indicated. Tobramycin has been used prophylactically against Pseudomonas infection for several decades. Although tobramycin is typically sprayed in the oropharynx, the authors began using it as an additive to nasal irrigation in the late 1980s. There appears to be a benefit.

Tobramycin, 20 mg in 50 ml of nasal irrigation solution, is used once daily. Stronger concentrations are irritating and will cause the ostia to scar shut. Bacterial resistance or patient sensitivities do not occur. Alternate antibiotics or cleaning agents have been suggested.

Gentamycin has been recommended as a less expensive alternative; however, it has not been investigated and it is not well tolerated. Betadine has also been recommended.

In the authors' experience, the addition of tobramycin for individuals with Pseudomonas infection, specifically those with cystic fibrosis, provides significant benefit to the patient. Whether the addition of Betadine, gentamycin, culture-directed antibiotics, or other chemicals is of value is hotly debated.

There are two forms of delivery of nasal irrigation even flow delivery and pulsatile delivery. Some physicians claim greater patient acceptance with an even flow or laminar delivery system; however, the authors prefer a pulsatile delivery system. Pulsatile irrigation appears to be superior to rinsing the mouth or using laminar irrigation, and it is superior for removing bacteria lodged in an open wound [23].

Pulsatile irrigation can be performed with an adjustable Waterpik (Water Pik Technologies, Inc., Fort Collins, CO); fixed pressure Waterpiks are too forceful. A solution of 500 ml body temperature tap water with 5 ml table salt is created. A nasal irrigator is attached to the Waterpik and the patient irrigates the nose using approximately half the volume in one side and half the volume in the other [17,24]. In some patients the solution irrigates through the nasal pharynx and comes out of the open mouth; in others the water irrigates in one nostril and out the other. In many patients it does one thing on one side and another on the contralateral side. An occasional patient will complain that the water is forced up the eustachian tube and causes otitis media. These patients are advised to discontinue nasal irrigation. Others will complain that the water finds its way into their sinuses and then gushes out hours later. This is often inconvenient and embarrassing. For these people the nasal irrigation needs to be timed so that any later discharge does not occur at work or at important social events.

NASAL HYPERTHERMIA

Nasal hyperthermia has recently gained attention for treatment of nasal disease. This method involves the delivery of heated mist of varying particle sizes to the nasal mucosa. It has been recommended for years to treat nasal symptoms attributable to various causes including chronic rhinosinusitis, allergic rhinitis, and the common cold [1–6, 7•, 8••, 9•, 10•,17–34]. Georgitis demonstrated that local hyperthermia was superior to nasal irrigation in significantly reducing nasal symptom scores and increasing nasal airflow in patients with perennial allergic rhinitis [25]. However, patients in this group were required to perform irrigation for a total of 15 minutes, far longer than the 2 to 3 minutes usually required in most current protocols. This may account for the large preference of patients for nasal hyperthermia over irrigation. Other studies have found no beneficial effects of steam inhalation on common cold symptoms [33]. Given current evidence, further inquiry regarding nasal hyperthermia is indicated.

REVIEW OF NASAL IRRITATION PRODUCTS

There are various nasal irrigation products with a broad range in cost and complexity. No single product has been demonstrated to be superior; the choice of device should be catered to the individual's needs and preference. The currently available products are described in Table 19-2.

RHINOLOGIC ILLNESSES
The common cold

For patients with experience in nasal irrigation, the nasal irrigator will provide symptomatic relief for the rhinitis associated with a common cold and acute sinusitis. However, for patients not experienced in nasal irrigation, this is more often traumatic than successful and it is therefore not recommended.

Allergic rhinitis

Our standard treatment for allergic rhinitis is nasal irrigation, environmental control, and nasal steroids. It is assumed that the allergens collect on the nasal mucosa, and the allergic load is diminished by irrigating the mucous blanket twice a day.

Crusty nasal conditions

All crusty nasal conditions respond favorably to nasal irrigation. Nasal irrigation removes the crusts, promotes healing, and diminishes infection and bleeding. This may or may not be beneficial for the occasional anterior Kiesselbach's plexus epistaxis. However, many patients with recurrent nosebleeds do have crusting. To whatever degree irrigating the crusts diminishes the cycle leading to recurrent epistaxis, the nasal irrigation is of benefit.

Nasal tip infections, most commonly staphylococcal vestibulitis, respond best to bacitracin ointment; however, the nasal irrigation will remove some of the crusts and may provide some benefit.

Aging rhinitis

Aging rhinitis is caused by diminished hormones. The nasal mucosa atrophies, secretions thicken, and nasal mucus becomes tenacious. This is recognized most typically in elderly men, with constant postnasal drip, cough, and a gravelly voice. As aging rhinitis progresses this can become crusty and infected. The aging nose is virtually cured by twice daily nasal irrigation. This common problem is easily treated and responds to no

---

TABLE 19-2. REVIEW OF NASAL IRRIGATION PRODUCTS

Sinus Rinse (NeilMed Products, Santa Rosa, CA): This saline nose wash kit includes an irrigation bottle and 50 packets of a sodium chloride mixed with sodium bicarbonate. www.nasalrinse.com

SaltAire (The New York Sinus Center, New York, NY): The SaltAire irrigating solution is composed of purified water, sodium chloride, sodium bicarbonate, dibasic sodium phosphate, trisodium EDTA, and thimerosal. The product comes prepared in either a 12.5 oz irrigating bottle or a 32 oz refill bottle. www.saltairsinus.com

Neti Pot (Health & Yoga, New Delhi, India): This product includes a stainless steel pot with a conical end that is filled with warm, slightly salted water. The spout of the pot is inserted into one nostril and the position of the head and pot are adjusted to allow the water to flow out of the other nostril (see Fig. 19-3). www.healthandyoga.com

Pretz Nasal Products (Parnell Pharmaceuticals, Larkspur, CA): This company provides an irrigating solution that includes glycerin and saline formula with an added organic compound called yerba santa. Yerba santa has not been demonstrated in the medical literature to provide benefit in nasal irrigation. www.parnellpharm.com/pretz.htm

Waterpik (Water Pik Technologies, Inc., Fort Collins, CO): A pulsating liquid delivery system formerly engineered for use as an oral irrigator is currently being used for nasal irrigation. Only the adjustable flow model is recommended. This product requires the use of a nasal adapter that can be purchased from several companies including Ethicare (Ft. Lauderdale, FL), Kenwood Therapeutics (Fairfield, NJ), and HydroMed Inc. (Sherman Oaks, CA) (see Fig. 19-4). www.waterpik.com

ENTSol (Kenwood Therapeutics, Fairfield, NJ): This line of nasal irrigation products includes an ENTSol reusable 8 oz. bottle for use as a nasal wash irrigation device that can be used with powdered solutions such as ENTSol Packets or ENTSol Solution (see Fig. 19-5). www.entsolwash.com

Hydro-Flo (Ethicare, Ft. Lauderdale, FL): This delivery system is motorized and provides a steady (non-pulsatile) flow of irrigating solution from a sealed 1.5 liter container. Flow rate can be controlled during irrigation. www.ethicare.com

Grossan Sinus Irrigator (HydroMed Inc., Sherman Oaks, CA): The irrigating device employs pulsating irrigation delivered through a cone-shaped silicon nasal tip adapter attached to a Waterpik oral irrigator. www.sinus-relief.com/whatsirr.html

Lavage (Lavage Inc., Oakland, CA): This product provides a simple irrigation bottle and a useful mixing bowl. No premade solution is provided and normal saline is recommended. www.nasalcare.com

other treatment paradigm. It is worsened by antihistamines and is unchanged by nasal steroids.

Atrophic rhinitis

Atrophic rhinitis, also known as ozena, is a condition that can be caused by Klebsiella, but is also caused by excessive drying, crusting, and infection. This is seen most commonly in the United States as a condition called *empty nose syndrome*. Some nasal surgery removes excessive nasal tissue, particularly procedures that remove the inferior turbinate and especially procedures that remove both the inferior and middle turbinates. These patients develop crusting, discharge, pain, and infection. On examination it is evident that the nose is empty. Patients who have lost the nasal resistance of inspiration will often complain that they cannot breathe. Because inspiration is measured by trigeminally monitored resistance, a widely patent nose has no trigeminal stimulation and is mistakenly interpreted as nasal obstruction. This is atrophic rhinitis and responds to nasal irrigation. If the condition is chronic and severe, patients may need to irrigate 3 or 4 times a day

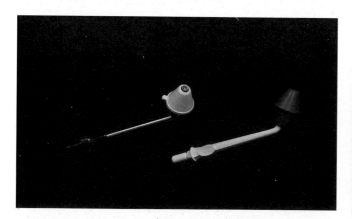

FIGURE 19-3.
Neti Pot (Health & Yoga, New Delhi, India) nasal irrigation device.

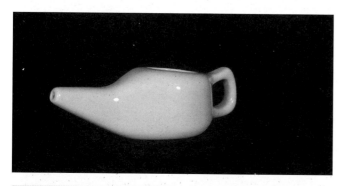

FIGURE 19-4.
Nasal adapters for the Waterpik (Water Pik Technologies, Inc., Fort Collins, CO).

and may need to do this for a 4 to 8 weeks before they see improvement. From then on they can typically irrigate twice daily.

Endoscopic sinus surgery

Nasal irrigation is extremely useful as an adjunct to healing endoscopic sinus surgery. Once the nose is healed and the packing is absorbed, one must either clean the nose endoscopically, 2 or 3 times a week for 6 weeks, or teach the patient how to perform nasal irrigation. Outpatients are instructed to use nasal irrigation twice daily for 6 weeks. Crusting, scarring, and adhesions do not occur and patients recover quickly. Many patients find the treatment so beneficial that they continue the nasal irrigation for extended periods.

Cystic fibrosis

Cystic fibrosis is almost always accompanied by changes in the nose and paranasal sinuses. Some patients will develop polyps. A maxillofacial computed tomographic scan will demonstrate underdeveloped paranasal sinuses, and these are invariably opacified and filled with a thick, viscous, yellow secretion. If cultured, the secretion will grow Pseudomonas. For pulmonary and nasal health, patients are recommended for endoscopic sinus surgery followed by twice daily nasal irrigation. Endoscopic sinus surgery does very little to improve nasal health because the inspissated secretions are simply too thick for the mucociliary system to manage. However, the surgery creates a tunnel or common chamber of the nose and paranasal sinuses, which can then be successfully irrigated. Twice daily nasal irrigation following endoscopic sinus surgery has been shown to have tremendous benefit.

HIV

A thick, tenacious nasal secretion marks HIV illness, particularly in its advanced stages. Pansinusitis occurs

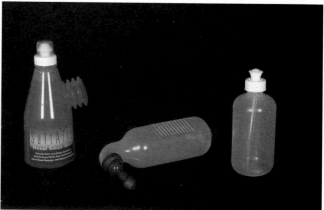

FIGURE 19-5.
Different types of nasal irrigation bottles.

in 75% or more of patients with HIV, and this illness contributes to diminished quality of life. These patients are also recommended for endoscopic sinus surgery. The surgery is designed to drain the sinuses as well as to create a tunnel that can be irrigated. Patients are advised to irrigate twice daily, not only during their recovery but also for the remainder of their lives. Tobramycin may be added to the irrigation solution for those with chronic infections.

Chronic sinusitis

The role of nasal irrigation in the management of chronic sinusitis has not been well defined. Some patients benefit from long-term, twice daily nasal irrigation, particularly after endoscopic sinus surgery. For those who can irrigate successfully, the addition of tobramycin may provide additional benefit.

Nasal irrigation may also play a role in the management of the fungal etiology of chronic sinusitis. Initial data from a group of 51 patients with chronic sinusitis treated with amphotericin B nasal irrigation showed that 38 (75.5%) of the patients demonstrated improved symptoms and improvement in the endoscopic examination of the nose. Of the 38 patients, 16 used topical and systemic steroids. Five of these 16 patients (31%) were able to reduce their systemic steroid use while 8 of 16 patients (50%) were able to entirely stop systemic steroid use. Nasal irrigation with amphotericin B appears to be safe and effective for treatment of chronic sinusitis [34].

CONCLUSIONS

Nasal irrigation is a practical and inexpensive practice that has been documented to improve nasal function and health.

REFERENCES AND RECOMMENDED READING

Papers of particular interest, published recently, have been highlighted as:
• Of importance
•• Of major importance

1. Burns JL: Nasal lavage. *J Otolaryngol* 1992, 21:83.

2. Staley P, MacWilliam L, Greenstone M, *et al.*: Efficacy of saccharin test for screening to detect abnormal mucociliary clearance. *Br J Dis Chest* 1984, 78:62–65.

3. Luk CKA, Dulfano MJ: Effect of pH, viscosity and ionic strength changes on ciliary beating frequency of human bronchial explants. *Clin Sci* 1983, 64:449–451.

4. Houtmeyers E, Gosselink R, Gayan-Ramirez G, Decramer M: Effects of drugs on mucus clearance. *Eur Respir J* 1999, 14:452–467.

5. Stammberger H: *Functional Endoscopic Sinus Surgery: The Messerklinger Technique.* Philadelphia: BC Decker; 1991:18–19.

6. Houtmeyers E, Gosselink R, Gayan-Raminez G, Decramer M: Regulation of mucociliary clearance in health and disease. *Eur Respir J* 1999, 13(5):1177–1188.

7.• Homer JJ, Dowley AC, Condon L, *et al.*: The effect of hypertonicity on nasal mucociliary clearance. *Clin Otolaryngol* 2000, 25:558–560.
This study observes the effect of hypertonicity on saccharin clearance time and demonstrates an increase in mucociliary clearance at 5% tonicity compared to 0.9% tonicity.

8.•• Tomooka LT, Murphy C, Davidson TM: Clinical study and literature review of nasal irrigation. *Laryngoscope* 2000, 110:1189–1193.
This report provides a good literature review on nasal irrigation and Waterpik applications. A self-administered quality of well-being questionnaire before and after nasal irrigation with the Waterpik demonstrated a general improvement in patient quality of life.

9.• Talbot AR, Herr TM, Parsons DS: Mucociliary clearance and buffered hypertonic saline solution. *Laryngoscope* 1997, 107:500–503.
This study indicates a benefit from buffered normal saline compared to normal saline. However, the authors did not take into account the effect of hypertonicity from the buffered solution. It is likely that the results would be different in a better-controlled study.

10.• Homer JJ, England RJ, Wilde AD, *et al.*: The effect of pH of douching solutions on mucociliary clearance. *Clin Otolaryngol* 1999, 24:312–315.
This well-written review compares douching solutions of variable pH using the saccharin clearance time. Buffered solutions were not found to be of benefit.

11. Zeiger RS: Prospects for ancillary treatment of rhinosinusitis in the 1990s. *J Allergy Clin Immunol* 1992, 90:478–495.

12. Mabry RL: Therapeutic agents in the medical management of rhinosinusitis. *Otolaryngol Clin North Am* 1993, 26:561–571.

13. Ferguson BJ: Allergic rhinitis: options for pharmacotherapy and immunotherapy. *Postgrad Med* 1997, 101:117–126.

14. Parikh A, Scadding GK: Seasonal allergic rhinitis. *BMJ* 1997, 314:1392–1395.

15. Grossan M: Irrigation treatment of throat infections. *EENT Monthly* 1972, 51:38–42.

16. Shoseyov D, Bibi H, Shai P, *et al.*: Treatment with hypertonic saline versus normal saline wash of pediatric chronic rhinosinusitis. *J Allergy Clin Immunol* 1998, 101:602–605.

17. Boek WM, Keles N, Graamans K, *et al.*: Physiologic and hypertonic saline solutions impair ciliary activity in vitro. *Laryngoscope* 1999, 109:396–399.

18. Stanley PJ, Wilson R, Greenstone MA, *et al.*: Abnormal nasal mucociliary clearance in patients with rhinitis and its relationship to concomitant chest disease. *Br J Dis Chest* 1985, 79:77–82.

19. Fabricant ND: Significance of the pH of nasal secretions in situ. *Arch Otolaryngol* 1941, 33:150–163.

20. Shaikh WA: Ephedrine-saline nasal wash in allergic rhinitis. *J Allergy Clin Immunol* 1995, 96:597–600.

21. Ferguson BJ: Allergic rhinitis: options for pharmacotherapy and immunotherapy. *Postgrad Med* 1997, 101:117–126.

22. Mabry RL: Therapeutic agents in the medical management of rhinosinusitis. *Otolaryngol Clin North Am* 1993, 26:561–571.

23. Anglen JO, Apostoles S, Christensen G, Gainor B: The efficacy of various irrigation solutions in removing slime-producing staphylococcus. *J Orthop Trauma* 1994, 8:390–396.

24. Davidson TM: Handbook of nasal disease. Available at: http://www.drdavidson.org. Accessed May 22, 2001.

25. Georgitis JW: Local hyperthermia and nasal irrigation for perennial allergic rhinitis: effect on symptoms and nasal airflow. *Ann Allergy* 1993, 71:385–389.

26. Wills PJ, Hall RL, Chan W, *et al.*: Sodium chloride increases the ciliary transportability of cystic fibrosis and bronchiectasis sputum on the mucus-depleted bovine trachea. *J Clin Invest* 1997, 99:9–13.

27. Davidson TM, Murphy C: Rapid clinical evaluation of anosmia: the alcohol sniff test. *Arch Otolaryngol Head Neck Surg* 1997, 123:591–594.

28. Adam P, Stiffman M, Blake RL: A clinical trial of hypertonic saline nasal spray in subjects with the common cold or rhinosinusitis. *Arch Fam Med* 1998, 7:39–43.

29. Yerishalmi A, Karman S, Lwoff A: Treatment of perennial allergic rhinitis by local hyperthermia. *Proc Natl Acad Sci USA* 1982, 79:4766–4769.

30. Tyrell D, Barrow I, Arthur J: Local hyperthermia benefits natural and experimental colds. *BMJ* 1989, 298:1280–1283.

31. Mackinin ML, Matthew S, VanderBrijg-Medendorp S: Effect of inhaling heated vapor on symptoms of the common cold. *JAMA* 1990, 264:989–991.

32. Georgitis JW: Nasal hyperthermia and simple irrigation for perennial rhinitis: changes in inflammatory mediators. *Chest* 1994, 106:1487–1492.

33. Anderson JP, Bush JW, Berry CC: Classifying function for health outcome and quality-of-life evaluation: self versus interviewer modes. *Med Care* 1986, 24:454–469.

34. Cody DT 2nd, Neel HB 3rd, Ferreiro JA, Roberts GD: Allergic fungal sinusitis: the Mayo Clinic experience. *Laryngoscope* 1994, 104:1074–1079.

CHAPTER 20

Referral of Patients with Rhinitis or Sinusitis

Michael A. Kaliner

RHINITIS

An estimated 35 to 45 million Americans suffer from allergic rhinitis [1]. Hay fever is the most commonly reported chronic condition among teenagers, with 64.6 cases per 1000 persons [2]. In 1990, the medical costs of rhinitis were estimated to exceed $1.8 billion dollars, increasing to more than $6 billion by 1999 [3]. The potential costs of lost work days and impaired productivity may be over $11 billion, or $1000 per worker per year [4]. Nonallergic rhinitis is also extremely prevalent, with an estimated patient base of more than 10 million people, mostly adult females.

The point at which a physician asks for advice from another doctor varies enormously. Some busy clinicians are always willing to get a second opinion, whereas others have a difficult time initiating referrals. In fact, many patients are self-referred to the specialist because their primary care physicians are unwilling to refer them. Thus, specialists receive referrals of patients with conditions ranging from standard medical problems to extremely complex conditions. Some of these patients could be managed by knowledgeable primary care physicians; others have such complex disease that they can be managed only by the most competent specialist.

In 1997 general criteria were established for the patients who might benefit from a referral [5••]. It then became apparent that for a physician to get the most from a referral, expectations of what the specialist should provide also needed to be documented. Not every patient with allergies requires allergy injection therapy, and just as likely, not every sinusitis patient requires surgery.

A patient should be referred to a specialist when rhinitis or its treatment is interfering with a patient's performance, causing significant absence from school or work, or when the patient's quality of life is significantly affected; when the patient develops complications of rhinitis, such as sinusitis, otitis, hearing loss, dental or facial malformations, asthma, or bronchitis; when the patient requires systemic corticosteroids or prolonged nasal high-dose corticosteroids to control their disease; or when a patient is symptomatic 4 to 6 months each year [6••].

The specialist should provide the referring physician with identification of specific allergens or other triggers for the patient's condition; advice on how to avoid exposure to these triggers; clarification of allergic or other etiologic basis for the patient's condition; assistance in developing an effective treatment plan, including allergy avoidance, pharmacotherapy, and immunotherapy; and specialized services, such as preparation of allergy extracts and provision of immunotherapy [6••].

SINUSITIS

Sinusitis is as prevalent as rhinitis and can cause serious complications if inadequately treated. It is possible to treat acute sinusitis with complete resolution of the disease. However, for patients with recurrent or chronic sinusitis, it is critical to identify and treat the underlying condition responsible for sinusitis. Once the underlying allergic, immunologic, infectious, or anatomical problems are identified, treatment of the disease can be addressed in a systematic fashion and the sinusitis can be resolved.

In the past acute, chronic, or recurrent sinusitis was managed by the primary care physician, who consulted an otolaryngologist for surgical intervention if the therapy was not effective. However, over the past decade, more patients with sinusitis are being referred to allergists to take advantage of their training in medicine or pediatrics and their knowledge of nasal physiology, microbiology, and pathology.

A patient should be referred to a specialist when sinusitis or its treatment is interfering with the patient's performance, causing significant absence from school or work on a chronic or recurrent basis, or when the patient's quality of life is significantly affected; when the patient develops frequent or disabling sinus infections or when there are complications of sinusitis, such as otitis, asthma, or bronchitis; when an allergic or immunologic cause for sinusitis is suspected; or when sinusitis persists for several months, becomes chronic, or recurs 2 to 4 times per year, despite treatment [7••].

The specialist should provide the referring physician with confirmation of the diagnosis of sinusitis or an alternative explanation of the cause of the symptoms; clarification of allergic, immunologic, or anatomical basis for the patient's condition; identification of specific allergens or other triggers for the patient's condition, and education in ways to avoid exposure to these triggers; assistance in developing an effective treatment plan, including allergy avoidance, pharmacotherapy,

anti-infectious therapy, nasal hygiene, and immunotherapy, if appropriate; and specialized services, such as prescribing immunoglobulin replacement therapy, prophylactic immunizations, preparation of allergy extracts, and provision of immunotherapy [7••].

Close cooperation among the referring physician, otolaryngologist, and allergist is appropriate. Allergic, immunologic, and medical approaches to sinusitis should be provided by the medical provider with the greatest expertise. It is imperative that anyone providing care for patients with sinusitis be capable of determining if allergic or nonallergic processes are predisposing the patient to sinusitis. Surgical intervention is appropriate for some patients, but others can and should be managed medically.

REFERENCES AND RECOMMENDED READING

Papers of particular interest, published recently, have been highlighted as:
- • Of importance
- •• Of major importance

1. National Institutes of Allergy and Infectious Diseases: *Allergic Diseases.* Bethesda, MD: US Department of Health and Human Services; 1991. NIH Publication 91-3221.

2. National Institutes of Allergy and Infectious Diseases: *Allergic Diseases.* Bethesda, MD: US Department of Health and Human Services; 1993. NIH Publication 93-493.

3. McMenamin P: Costs of allergic rhinitis in the United States. *Ann Allergy* 1994, 73:35–39.

4. Ross RN: Hay fever: a costly disease for American business. *Diseases management forum: allergy.* Boston: Managed Care Communications, Inc., 1995:144.

5.•• Kaliner MA: Allergy care in the next millennium: Guidelines for the specialty. *J Allergy Clin Immunol* 99:729–734, 1997.
This important paper outlines referral guidelines for patients with rhinitis, sinusitis, and asthma.

6.•• Dykewicz MS, Fineman S, Skoner DP, *et al.*: Diagnosis and management of rhinitis: complete guidelines of the Joint Task Force on Practice Parameters in Allergy, Asthma and Immunology. *Ann Allergy Asthma Immunol* 1998, 81:478–518.
This paper is the official position statement of allergists regarding rhinitis.

7.•• Joint Task Force on Practice Parameters: Parameters for the Diagnosis and Management of Sinusitus. *J Allergy Clin Immunol* 1998, 6:107–114.
This paper is the official position statement of allergists regarding sinusitis.

Index

The letters f and t indicate figures and tables, respectively.